FIRST AID FOR THE® USMLE STEP 2 CS

Fourth Edition

TAO LE, MD, MHS
Associate Clinical Professor of Medicine and Pediatrics
Chief, Section of Allergy and Immunology
Department of Medicine
University of Louisville

VIKAS BHUSHAN, MD
Diagnostic Radiologist

MAE SHEIKH-ALI, MD
Assistant Professor of Medicine
Assistant Program Director, Endocrinology Fellowship Program
Division of Endocrinology, Diabetes and Metabolism
University of Florida College of Medicine–Jacksonville

FADI ABU SHAHIN, MD
Gynecologic Oncology
Florida Gynecologic Oncology

Medical

New York / Chicago / San Francisco / Lisbon / London / Madrid / Mexico City
Milan / New Delhi / San Juan / Seoul / Singapore / Sydney / Toronto

First Aid for the® USMLE Step 2 CS, Fourth Edition

Copyright © 2012, 2010, 2007, 2004 by Tao Le. All rights reserved. Printed in the United States of America. Except as permitted under the United States Copyright Act of 1976, no part of this publication may be reproduced or distributed in any form or by any means, or stored in a data base or retrieval system, without the prior written permission of the publisher.

First Aid for the® is a registered trademark of The McGraw-Hill Companies, Inc.

3 4 5 6 7 8 9 0   QVR   17 16 15 14 13

ISBN 978-0-07-176050-8
MHID 0-07-176050-4
ISSN 1930-5354

NOTICE

Medicine is an ever-changing science. As new research and clinical experience broaden our knowledge, changes in treatment and drug therapy are required. The authors and the publisher of this work have checked with sources believed to be reliable in their efforts to provide information that is complete and generally in accord with the standards accepted at the time of publication. However, in view of the possibility of human error or changes in medical sciences, neither the authors nor the publisher nor any other party who has been involved in the preparation or publication of this work warrants that the information contained herein is in every respect accurate or complete, and they disclaim all responsibility for any errors or omissions or for the results obtained from use of the information contained in this work. Readers are encouraged to confirm the information contained herein with other sources. For example and in particular, readers are advised to check the product information sheet included in the package of each drug they plan to administer to be certain that the information contained in this work is accurate and that changes have not been made in the recommended dose or in the contraindications for administration. This recommendation is of particular importance in connection with new or infrequently used drugs.

This book was set in Goudy Old Style by Rainbow Graphics.
The editors were Catherine A. Johnson and Peter J. Boyle.
Project management was provided by Rainbow Graphics.
The production supervisor was Jeffrey Herzich.
The designer was Mary McKeon.
Quad/Graphics was printer and binder.

This book is printed on acid-free paper.

McGraw-Hill books are available at special quantity discounts to use as premiums and sales promotions, or for use in corporate training programs. To contact a representative please e-mail us at bulksales@mcgraw-hill.com.

DEDICATION

To the contributors of this and past editions, who took time to share their experience, advice, and humor for the benefit of future physicians.

and

To our families, friends, and loved ones, who supported us in the task of assembling this guide.

CONTENTS

Contributors ix

Faculty Reviewers xi

Preface...xiii

Acknowledgments..xv

How to Contribute..xvii

SECTION 1   GUIDE TO THE USMLE STEP 2 CS   1

Introduction 2

USMLE Step 2 CS—The Basics.. 2

Preparing for the Step 2 CS.. 7

Test-Day Tips 10

First Aid for the IMG 12

Supplement—The USMLE Step 2 CS Travel Guide....................... 19

SECTION 2   THE PATIENT ENCOUNTER   37

Introduction 38

Doorway Information... 39

Taking the History.. 42

The Physical Exam 52

Closure 61

How to Interact with Special Patients...................................... 63

Challenging Questions and Situations 64

Counseling 71

The Patient Note 74

SECTION 3   MINICASES   79

Headache 81

Confusion/Memory Loss... 83

Depressed Mood.. 85

Psychosis 86

Dizziness.. 87

Loss of Consciousness 89

Numbness/Weakness 90

Fatigue and Sleepiness 91

Night Sweats 93

Insomnia 93

Sore Throat 94

Cough/Shortness of Breath 95

Chest Pain 97

Palpitations 99

Weight Loss 100

Weight Gain 101

Dysphagia 101

Nausea/Vomiting 102

Abdominal Pain 103

Constipation/Diarrhea 107

Upper GI Bleeding 109

Blood in Stool 110

Hematuria 111

Other Urinary Symptoms 112

Erectile Dysfunction 113

Amenorrhea 114

Vaginal Bleeding 116

Vaginal Discharge 117

Dyspareunia 118

Abuse 118

Joint/Limb Pain 119

Low Back Pain 122

Child with Fever 123

Child with GI Symptoms 124

Child with Red Eye 126

Child with Short Stature 126

Behavioral Problems in Childhood 127

SECTION 4   PRACTICE CASES   129

Case 1   48-Year-Old Woman with Abdominal Pain 132

Case 2   21-Year-Old Woman with Abdominal Pain 139

Case 3   74-Year-Old Man with Right Arm Pain 147

Case 4   21-Year-Old Man with Sore Throat 154

Case 5   55-Year-Old Man with Bloody Stool 161

Case 6   46-Year-Old Man with Chest Pain 168

Case 7   7-Month-Old Boy with Fever 175

Case 8   18-Month-Old Girl with Fever 181

Case 9   26-Year-Old Man with Cough 187

Case 10   54-Year-Old Woman with Cough 194

Case 11   52-Year-Old Woman with Jaundice 202

Case 12   65-Year-Old Woman with Forgetfulness and Confusion 209

Case 13   56-Year-Old Man Presents for Diabetes Follow-up 216

Case 14   53-Year-Old Man with Dizziness 223

Case 15   46-Year-Old Man with Fatigue 230

Case 16   32-Year-Old Woman with Fatigue 237

Case 17   61-Year-Old Man with Fatigue 244

Case 18   35-Year-Old Woman with Headaches 251

Case 19   57-Year-Old Man with Bloody Urine 258

Case 20   54-Year-Old Man Presents for Hypertension Follow-up 265

Case 21   33-Year-Old Woman with Knee Pain 272

Case 22   66-Year-Old Man with Tremor 280

Case 23   49-Year-Old Man with Loss of Consciousness 288

Case 24   30-Year-Old Woman with Weight Gain 295

Case 25   36-Year-Old Woman with Menstrual Problems 302

Case 26   28-Year-Old Woman with Pain During Sex 309

Case 27   51-Year-Old Man with Back Pain 316

Case 28   6-Month-Old Girl with Diarrhea 322

Case 29   75-Year-Old Man with Hearing Loss 328

Case 30   8-Year-Old Boy with Bed-Wetting 335

Case 31   25-Year-Old Man Presents Following Motor Vehicle Accident 341

Case 32   25-Year-Old Woman Presents Following Sexual Assault 349

Case 33   28-Year-Old Woman Presents with Positive Pregnancy Test 356

Case 34   20-Year-Old Woman with Sleeping Problems 363

Case 35   27-Year-Old Man with Visual Hallucinations 370

Case 36   10-Year-Old Girl with New-Onset Diabetes 377

Case 37   35-Year-Old Woman with Calf Pain 384

Case 38   31-Year-Old Man with Heel Pain 391

Case 39   5-Day-Old Boy with Jaundice 399

Case 40   2-Year-Old Girl with Noisy Breathing 405

Case 41   32-Year-Old Man Presents for Preemployment Physical.............. 411

Case 42   62-Year-Old Man with Hoarseness 418

Case 43   67-Year-Old Woman with Neck Pain 425

Case 44   11-Month-Old Girl with Seizures 431

SECTION 5   TOP-RATED REVIEW RESOURCES   437

How to Use the Database 438

Appendix... 445

Index.. 449

About the Authors.. 461

CONTRIBUTORS

Mohammad Aldaas, MD
Clinical Research Associate
Texas Heart Institute

Kevin Day
Northwestern University Feinberg School of Medicine
Class of 2012

Michael King, MD
Resident, Department of Medicine
Albert Einstein Medical Center

Kachiu Cecilia Lee, MD, MPH
Resident, Department of Dermatology
Brown University

Ruba Sheikh-Ali, MD
Damascus University School of Medicine
Class of 2011

Amy Yin, MD
Resident, Department of Physical Medicine & Rehabilitation
Harvard Medical School/Spaulding Rehabilitation Hospital

FACULTY REVIEWERS

Irene Alexandraki, MD, MPH, FACP
Assistant Professor of Medicine
University of Florida College of Medicine–Jacksonville

Carlos Palacio, MD
Associate Professor of Medicine
University of Florida College of Medicine–Jacksonville

The USMLE Step 2 CS can be a source of stress and anxiety, especially among international medical graduates (IMGs), who find themselves at a disadvantage because of their non-US training background. *First Aid for the USMLE Step 2 CS* is our "cure" for this exam. This book represents a virtual medicine bag of high-yield tools for students and IMGs, including:

- A thorough exam preparation guide for the USMLE Step 2 CS. It includes proven study and exam strategies for the clinical encounters based on the patient-centered interview.
- A new color design to enhance efficient study.
- Step-by-step strategies for interacting with standardized patients, including "difficult" patients.
- Detailed descriptions of high-yield physical exam maneuvers that will win you points without costing time.
- A revised and expanded set of minicases representing common complaints designed to help you rapidly develop a working set of differential diagnoses.
- Forty-four full-length practice cases that allow you to simulate the real exam. They include all-new pediatric and telephone interviews as well as suggested "closing statements" for each case.

This book would not have been possible without the suggestions and feedback of medical students, IMGs, and faculty members. We invite you to share your thoughts and ideas to help us improve *First Aid for the USMLE Step 2 CS*. See How to Contribute, p. xvii.

Louisville	Tao Le
Los Angeles	Vikas Bhushan
Jacksonville	Mae Sheikh-Ali
Fort Myers	Fadi Abu Shahin

ACKNOWLEDGMENTS

We owe special thanks to the attendings, fellows and residents, and students who helped with this edition. Attendings—From University of Florida College of Medicine: Arshag D. Mooradian, MD; Malcom Foster, MD; Joe Chehade, MD; Kent Wehmeier, MD; Senan Sultan, MD. From Mayo Clinic: Shon E. Meek, MD. From University of Virginia Medical Center: Kurt P. Miceli, MD. From Drexel University College of Medicine: Joseph M. Boselli, MD; Howard A. Miller, MD. From Lankenau Hospital: Rita El-Hajj, MD. From University of Damascus: Halla Sheikh-Ali, MD. Fellows and residents—From University of Florida College of Medicine: Emad Naem, MD; Rosalyn Alcalde, MD; Sandra Mesliniene, MD; Margret Gladysz, MD. Students—From University of Damascus: Ayman Albakour, MD; Raeda Alshantti, MD; Ruba Barber, MD. Special thanks to Salam Sheikh-Ali, MD, for her help in editing.

Thanks to our editor, Catherine Johnson, for her enthusiasm, support, and commitment to the *First Aid* series. Thanks to Carol Ayres, our developmental editor, for her dedication to our projects, and to Selina Franklin and Louise Petersen for their organization and administrative assistance. Also, a special thanks to Rainbow Graphics, especially David Hommel and Susan Cooper, for remarkable editorial and production work. For support and encouragement throughout the process, we are grateful to Thao Pham and Jonathan Kirsch.

Louisville	Tao Le
Los Angeles	Vikas Bhushan
Jacksonville	Mae Sheikh-Ali
Fort Myers	Fadi Abu Shahin

HOW TO CONTRIBUTE

First Aid for the USMLE Step 2 CS incorporates many contributions from students and faculty. We invite you to participate in this process. Please send us:

- Study and test-taking strategies for the Step 2 CS exam
- High-yield case topics that may appear on future Step 2 CS exams
- Personal comments on review books that you have examined

For each entry incorporated into the next edition, you will receive up to a $20 Amazon.com gift certificate and a personal acknowledgment in the next edition. Significant contributions will be compensated at the discretion of the authors. The preferred way to submit entries, suggestions, or corrections is via our blog:

www.firstaidteam.com

Otherwise, you can e-mail us directly at:

firstaid@usmlerx.com

Contributions sent earlier will receive priority consideration for the next edition of *First Aid for the USMLE Step 2 CS*.

NOTE TO CONTRIBUTORS

All entries are subject to editing and reviewing. Please verify all data and spellings carefully. In the event that similar or duplicate entries are received, only the first entry received will be used. Please follow the style, punctuation, and format of this edition as much as possible. All contributions become property of the authors.

INTERNSHIP OPPORTUNITIES

The author team of Le and Bhushan is pleased to offer part-time and full-time paid internships in medical education and publishing to motivated medical students and physicians. Internships may range from two to three months (eg, a summer) up to a full year. Participants will have an opportunity to author, edit, and earn academic credit on a wide variety of projects, including the popular *First Aid* series. Writing/editing experience, familiarity with Microsoft Word, and Internet access are required. For more information, e-mail a résumé or a short description of your experience along with a cover letter and writing sample to **firstaid@usmlerx.com.**

Guide to the USMLE Step 2 CS

Introduction

USMLE Step 2 CS—The Basics

Preparing for the Step 2 CS

Test-Day Tips

First Aid for the IMG

Supplement—The USMLE Step 2 CS Travel Guide

INTRODUCTION

Since 2004, all US and Canadian medical students as well as international medical graduates (IMGs) have been required to pass a clinical skills exam known as the United States Medical Licensing Examination (USMLE) Step 2 Clinical Skills (CS)—a test involving clinical encounters with "standardized patients"—as a prerequisite to entering residency training in the United States.

Even if you are a pro at taking standardized exams, such as the USMLE Step 1 and Step 2 Clinical Knowledge (CK), you may find it challenging to prepare for the USMLE Step 2 CS—which, like the Clinical Skills Assessment (CSA) it has replaced, uses live patient actors to simulate clinical encounters. Common mistakes medical students and IMGs make in preparing for the Step 2 CS include the following:

- Panicking because of the unfamiliar format of the test
- Not practicing enough with mock patient scenarios before the actual exam
- Not developing a logical plan of attack based on patient "doorway information"
- Failing to understand the required objectives for each patient encounter
- Managing time poorly during patient encounters
- Becoming flustered by challenging questions or situations
- Taking unfocused histories and physical exams
- Failing to understand how to interact with a patient appropriately
- Neglecting to carry out easy but required patient interactions

This book will guide you through the process of efficiently preparing for and taking the Step 2 CS with four organized sections:

- **Section 1** introduces you to the USMLE Step 2 CS.
- **Section 2** reviews critical, high-yield steps to take during the patient encounter.
- **Section 3** provides high-yield minicases for common doorway chief complaints to help you rapidly develop focused differentials during the exam.
- **Section 4** offers full-length practice cases to help you simulate the real thing.
- **Section 5** rates other resources that help you prepare for the Step 2 CS.

USMLE STEP 2 CS—THE BASICS

What Is the USMLE Step 2 CS?

The USMLE Step 2 CS is a one-day exam whose objective is to ensure that all US and Canadian medical students seeking to obtain their medical licenses—as well as all IMGs seeking to start their residencies in the United States—have the communication, interpersonal, and clinical skills necessary to achieve these goals. To pass the test, all examinees must show that they can speak, understand, and communicate in English as well as take a history and perform a brief physical exam. Examinees are also required to exhibit competence in written English and to demonstrate critical clinical skills by writing a brief patient note (PN), follow-up orders, and a differential diagnosis.

The Step 2 CS simulates clinical encounters that are commonly found in clinics, physicians' offices, and emergency departments. The test makes use of "standardized patients" (SPs), all of whom are laypersons who have been extensively trained to simulate various clinical problems. The SPs give the same responses to all candidates participating in the assessment. When you take the Step 2 CS, you will see 11–12 SPs, but cases will be mixed in terms of age, gender, ethnicity, organ system, and discipline. For quality assurance purposes, a video camera will record all clinical encounters, but the resulting videotapes will not be used for scoring. The cases used in the Step 2 CS represent the types of patients who are typically encountered during core clerkships in the curricula of accredited US medical schools. These clerkships are as follows:

- Internal medicine
- Surgery
- Obstetrics and gynecology
- Pediatrics
- Psychiatry
- Family medicine
- Emergency medicine

Examinees do **not** interact with children during pediatric encounters. Instead, SPs assuming the role of pediatric patients' parents recount patients' histories, and no physical exam is required under such circumstances.

> There is no physical exam in pediatric or phone encounters. Instead, you should focus on obtaining a thorough history.

How Is the Step 2 CS Structured?

Before entering a room to interact with an SP, you will be given the opportunity to review some preliminary information. This information, which is posted on the door of each room (and hence is often referred to as "doorway information"), includes the following:

- Patient characteristics (name, age, sex)
- Chief complaint and vitals (temperature, respiratory rate, pulse, blood pressure)

You will be given 15 minutes (with a warning bell sounded after 10 minutes) to perform the clinical encounter, which includes reading the doorway information, entering the room, introducing yourself, obtaining an appropriate history, conducting a focused physical exam, formulating a differential diagnosis, and planning a diagnostic workup. You will also be expected to answer any questions the SP might ask; discuss the diagnoses being considered; and advise the SP about follow-up plans. After leaving the room, you will have 10 minutes to type a PN. *Note:* Starting July 17, 2011, all examinees taking the Step 2 CS will be required to type the patient note. Examinees will not be permitted to handwrite the note, unless technical difficulties on the test day make the PN typing program unavailable.

> Many students choose to use a bullet-style format when typing the PN.

How Is the Step 2 CS Scored?

Of your 11–12 patient encounters, 10 will be scored. Two people will score each encounter: the SP and a physician. The SP will evaluate you at the end of each encounter by filling out three checklists: one for the history, a second for the physical exam, and a third for communication skills. The physician will evaluate the PN you write after each encounter. Your overall score, which will be based on the clinical encounter as a whole and on your overall communication skills, will be determined by the following three components:

- **Integrated Clinical Encounter (ICE) score.** The skills you demonstrate in the clinical encounter are reflected in your ICE score. This score consists of a **data-gathering (DG) score** and a **PN score.**
    - **DG score.** To determine your DG score, SPs will document your ability to gather data pertinent to the clinical encounter. Specifically, SPs will note whether you asked the questions listed on their checklists, successfully obtained relevant information, and correctly conducted the physical exam (as indicated by your performance of the procedures on their checklists). Your final DG score will represent an average of your performance with all 10 SPs. If you asked questions or performed procedures that are not on an SPs checklist, you will not receive credit—but at the same time will not lose credit—for having done so.
    - **PN score.** A physician will score your PN according to predefined criteria, including organization, quality of information, data interpretation, and the absence of inappropriate or dangerous actions. Your final PN score will then represent the average of your individual PN scores over all 10 clinical encounters. Your ICE score will represent the sum of your DG and PN scores (ICE = DG + PN).
- **Communication and Interpersonal Skills (CIS) score.** In addition to assessing your DG skills, SPs will evaluate your interpersonal skills (IPS). These include rapport, interviewing skills, personal manner, and counseling. Your overall CIS score will be the sum of your averaged IPS scores and your spoken English proficiency rating.
- **Spoken English Proficiency (SEP) score.** This component scores you on listening effort, pronunciation, and word choice.

> You must pass all three components to pass the exam.

The grade you receive on the USMLE Step 2 CS will be either a "pass" or a "fail." To pass the Step 2 CS, candidates must pass all three components. Early results indicate that most US and Canadian medical students pass (see Table 1-1). The failure rate is higher among IMGs, with nearly one in four examinees failing.

TABLE 1-1. Step 2 CS Pass Rates				
	July 2007–June 2008		July 2008–June 2009	
	No. Tested	Passing	No. Tested	Passing
US/Canadian	17,350	97%	17,637	97%
IMGs	17,223	70%	17,017	71%

US students rarely fail the SEP subcomponent. If they do fail, it is most likely because of poor ICE scores. Relatively few US students fail both ICE and CIS. For IMGs, CIS is the most likely component to cause failure. SEP is more of a challenge but is still the least likely component to cause failure. Few IMGs fail all three subcomponents.

Your report will include a graphic representation of your strengths and weaknesses on the three components of the exam. Since October 2008, feedback on the CIS component of the exam has been expanded to encompass three additional categories: questioning skills, information-sharing skills, and professional manners and rapport.

Among students who fail Step 2 CS, US students are most likely to fail because of ICE scores, and IMGs are most likely to fail because of CIS.

Anticipated Changes to the Step 2 CS

The NBME has indicated indicated that changes to the Step 2 CS may be made in 2012. Please go to www.usmle.org or www.firstaidteam.com for the latest updates. Some of the expected changes are as follows:

1. **Patient note.** Potential changes to this section include asking examinees to document their analysis of a patient's possible diagnoses and how such diagnoses are supported or refuted by the evidence obtained from the history and physical examination.
2. **Assessment of communication skills.** Currently, the Step 2 CS measures an examinee's ability to effectively gather and share information and to establish a professional rapport with the SP. In the future, examinees will be also be evaluated on their ability to tailor their questions and responses to the specific needs of the case presented and on their ability to react to the entire range of the patient's concerns. This addition focuses on the ability of the examinee to conduct a *patient-centered interview* (discussed at length later in this section), in which he or she identifies and responds to the broader scope of the patient's concerns—beyond just the diagnosis. The system of scoring communication skills will adapt to reflect this change. Examinees who demonstrate a broader and deeper range of communication skills and approach the encounter in a focused manner will be rewarded with a higher score. More information about the modifications to the assessment of communication skills is available in the National Board of Medical Examiners' (NBME) Fall/Winter 2010 Newsletter (Volume 57, number 2; www.nbme.org/PDF/2010_FallWinterExaminer.pdf).

How Do I Register to Take the USMLE Step 2 CS?

Applicants can register directly for the Step 2 CS without having passed any other USMLE Step. However, registration information and procedures are constantly evolving. For the most current information on registering for the Step 2 CS, go to www.usmle.org or check with your dean's office. IMGs should also refer to the Web site of the Educational Commission for Foreign Medical Graduates (ECFMG) at www.ecfmg.org.

US students must register using the NBME's interactive Web site for applicants and examinees (click the appropriate link at www.nbme.org). IMGs can either apply online using the ECFMG's Interactive Web Application (IWA) at https://iwa2.ecfmg. org/gradoverview.asp or download the paper application from the ECFMG Web site and mail it to the ECFMG with the registration fee. Although there is no specific application deadline, you should apply early to ensure that you get your preferred test date and center.

After your application has been processed, you will receive a scheduling permit by e-mail. Orientation manuals and videos of sample encounters are available at www. usmle.org or can be obtained on CD when you register. The video is an excellent preparation resource that shows exactly how the Step 2 CS is administered as well as how to conduct yourself during the exam. Once you have received your scheduling permit, you are eligible to take the Step 2 CS for one year, starting from the date your application was processed. Your scheduling permit will list your eligibility period, scheduling instructions, and identification requirements for admission to the exam. You can schedule the test through the NBME or ECFMG Web sites or by telephone. Access information will be included with your registration materials. Note that test centers offer both morning and afternoon sessions. You may be offered an afternoon session if you select a date and center for which morning sessions are already filled. Try to select a date and center that offer you a morning session (when you are fresher and more relaxed).

Although you cannot extend your eligibility period for the Step 2 CS, you can cancel or reschedule your exam date. You will not be charged a fee if you cancel or reschedule 14 calendar days before your scheduled test date, not including the day of the test. However, a fee of $150 will be levied if you cancel or reschedule at any time during the 14-day period before (but not including) your scheduled test date. You will need to pay $400 if you miss an appointment without canceling or rescheduling.

Finally, a word of caution regarding the exchange of scheduled test dates. Some applicants have been known to post requests on online forums to swap their appointment with another applicant. The Step 2 CS scheduling system does not allow anyone to schedule or reschedule an appointment on behalf of another applicant. In addition, the system works on a "first come, first served" basis—so if you cancel your appointment in anticipation of such an exchange, your test date might be claimed by someone else who happens to be logged onto the system at the same time. Applicants are therefore advised to avoid such exchanges and instead to reschedule test dates only within the formal protocols.

Where Can I Take the Exam?

The Step 2 CS will be administered at five regional sites called Clinical Skills Evaluation Collaboration centers (see Figure 1-1). Additional centers are currently under consideration.

For detailed information about cities, hotels, and transportation, please refer to the USMLE Web site (www.usmle.org), the ECFMG Web site (www.ecfmg.org), and the Section 1 Supplement of this text.

FIGURE 1-1. Step 2 CS Test Centers

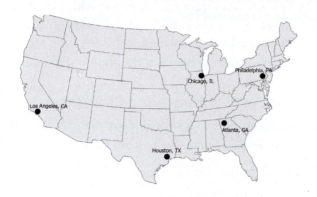

How Long Will I Wait to Get My Scores?

Step 2 CS results are posted to your On-line Applicant Status and Information System (OASIS) account on the ECFMG/NBME Web site. An e-mail is sent to you once your score report has been uploaded onto your account page. A fixed schedule of score-reporting periods is published on the USMLE Web site well in advance of your test date. The majority of examinees who take the Step 2 CS receive their scores on the first day of the corresponding reporting period, which is usually 1–3 months from the date of the test. If you do not receive your results within that time, you must send a written request for a duplicate report to the NBME or the ECFMG. Again, the score report you receive indicates only whether you passed or failed the exam. Your numerical score is not disclosed to you or to any of the programs to which you apply. Once you pass the Step 2 CS, your passing score remains valid for the purpose of applying for residency training.

What If I Fail?

If you fail the Step 2 CS, you can retake it, but not more than three times within any 12-month period. In addition, each time you take the exam, you must submit a new application and appropriate fee.

If for some reason you think that you received a failing score unfairly, you may be able to appeal and request a rescoring of your exam. However, doing so is unlikely to change your overall exam results. Check your orientation manual or the USMLE and/or ECFMG Web sites for the latest reexamination and appeal policies.

PREPARING FOR THE STEP 2 CS

In preparing for the Step 2 CS, keep in mind that you will need to demonstrate certain fundamental but critical clinical skills to pass. These skills include the following:

- Interacting with patients in a professional way
- Taking a good medical history

- Performing an appropriate physical exam
- Counseling and delivering information
- Typing a logical and organized PN

In this section, we briefly explore a few of these skills. Section 2 reviews these skills in greater detail in addition to the mechanics of the clinical encounter and PN.

Ability to Interact with Patients in a Professional Way

There are several elements of the CIS component that you must incorporate into each encounter. These are simple and easy to learn but require practice.

- **Introduce yourself to the patient.** When you first meet a patient, be sure to smile, address the patient by his or her last name (eg, "Mr. Jones"), introduce yourself clearly, shake hands firmly, and establish good eye contact.
- **Actively listen to the patient.** Allow the patient to list his/her concerns without interrupting or interjecting your own thoughts. Your demeanor should be curious, nonjudgmental, and compassionate.
- **Use "draping manners."** Always keep the patient well draped. You can cover the patient at any time before the physical exam, but it is better to do so at the beginning of the encounter. Do not expose large portions of the patient's body at the same time; instead, uncover only the parts that need to be examined, and only one at a time. Be sure to ask permission before you uncover any part of the body and explain why you are doing so. You should also ask permission to untie the patient's gown and should tie the gown again when you are done.
- **Be mindful of appearance.** In your encounters, you should appear confident, calm, and friendly as well as serious and professional. You will wear a clean white lab coat over professional-looking but comfortable clothes. Do not wear shorts or jeans. Men should wear slacks, a shirt, and a tie. Women should consider slacks and low-heeled shoes and should avoid wearing skirts above the knee.
- **Maintain appropriate body language.** During the clinical encounter, look the patient in the eye, smile when appropriate, and show compassion. When trying to console a patient, you may place your hand on his or her shoulder or arm but not on the leg or hand. Do not exaggerate your facial expressions in an effort to convince the patient that you empathize with him or her. Never talk to a patient while standing somewhere he or she cannot see you, especially during the history and closure.
- **Focus your concentration on the patient.** Ask permission before you examine any part of the patient's body and explain what you intend to do. Pay attention to everything the patient says and does, because it is most likely purposeful. You can show concern by doing the following:
  - **Keep the patient comfortable.** Help the patient sit up, lie down, and get onto and off the examination table. Do not repeat painful procedures.

- **Show compassion for the patient's pain.** If the patient does not allow you to touch his or her abdomen because of severe pain, say, "I know that you are in pain, and I want to help you, but I need to examine you to be able to locate the source of pain and give you the right treatment."

- **Show compassion for a patient's sadness.** To demonstrate empathy, you may take a brief moment of silence and place your hand lightly on the patient's shoulder or arm. You may then say something like, "You must feel sad. Would you like to tell me about it?"

- **Respect the patient's beliefs.** Do not reject a patient's beliefs even if they sound incorrect to you. A patient may tell you, "I am sure that the pain I have is due to colon cancer." You may respond to this with something like, "That may be one possibility, but there are others that we need to consider as well."

> *IMGs should focus on communication and interpersonal skills. US medical students should be careful not to use complex language or medical jargon.*

Ability to Take a Good Medical History

The interviewing techniques you use should allow you to collect a thorough medical history. It is true that you can prepare a list of questions to use for every system or complaint. However, be aware that you will not be able to cover everything. Therefore, you should ask only those questions that are relevant to the specific case; your goal is to direct each interview toward exploring the chief complaint and uncovering any hidden complaints.

If you feel that a patient is not following your line of questioning, be careful, as this may indicate that you are drifting away from the correct diagnosis. You should also bear in mind that physical findings may be simulated and may not look the same as real ones (eg, simulating wheezes during chest auscultation). In such circumstances, you should pretend that the findings are real.

Do not be intimidated by angry patients. Remember that SPs are only actors, so stay calm, firm, and friendly. Ask about the reason for a patient's anger or complaint, and address it appropriately. Do not be defensive or hostile. If you do not understand what a patient has said or recognize a drug that has been prescribed, do not hesitate to ask, "Can you please repeat what you said?" or "What is the name of that drug again?"

Finally, remember to use the **summary technique** at least once during the interview. This technique, which involves briefly summarizing what the patient has just told you, often using the patient's own words, may be used either after you finish taking the history or after the physical exam. Summarizing will help ensure that you remember the details of the history before you leave the room to write the PN.

> *The summary technique is an excellent patient communication strategy.*

Ability to Counsel and Deliver Information

At the end of each encounter, you will be expected to tell the patient about your findings, offer your medical opinion (including a concise differential diagnosis), describe the next step in diagnosis, and outline possible treatments. In doing so, you should always be clear and honest. Tell the patient only the things you know, and do not try to render a final diagnosis. Make sure the patient understands what you are saying, and avoid the use of complex medical terms. Before you leave, ask the patient if he or she still has any questions. After you respond, follow up by asking, "Did that answer your question?"

When counseling a patient, always be open. Tell the patient what you really think is wrong, and explain that the final diagnosis can be made only after some tests have been taken. You should also explain some of the tests you are planning to conduct. Address any concerns the patient may have in a realistic manner, and never offer false reassurances.

TEST-DAY TIPS

The Step 2 CS is a one-day exam. You will be scheduled for either the morning or the afternoon session. The duration of the Step 2 CS, including orientation, testing, and breaks, is approximately 8 hours. Once you have entered the secured area of the assessment center for orientation, you may not leave that area until the exam has been completed. During this time, the following conventions should be observed:

- You may not use watches (analog or digital), cell phones, or beepers at any time during the exam.
- The morning session starts at 8 A.M. and the afternoon session at 3 P.M. Test proctors will generally wait up to 30 minutes for latecomers, so the actual exam usually does not begin until 8:30 A.M. or 3:30 P.M. Nonetheless, you should plan to arrive 30 minutes before your session is scheduled to begin.
- Do not come to an afternoon session early in an attempt to meet candidates from the morning session, as they are not allowed to leave until you are locked in.
- Bring a government-issued photo ID (eg, a US driver's license or a passport) that carries your signature.
- Be sure to bring your admission permit! You will not be admitted to the test center without it.

> No watches of any kind, either analog or digital, are allowed in the test area. Neither are pens/pencils or scratch paper.

After the 30-minute waiting period has ended, the staff will give you a name tag, a numbered badge to be worn around your arm, a pen, and a clipboard. There is no need to bring a pen of your own; in fact, you are not allowed to use anything other than the pen provided at the exam site.

> Don't bring your luggage to the test center. Check it with the hotel front desk.

If you are traveling with luggage, do not bring it to the test site, as the staff cannot store it for you. You will be provided only a coat rack and a small storage locker for belongings that you are not allowed to carry during the encounter, such as watches, cell phones, purses, and handbags. If you are planning to travel immediately after the exam, you can keep your luggage at the front desk of your hotel.

At the beginning of your session, you will be asked to sign a confidentiality agreement. An orientation session will then be held to introduce you to the equipment that you will find in the examination rooms. Examine and become familiar with the equipment, especially the bed, foot extension, and head elevation. Do not hesitate to try every piece of equipment made available to you during this session.

You will be given two breaks during the exam. The first break lasts 30 minutes and takes place after the fourth encounter. During this break, the staff will serve you a meal. The second break lasts 15 minutes and takes place after the eighth encounter. Use the bathroom during these breaks, as you will not have time to do so during the encounters. Finally, remember that smoking is strictly prohibited not only during the exam but also during breaks. You cannot leave the center during break periods.

In the break room, you will be assigned a seat and a desk. You can keep your food or drink on this desk so that it will be accessible during break time. Although the testing staff will provide you with one meal, you may want to bring some high-energy snacks for your breaks. Also remember that your personal belongings will not be accessible to you until the end of the exam—so if you do plan to bring food with you, keep it on your assigned desk, not in the storage area.

> *Bring water or energy snacks to keep at your desk if you need them.*

The Step 2 CS is not a social event, so when you meet with other candidates during breaks, do not talk about the cases you encountered. During breaks (and, of course, during the encounters), speak only in English; doing otherwise is considered irregular and may be questioned.

Finally, remember that, even though all your encounters are videotaped, these tapes are not used for scoring purposes. They are used only to ensure the safety of the SPs and candidates and to ensure quality. So, don't worry about the camera, and don't try to look for it during the encounters. Act as you would on a regular clinic day.

Some Final Words

The following general principles will help you excel on the Step 2 CS:

- **Think about the present, not the past.** Clear your head when moving to the next encounter. Thinking about what you should have done or should have asked will only distract you from your current encounter.
- **Passing does not require perfection.** You need not be perfect. In fact, given the time constraints involved, the Step 2 CS rewards efficiency and relative completeness over perfection.
- **There is a reason for everything you see.** If a patient is wearing a peculiar Mexican hat, inquire why this is the case. He might have been in Mexico, and the diarrhea he presents with may thus be a simple traveler's diarrhea.

> *Go for efficiency, not perfection.*

FIRST AID FOR THE IMG

If you are an IMG candidate seeking to pass the Step 2 CS, you must take a number of variables into account, from plotting a timetable to mastering logistical details to formulating a solid test preparation strategy.

Determining Eligibility

Before contacting the ECFMG for a Step 2 CS application, you must first take several preliminary steps. Begin by ascertaining whether you are eligible (see Table 1-2). Check the ECFMG Web site for the latest eligibility criteria.

TABLE 1-2. IMG Eligibility for the USMLE Step 2 CS[a]	
Medical Students	**Medical School Graduates**
You must be enrolled in a foreign medical school listed in the International Medical Education Directory (IMED, http://imed.ecfmg.org) both at the time you apply and at the time you take the assessment. You must also be within 12 months of graduation when you take the exam.	You must be a graduate of a medical school that was listed in the IMED at the time of your graduation.

[a] You are **not** required to have passed the English-language proficiency test or the Test of English as a Foreign Language to be eligible for the Step 2 CS.

> *Ideally, you should get your ECFMG certificate before you submit your residency applications.*

Once you have established your eligibility to take the exam, you will need to factor in the residency matching process (the "Match"). If you are planning to apply for a residency in the United States, your timetable should reflect that and should be carefully planned at least one year in advance.

You are allowed to **register** (pay the fee) for the Match regardless of your ECFMG status. To **participate** in the Match, however, the National Residency Matching Program (NRMP) requires that you be ECFMG certified (or that you meet ECFMG requirements for certification even if you have not received your certificate) by the rank-order-list deadline (typically in February of each year). Applicants who do not meet these requirements will be automatically withdrawn from the Match. Therefore, you should take the Step 2 CS no later than October in the year before your target Match Day (see Figure 1-2).

There is a significant advantage to obtaining ECFMG certification by the time you submit your application for residency in the fall. Should you do so, residency programs are apt to consider you a ready applicant and may favor you over other candidates who have yet to take the Step 2 CS—even if such candidates have more impressive applications. In addition, if you are certified early, you can take the Step 3 and get your results back before the rank-order-list deadline. A good score on Step 3 can provide a perfect last-minute boost to your application and may also make you eligible for the H-1B visa. In sum, take the Step 2 CS as soon as you are eligible (see Table 1-2) but not before you are confident that you are fully prepared. Remember

FIGURE 1-2. Typical Step 2 CS Timeline for IMGs

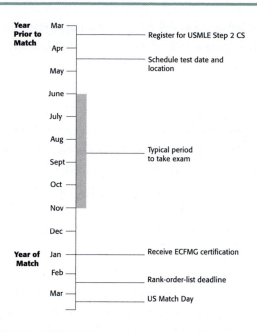

that, to get ECFMG certification, you need to pass the Step 1, Step 2 CK, and Step 2 CS within a seven-year period. In deciding when to apply for the Step 2 CS, when to take it, and whether you are ready for it, keep the following points in mind:

- Scheduling your test date can be difficult during busy seasons. Apply at least three months before your desired examination date. Ideally, you should aim to take the Step 2 CS in June or July to be certified when you apply for residency.
- Schedule your exam on the date that you expect to be fully prepared for it. For IMGs, preparation for the exam typically requires anywhere between 1 and 12 weeks, factoring in your level of English proficiency as well as your medical knowledge and skills.
- If you choose to apply for the Step 2 CS using a paper application, it will take up to four weeks to receive your notification of registration, but it may take as few as 10 days to receive this information if you use the ECFMG's IWA.

Some residency programs use the Step 2 CS as a screening tool to select IMG applicants for interviews, so it is ideal to meet the deadline for the Match.

If you are an IMG living outside the United States, you must also factor in the time it may take to obtain a visa. You do not need a visa to come to the United States if you are a US or Canadian citizen or a permanent resident. Citizens of countries participating in the Visa Waiver Program (such as European Union countries) may not need to obtain a visa either. You are responsible for determining whether you need a visa (usually H-1B or H-2B) and, having done so, for obtaining that visa (regardless of how time-consuming and difficult this process may be). Before you apply to take the Step 2 CS, you should therefore complete the following tasks:

> *All the USMLE exams need to be passed within a seven-year period for ECFMG certification.*

- Check with the US embassy in your country to determine whether you need a visa.
- Determine how long it will take to get an appointment at the embassy.
- Find out how long it will take to get the visa and whether a clearance period is required.
- Check travel availability to the cities in which the exam centers are located.

As proof of the reason for your visit to the United States, the ECFMG will send you a letter to present to the US consulate in your country. This letter will be sent to you only after you apply to take the Step 2 CS (ie, after you have paid the fee) and will not guarantee that you will be granted a visa. For this reason, it is wise not to schedule your actual exam day until you have arrived in the United States or have at least obtained your visa.

Application Tips

When you receive your application to take the Step 2 CS, be sure to read it carefully before filling it out. You do not want your application returned to you—thus wasting valuable time—simply because you forgot to answer a question or made a careless mistake. Applications that contain the following errors will be returned; they are common, so do everything you can to avoid them:

- An application that is not written in ink or is illegible
- An incomplete application
- An application that is not the original document (ie, a faxed or photocopied application)
- An application that contains a nonoriginal signature or photograph
- An application that contains a photograph of the applicant that was taken more than six months before the date the application was submitted
- An application in which the signature of the medical school official or the notary public is more than four months old
- An application in which the medical school or notary public seal or stamp does not cover a portion of your photograph
- An application that does not explain why it was signed by a notary public but not by your medical school official
- An application that does not include full payment

> *Use the ECFMG's IWA to minimize delays and errors.*

Commonly encountered errors specific to IMGs include the following:

- Failure to send the ECFMG a copy of your medical school diploma with two full-face photographs
- Failure to send the ECFMG an English translation of your medical school diploma if the original is not in English
- Failure to staple together your medical school diploma and its English translation or to ensure that the translator's stamp covers both the original and the translation

Once you have completed your application and have double-checked it for errors, make every effort to send it by express mail or courier service. To check the status of your application on-line, you can use OASIS (https://oasis2.ecfmg.org).

Improving Your English Proficiency

For many IMGs taking the Step 2 CS, a critical concern lies in the demonstration of proficiency in spoken English. In Step 2 CS terms, this refers to the ability to speak English clearly and comprehensibly and to understand English when the SP speaks to you.

You may not have a problem with English proficiency if you are a native English speaker, have studied in a US or other English-speaking school, have learned medicine in English in your medical school, or have spent at least a few months or years of your life in an English-speaking country. English proficiency may, however, be the main obstacle facing IMGs at the other end of the spectrum. The good news is that most IMGs who have already passed the USMLE Step 1 have the basic English language skills needed to pass the Step 2 CS. For such candidates, the key to passing the Step 2 CS lies in organizing these skills and practicing. Your spoken English proficiency is based on the following components:

- **The ability to speak in a manner that is easy for the SP to follow and understand.** To this end, choose phrases that are simple, direct, and easy both for you to remember and for the SP to understand. Speaking slowly will also make it easier for SPs to understand you and will minimize the effect your accent has on your comprehensibility.

- **The correct use of grammar.** The key to mastering this element is to be familiar with commonly used statements, transitions, and questions and to practice them as much as possible. This will minimize the probability that you will make significant grammatical errors.

- **Comprehensible pronunciation.** Again, the key to good pronunciation lies in practicing common statements and questions, repeating them to yourself aloud, and asking someone (preferably a native English speaker) to listen to you and correct your mistakes. The more you practice, the better your chances will be of reaching an acceptable and even a superior level of clear, comprehensible English.

- **The ability to correct and clarify your English if necessary.** You may find it difficult to prepare for a situation in which an SP does not understand you and asks you for the meaning of something you have just said. Here again, however, you can avoid this situation by practicing common statements, questions, and transitions; speaking as slowly and clearly as possible; and using nontechnical words instead of complicated medical terminology. If an SP still cannot understand something you have said, simply repeat the phrase or question, or restate it in simple lay terms.

> *The key to better spoken English is practicing commonly used statements, transitions, and questions.*

Make every effort to remain calm throughout your clinical encounters. Nervousness can cause you to mumble, making it difficult for the SP to understand you. Likewise, if you become nervous and start looking at the clock and rushing, you will further increase the likelihood of making mistakes. So, remain calm, concentrate, and take your time.

Fifteen minutes may seem like a short time to do and say all the things you think are necessary, but it will be more than enough if you follow an organized plan. Most of the things you have to say in the exam are the same in each encounter, so by thoroughly studying common cases and medical conditions (see Sections 3 and 4), you can minimize this obstacle.

If you are still unsure about your English proficiency, the ECFMG suggests that you take the Test of Spoken English (TSE) to get a measure of your abilities. If you score higher than 35 on this exam, you have likely attained the level of English proficiency necessary for the Step 2 CS. You may also consider taking the Test of English as a Foreign Language (TOEFL) before you take the Step 2 CS. However, doing so is no longer a prerequisite to taking the Step 2 CS or to ECFMG certification. For more information about the TSE and the TOEFL, contact:

TOEFL/TSE Services
PO Box 6151
Princeton, NJ 08541-6151
609-771-7100
toefl@ets.org
www.toefl.org

Getting Clinical Rotations and Observerships

Many IMGs may lack basic familiarity with the workings of US medical schools. A clinical rotation or observership in the United States can prepare IMGs for the Step 2 CS by introducing them to the US system and, in the process, immersing them in the "American way" of taking a history, performing a physical exam, and writing PNs. Clinical rotations are also good to have on your curriculum vitae when you apply for residency programs. Furthermore, performing well on your rotation can earn you strong letters of recommendation, which are the most important part of your application after your USMLE scores. The more time you spend in such a rotation, the better.

> Internal medicine and emergency medicine are the best rotations for Step 2 CS preparation.

If you are still a **medical student,** it should not be difficult for you to find a clinical rotation. Check the Web sites of the universities in which you are interested and e-mail or write the program director and chairman of each. If you are already in the United States, call the relevant departments and make appointments to meet with the personnel responsible for the rotations. Most of the time, such personnel will send you an application by mail. For the purposes of your residency application, however, it is highly recommended that you also do a rotation in the specialty in which you are interested.

If you are a **medical graduate,** your mission is more difficult but not impossible. You are no longer eligible for clinical elective rotations (clerkships), but you can still apply for observerships and externships.

The observership is perhaps the least active function you can fill in a hospital, but it can still be highly useful. Getting an observership is not an easy task because most hospitals do not have any such formal rotation or training program. Nonetheless, here is some advice that may help you:

- Prepare a list of hospitals in your area or any area that interests you. Include all types of teaching hospitals: university, community, and Veterans Affairs medical centers.
- Contact people (attendings, senior residents, secretaries, administrators) whom you may know. Connections are an important way to uncover these unofficial rotations.
- Send e-mails and/or letters to the chairman and program director of each hospital.
- Call the office of the chairman or program director and try to set an appointment to meet him/her.
- Seek out people (attendings, residents, secretaries, administrators) from your country who may be able to help you. Inform them that you would be willing to pay for your malpractice insurance if necessary.
- Talk to other physicians who are doing or have done observerships and ask them where they did so and how to apply.

During your rotation, you will "officially" be an observer, which means that you cannot touch a patient or write on charts. The only things you are officially allowed to do are observe, do rounds with your team, answer an occasional question, present some topics, and attend conferences. On rare occasions, you may be able to examine some patients and write some notes. Here is some advice for making the most of your observership:

- Show a high level of enthusiasm.
- Come early and stay late (not very late, though).
- Follow up on patients your team is taking care of and learn everything you can about them.
- Read about the cases your team is managing.
- Chat and spend time with the patients, but always let them know that you are an observer. This is the best way to practice taking histories and to improve your language skills.
- Write your own PNs and orders, ask your residents to correct them, and compare them to the official notes.
- Talk to the nurses, secretaries, and support staff. This will improve your communication skills.
- If you do not get a chance to examine patients, carefully observe the residents and medical students during the physical exam.
- Do as many presentations as you can.

Here is a partial list of hospitals that have been known to offer observerships or externships:

- DC General Hospital, Washington, DC
- Emory University, Atlanta, GA
- Harbor Hospital, Baltimore, MD
- Providence Hospital, Washington, DC
- Veterans Administration Medical Center, Washington, DC
- University of Miami, Miami, FL
- Mayo Clinic, Rochester, MN (visiting physicians program)
- Mount Sinai Hospital, Miami, FL
- Hospital of St. Raphael, New Haven, CT
- Hahnemann Hospital, Philadelphia, PA
- Maricopa Medical Center, Phoenix, AZ

Some Final Tips

There are a few final practical measures you can take to help ensure your success on the Step 2 CS:

- Check and recheck the ECFMG and USMLE Web sites for the latest information about the Step 2 CS. This will help you get a clear idea about regulations, requirements, registration, examination dates, and all other details concerning the Step 2 CS.
- Carefully prepare for the exam using the preparation materials included in this book.
- Check other Web sites and discussion forums. They can be a good source of information.
- Review the steps of history taking (see Section 2). Choose and prepare common questions and cases (see Sections 3 and 4).
- Review the steps of the physical exam (see Section 2). Practice the physical exam as if you were performing the real exam.
- Practice writing PNs (see Section 4).

The USMLE Step 2 CS Travel Guide

Traveling to the United States

Atlanta ("The Big Peach")

Chicago ("The Windy City")

Houston ("Space City")

Los Angeles ("The City of Angels")

Philadelphia ("The City of Brotherly Love")

Useful Web sites

After you've worked hard to prepare for the Step 2 CS, the last thing you need is extra travel stress—or, worse still, problems on test day. The best way to ensure that everything goes as smoothly as possible is to plan ahead. Getting all the details in place well in advance of your trip will help you focus on what's really important: doing a great job on the exam!

The following quick guide can be used as a planning tool both before and during your travels. For each of the five cities with a Step 2 CS testing center (called Clinical Skills Evaluation Collaboration, or CSEC, centers), we have provided details on the best ways to get to your destination and some things to do once you have arrived. Since most of you will be flying, we have placed special emphasis on distances to the CSEC test sites and routes from the airports. Also listed are a number of nearby hotels, most of which are reasonably priced and within walking distance of the CSEC centers. As a cheaper option, we have included one youth hostel for each city. Finally, we have recommended a few well-known restaurants and tourist attractions for each destination. All five CSEC destinations are amazing cities, and we do not want you to miss out on what they have to offer. Although you should not let sightseeing get in the way of your test, you might want to schedule at least a few hours to see the sights. Even better, think about giving yourself an extra day or two after the exam to relax and really enjoy yourself in a new and exciting city.

With that said, make sure to confirm the details of the destinations we've presented before you start your trip. We have compiled a broad range of suggestions for you, but by the time you get to your destination, some of the details may well have changed. Another great source of information is the travel section on the USMLE Web site. Also note that the Association of American Medical Colleges (AAMC) has negotiated reduced hotel rates with many nearby hotels for the Step 2 CS. We have included many of these hotels here, but be sure to check the updated list online. Links to these sites are provided at the end of this section.

TRAVELING TO THE UNITED STATES

We know that many of you who are planning to take the Step 2 CS may be coming to the United States for the first time—so here are a few things to keep in mind to help minimize travel hassles.

Arrange your documents. Generally, the most important document you will need for the Step 2 CS is your **scheduling permit.** However, other documents may be required as well, especially if you're coming from another country. These may include the following:

- Your **passport**
- A US **tourist visa** (usually a H-1B/H-2B visa; apply at the nearest US embassy in your country)
- An **international driver's license** (consider getting one if you're planning to drive to your testing center)

Make sure your travel plans are in place. Be sure to make your reservations well in advance, and think about how you're going to get around in the test city. Once you've arrived at your destination, make sure you know how to get to the CSEC center on the day of your test, especially if you're planning to stay a bit farther away.

Consider travel safety. When traveling abroad, particularly in major US population centers, it's important to follow a few general guidelines to ensure your safety:

- In general, Americans are friendly and willing to help; however, not everyone has the best intentions. Be particularly alert to individuals who seem a bit too eager to help or who go out of their way for you.
- Keep an eye on your baggage while traveling by taxi, train, or any form of public transportation. Pickpockets and petty thieves tend to target visitors.
- Never carry anything in your baggage that doesn't belong to you. You are responsible for the contents of your baggage, including anything illegal that might have been placed there by someone else.
- Dress like the locals.
- Avoid walking alone in deserted streets at night.

Pack appropriately. Packing before air travel requires a lot of preparation. Here are a few useful tips:

- There are many restrictions for carry-on luggage these days, particularly with regard to liquids. Check the US Transportation Security Administration's Web site (www.tsa.gov) for the most up-to-date information.
- Prepare for lost or delayed baggage. Do not keep your scheduling permit, lab coat, or stethoscope in your checked baggage. Also remember to put a copy of your itinerary in your baggage so that authorities can locate you in the event that your baggage is lost.
- Using a mobile phone or a camera, take a photograph of your baggage to give to the authorities in the event that your baggage is delayed or lost.
- Tag your baggage with brightly colored tape or a distinguishing mark so that you can easily identify it at baggage carousels.

Plan, plan, plan. Here are some guidelines for planning your visit and booking your hotel:

- Try to schedule your exam well in advance. Doing so will make it easier for you to get a good price on your tickets and accommodations.
- Before you book a hotel or a flight, compare prices at multiple Web sites and at each organization's Web site (see "Useful Web Sites" at the end of this supplement).
- Before you choose a hotel, be sure to factor in the distance to the testing center as well as the services each hotel offers—for example, whether it has a free airport shuttle, free breakfast, and access to Wi-Fi. Bear in mind that staying in a

youth hostel may save you money on hotel accommodations, but may increase travel time to the CSEC center on test day.

ATLANTA ("THE BIG PEACH")

Clinical Skills Evaluation Collaboration Center
Two Crown Center
1745 Phoenix Boulevard, Suite 500 (5th Floor)
Atlanta, GA 30349-5585

The Atlanta metro area has a population of more than five million and is the capital city of the great state of Georgia. Throughout history, Atlanta has served as a main north–south and east–west railway hub; in fact, its name was derived from the Atlanta-Pacifica railway that ran through the town in the 1840s. Today, Atlanta is home to the Centers for Disease Control and Prevention as well as the headquarters of Coca-Cola. We know you'll enjoy your time in this diverse and thriving city!

Getting There

- **Air:** Atlanta's major airport is the Hartsfield-Jackson Atlanta International Airport (ATL), located about 9 miles/14.5 kM south of downtown and only a few blocks from the CSEC center.
- **Ground:**
  - Greyhound, 232 Forsyth Street Southwest (www.greyhound.com): The main bus terminal is located downtown, about 12 miles/19.3 kM from the CSEC center, which is approximately 20 minutes by taxi for a flat rate of $25.
  - Amtrak, 1688 Peachtree Street Northwest (www.amtrak.com): The main train station is also located downtown, about 16 miles/25.7 kM from the testing center. Atlanta is on the Crescent Line, which runs between New Orleans and New York.

Getting Around When You Arrive

- **Shuttles:** Most hotels offer free shuttle service to and from the airport. There are also two airport shuttle services available from the airport. Both run into town on a regular basis; schedules are available online:
  - AAA Airport Express (www.aaaairportexpress.com)
  - Airport Metro Shuttle (www.airportmetro.com)
- **Taxis:** Taxis are available at the airport and at the bus/train terminals and cost $30–$35 from the airport to downtown. Local taxi companies include the following:
  - Atlanta Checker Cab: 404-351-1111
  - National: 404-752-6834
  - Night and Day: 404-767-7464
  - Yellow Cab: 404-521-0200

- **Rental cars:** Automobile rentals are available at the airport. The most popular companies are as follows:
  - Alamo (www.alamo.com): 800-462-5266
  - Avis (www.avis.com): 800-230-4898
  - Budget (www.budget.com): 800-527-0700
  - Dollar (www.dollar.com): 800-800-3665
  - Enterprise (www.enterprise.com): 800-261-7331
  - Hertz (www.hertz.com): 800-654-3131
  - National (www.nationalcar.com): 800-227-7368
  - Payless (www.paylesscarrental.com): 800-729-5377
  - Thrifty (www.thrifty.com): 800-847-4389
- **Public transportation:** Atlanta has a regional metro system called MARTA (Metropolitan Atlanta Rapid Transit Authority, www.itsmarta.com). You will need tokens to ride MARTA; they can be purchased at the MARTA Ride Store inside Airport station (located inside the western end of the airport's main terminal), from token machines in MARTA's stations, or at many retail outlets. A trip downtown will take approximately 15 minutes. For about $1.75, you can also get to the CSEC center from the airport on the southbound C-TRAN Route 503 bus. Board in the South Terminal ground transport area and expect a 10-minute ride.

CSEC Center Location

The Atlanta CSEC center is located a few minutes to the south of the Hartsfield-Jackson airport, about a 0.25 miles/0.4 kM east of the intersection of West Fayetteville Road and Phoenix Boulevard. The V-shaped brown brick building that houses the CSEC center should be visible from the I-285 highway. The center is on the fifth floor, and plenty of free parking is available.

Where to Stay

The following list includes a few hotels located close to the test site as well as a youth hostel in the area. Most are just outside the airport, but there are some highways around, so plan your walk carefully. Remember to ask hotels about their USMLE deals, listed on the AAMC Web site (marked with an asterisk below).

- ***Country Inn & Suites Atlanta Airport South ($$):** 1808 Phoenix Boulevard (0.3 miles/0.5 kM away); 770-991-1099. Just around the corner from the CSEC center, making it very convenient.
- ***Best Western Hotel & Suites Airport South ($$):** 1556 Phoenix Boulevard (about 0.7 miles/1.1 kM away); 770-996-5800.
- ***Comfort Inn & Suites Airport South ($$):** 2450 Old National Parkway (about 1.5 miles/2.4 kM away); 404-684-9898.
- ***Sheraton Gateway Atlanta Airport ($$):** 1900 Sullivan Road (2.0 miles/3.2 kM away); 770-997-1100.
- ***Hilton Garden Inn Atlanta Airport North ($$):** 3437 Bobby Brown Parkway (5.1 miles/8.2 kM away); 404-477-6600.

- **Atlanta Youth Hostel ($):** 223 Ponce de Leon Avenue Northeast (14 miles/22.5 kM away); 404-875-9449. A cheaper option with plenty of nightlife. A bit farther away from the CSEC center, but only a few blocks away from the MARTA North Avenue station.

Where to Eat and Play

Atlanta has amazing Southern food. Take advantage of this and enjoy some of our favorites:

- **The Varsity ($):** 61 North Avenue Northwest, Downtown; 404-881-1706. The world's largest drive-in restaurant, the Varsity is an Atlanta icon that has been serving burgers and hot dogs since 1928.
- **Sweet Auburn Curb Market ($):** 209 Edgewood Avenue Southeast, Downtown; 404-659-1665. A historic market with stalls that feature fresh produce and hot meals. Includes many small ethnic restaurants as well.
- **Fat Matt's Rib Shack ($):** 1811 Piedmont Avenue Northeast, Midtown; 404-607-1622. An Atlanta hot spot serving up Southern-style barbecue and playing live blues music every night.

What to See

Atlanta has much to see and do. Here are just a few places to consider seeing while you're in town:

- **Georgia Aquarium:** The world's largest aquarium, with more than 8.5 million gallons of water and 100,000 species of sea life.
- **World of Coca-Cola:** Come and celebrate the original home of this sugary drink in historic Piedmont Park.
- **Underground Atlanta:** A mall located under the streets in the Five Points neighborhood.
- **Sweet Auburn District:** Home to the Martin Luther King, Jr., National Historic Site.

For more information, check out:

- www.lonelyplanet.com/worldguide/usa/atlanta/
- www.atlanta.net

CHICAGO ("THE WINDY CITY")

Clinical Skills Evaluation Collaboration Center
8501 West Higgins Road, Suite 600
Chicago, IL 60631

Located on the shores of Lake Michigan, Chicago is the principal financial and cultural center of the Midwest and is currently the third-largest city in the United

States. Chicago is known for its gangster lore, blues clubs, and biting cold winters. With plenty of history, shopping, and culture, today's Windy City is bursting with life, so be sure to enjoy your stay!

Getting There

- **Air:** Chicago has two major airports. The larger is O'Hare International Airport (ORD), which is about 20 miles/32.2 kM northwest of downtown but only 5 miles/8 kM from the CSEC center. The other is Chicago Midway Airport (MDW), located about 12 miles/19.3 kM southwest of downtown and roughly 20 miles/32.2 kM from the testing center. Both have easy public transportation within the city but O'Hare may be more convenient given the closer proximity to the testing site.
- **Ground:**
  - Greyhound, 5800 North Cumberland Avenue (www.greyhound.com): The Chicago Cumberland Avenue Greyhound bus terminal is just a few blocks away from the CSEC center and is the closest of the six bus terminals in Chicago.
  - Amtrak, Canal Street between Adams and Jackson Boulevards (www.amtrak.com): The main train hub in Chicago is at downtown Union Station. This is a good choice, but you'll have to take public transportation or a taxi to get to the test site. The Chicago Transport Authority Blue Line runs to Cumberland Station from Union Station, taking you very close to the CSEC center.

Getting Around When You Arrive

- **Shuttles:** Most nearby hotels offer free shuttle service to and from the airport. You can also use either of the airport shuttle services. Schedules and up-to-date fares are available online:
  - Continental Airport Express (www.airportexpress.com): 888-284-3826
  - Omega Airport Shuttle (www.omegashuttle.com): 773-734-6688
- **Taxis:** As in any big city, taxis are usually the most direct way to get around Chicago. They cost roughly $30–$40 from O'Hare to downtown and about $10 from O'Hare to the CSEC center:
  - American United: 773-327-6161
  - Des Plaines Cab Service: 847-827-0110
  - Flash Cab: 773-992-0303
  - Yellow Cab: 312-225-7440
- **Rental cars:** Rental cars are available at the airport. The most popular companies are as follows:
  - Alamo (www.alamo.com): 800-462-5266
  - Avis (www.avis.com): 800-230-4898
  - Budget (www.budget.com): 800-527-0700
  - Dollar (www.dollar.com): 800-800-3665
  - Enterprise (www.enterprise.com): 800-261-7331
  - Hertz (www.hertz.com): 800-654-3131

- National (www.nationalcar.com): 800-227-7368
- Thrifty (www.thrifty.com): 800-847-4389
- **Public transportation:** Ride the famous Chicago "L," an easy-to-use and cheap light-rail system, or take a Chicago Transit Authority bus! Both the CSEC center and O'Hare are on the "L" Blue Line, and both connect to downtown. For the CSEC center, you'll want Cumberland Station (5800 North Cumberland Avenue). Single ride fares are $2.25, and multiday passes are also available. Fares are available at all stations. Check out fares and schedules online at www.transitchicago.com.

CSEC Center Location

The exam center is located on the northwest side of Chicago, about 15 miles/24.1 kM from downtown and just 5 miles/8 kM east of O'Hare along I-90 (Kennedy Expressway). From Cumberland Station, the CSEC center is a quick 0.8 miles/1.3 kM walk or cab ride to the north over the highway. The CSEC center is located within the First Midwest Bank Building. There should be plenty of free parking at the site. *Note for drivers:* The signs in the visitor lot indicate one-hour-only parking. This does **not** apply to Step 2 CS examinees, so you are still free to park there. You may park in the visitor lot for the duration of the exam, but do not park in spaces reserved for other tenants such as First Midwest Bank, Chicago Title, or Westwood College.

Where to Stay

The following hotels are good options near the testing center. Remember to ask hotels about their USMLE deals, listed on the AAMC Web site (marked with an asterisk below). If you have a car, you can also check out some of the hotels a bit farther west along I-90. You'll probably get a cheaper rate if you're willing to make a commute on the morning of the test.

- ***Marriott Chicago O'Hare ($$$):** 8535 West Higgins Road (0.02 miles/0.03 kM away); 773-693-4444. Right next door to the testing center!
- ***SpringHill Suites Chicago O'Hare ($$):** 8101 West Higgins Road (0.04 miles/0.6 kM away); 773-867-0000.
- ***Renaissance Chicago O'Hare Suites ($$$):** 8500 West Bryn Mawr Avenue (0.7 miles/1.2 kM away); 773-380-9600.
- ***Holiday Inn Chicago O'Hare ($$):** 5615 North Cumberland Avenue (0.8 miles/1.3kM away); 773-693-5800. Very close to the Cumberland Blue Line stop.
- ***Crown Plaza Chicago O'Hare ($$):** 5440 North River Road (2.08 miles/4.5 kM away); 847-671-6350.
- ***Sheraton Gateway Suites O'Hare:** 6501 North Manheim Road (2.8 miles/3.3 kM away); 847-699-6300.
- **Hostelling International Chicago ($):** 24 East Congress Parkway (15 miles/24.1 kM away); 312-360-0300. This large hostel is located downtown, about 15 miles/24.1 kM from the testing center, so plan at least an hour to make the trip on the Blue Line.

Where to Eat and Play

Chicago has hundreds of amazing restaurants of all varieties; here are just a few.

- **Giordano's World Famous Stuffed Pizza ($$):** 135 East Lake Street; 312-616-1200. Chicago is the town for pizza, and Giordano's delivers some of the best. There are branches all over the city, so find the one that works for you. This is likely to be the best and most filling meal you've had in a while.
- **Café Spiaggia ($$):** 980 North Michigan Avenue; 312-280-2750. Try lunch at the café. This relaxed restaurant is just next door to the world-famous Italian restaurant Spiaggia, which is known to be a favorite of the Obamas.
- **Blue Chicago ($$):** 736 North Clark Street; 312-642-6261. Check out one of Chicago's world-famous blues clubs, perhaps after you're done with the test.

What to See

Don't miss the sites of this amazing city just because you're staying near the airport and the testing center. After you're done taking the exam, think about booking a late flight and jumping on the "L" for an afternoon downtown.

- **Willis Tower:** Visit the Skydeck for amazing views from the tallest building in North America.
- **Navy Pier:** Features museums, shops, restaurants, and even a Ferris wheel on the shore of Lake Michigan.
- **Magnificent Mile:** The heart of the city, with upscale shopping and fantastic restaurants running along Michigan Avenue.

For more information, check out:

- www.lonelyplanet.com/worldguide/usa/chicago/
- www.choosechicago.com
- www.cityofchicago.org/tourism

HOUSTON ("SPACE CITY")

Clinical Skills Evaluation Collaboration Center
400 North Sam Houston Parkway, Suite 700
Houston, TX 77060

Houston was founded in 1836 on land near the Buffalo Bayou and was named after Sam Houston, then the president of the Republic of Texas. Today, Houston is one of the largest cities in the United States and is home to many major energy companies in addition to a substantial portion of the biomedical and aeronautical industries. It also boasts one of the best art festivals in the country, the Bayou City Art Festival, held here every spring and fall. Enjoy the show!

Getting There

- **Air:** Houston has two major airports: George Bush Intercontinental (IAH) and Hobby Airport (HOU). IAH is the larger of the two and is much closer to the CSEC center (8 miles/12.9 kM); HOU is smaller and farther away (27 miles/43.5 kM).
- **Ground:**
  - Greyhound, 2121 Main Street (www.greyhound.com): Houston has a terminal downtown. Outside of the station, there are plenty of taxis available. A ride to your hotel should take about 30 minutes.
  - Amtrak, 902 Washington Avenue (www.amtrak.com): Houston is on the Sunset Limited line, which runs all the way from Louisiana to California.

Getting Around When You Arrive

- **Shuttles:** Most hotels around the CSEC center offer free shuttle service. If your hotel doesn't provide service, check out the following: SuperShuttle (www.supershuttle.com): 713-523-8888
- **Taxis:** A number of taxi companies operate in Houston; below are just a few ($20–$40 to the CSEC center from the airport):
  - Liberty Cab: 713-695-6700
  - Square Deal Cab: 713-659-5105
  - United Cab: 713-699-0000
  - Yellow Cab: 713-236-1111
- **Rental cars:** Multiple rental car companies are available in Houston. The most popular companies are as follows:
  - Advantage (www.arac.com): 800-777-5500
  - Alamo (www.alamo.com): 800-462-5266
  - Avis (www.avis.com): 800-230-4898
  - Budget (www.budget.com): 800-527-0700
  - Dollar (www.dollar.com): 800-800-3665
  - Enterprise (www.enterprise.com): 800-261-7331
  - Hertz (www.hertz.com): 800-654-3131
  - National (www.nationalcar.com): 800-227-7368
  - Thrifty (www.thrifty.com): 800-847-4389
- **Public transportation:** If you're really adventurous, try Houston's Metro, which includes bus routes and light rail (www.ridemetro.org). Lines 102, 56, and 86 serve the area around the airport, the CSEC center, and hotels. Buses run every 10–45 minutes, depending on the route and time of day. The Metro also provides a direct shuttle between the IAH airport and the downtown transit center for $4.50. Visit their Web site for a trip planner, which will help you figure out the details.

CSEC Center Location

The CSEC center is located on the north side of Houston in a large office building at the intersection of Imperial Valley Drive and Beltway East Access Road. There is a parking garage with a large "400" on the side that is visible from the street. You'll see McDonald's and Arby's restaurants across the street. Free parking is available in the attached garage.

Where to Stay

The following hotels are located around the test site. You can walk from most, although the sidewalks aren't great. Remember to ask hotels about their USMLE deals, listed on the AAMC Web site (marked with an asterisk below).

- ***Baymont Inn & Suites ($):** 502 North Sam Houston Parkway East (0.2 miles/0.3 kM away); 281-820-2101. The Baymont gets high marks for cleanliness and service and is a great value.
- ***Settle Inn ($):** 500 North Sam Houston Parkway East (0.2 miles/0.3 kM away); 281-931-0101.
- ***Hyatt Place Houston/Greenspoint ($$):** 300 Ronan Park Place (0.7 miles/1.1 kM away); 281-820-6060. The Hyatt is a good deal, is close to the CSEC center, and is well recommended.
- ***Comfort Inn–Greenspoint ($$):** 12701 North Freeway (1.9 miles/3.1 kM away); 281-875-2000.
- ***Super 8–IAH West/Greenspoint ($):** 1230 North Sam Houston Parkway East (3.2 miles/5.1 kM away); 281-987-7100.
- ***Holiday Inn Houston Intercontinental Airport ($$):** 15222 JFK Boulevard (4.3 miles/6.9 kM away); 281-876-3888.
- ***Sheraton North Houston Hotel at Bush Intercontinental Airport ($$):** 15700 JFK Boulevard (4.5 miles/7.2 kM away); 281-442-5100.
- **Venetian Inn & Suites ($):** 6 North Sam Houston Parkway East (0.5 miles/0.8 kM away); 281-447-6888. Cheap, good service, but there is no shuttle from the airport.
- **Houston International Hostel ($):** 5302 Crawford Street (18 miles/28.9 kM away); 713-523-1009. The hostel is very cheap ($15/night in a dormitory) and is located about 30 minutes away from the CSEC center.

Where to Eat and Play

Houston has cuisine from all around the world but is especially well known for its Latin American fare. The restaurants we've listed aren't necessarily close to the test center, but we thought it might be fun for you to get out!

- **Americas ($$$):** 1800 Post Oak Boulevard; 713-961-1492. Americas serves Central and South American cuisine with flair.
- **Spanish Village Restaurant ($$):** 4720 Almeda Road; 713-523-2861. A restaurant that has been serving "Tex-Mex" food since 1953. Try their delicious margaritas.
- **Dry Creek Café ($):** 544 Yale Street; 713-426-2313. Relaxing and fun. Go for one of their "Bad Ass" burgers.

What to See

If your exam is over by early afternoon, you might have some extra time to enjoy the sights and sounds of Houston.

- **Theater district:** Located downtown with five great venues. Check out Bayou Place, with its many theaters, bars, and restaurants.
- **Museum district:** Located downtown near Rice University, with many museums and parks. It would be a shame to pass up the John C. Freeman Weather Museum.
- **Sports:** Check out an Astros (www.astros.com) or Rockets (www.rockets.com) game while you're there.

For more information, check out:

- www.houston-guide.com
- www.lonelyplanet.com/destinations/north_america/houston

LOS ANGELES ("THE CITY OF ANGELS")

Clinical Skills Evaluation Collaboration Center
100 North Sepulveda Boulevard, 13th Floor
El Segundo, CA 90245

LA is one of the best-known cities in the United States and is rich in cultural and ethnic diversity. One of its most notable attractions, of course, is Hollywood, the hub of the US motion picture industry. LA is also home to some amazing cultural sites, such as the Kodak Theatre, the Walt Disney Concert Hall, and all your favorite actors. Take in some stargazing while you're in town!

Getting There

- **Air:** Los Angeles is served by one major airport, Los Angeles International (LAX). It is one of the busiest airports in the world and is located only about 3 miles/4.8 kM from the CSEC center.
- **Ground:**
  - Greyhound, 1716 East 7th Street (www.greyhound.com): LA has a terminal near downtown. Plenty of taxis are available outside the station. A ride to your hotel should take about 30 minutes.
  - Amtrak, 800 North Alameda Street (www.amtrak.com): LA is on multiple rail routes that connect it to cities like New Orleans, Chicago, and Seattle.

Getting Around When You Arrive

- **Shuttles:** Many hotels around the CSEC center offer free shuttle service from LAX. If your hotel doesn't provide such service, check out the following:
  - SuperShuttle (www.supershuttle.com): 800-258-3826
  - Prime Time Shuttle (www.primetimeshuttle.com): 800-733-8267

- **Taxis:** A number of taxi companies operate in LA; below are just a few ($10–$15 from airport to CSEC center):
  - Beverly Hills Cab: 310-273-6611
  - Independent Taxi Owners Association: 800-521-9294
  - LA Taxi/United Checker Cab: 213-627-7000
- **Rental cars:** Multiple rental car companies are available in the area. These include Advantage, Alamo, Avis, Dollar, Enterprise, Hertz, and National. For a full list of rental companies, visit www.lawa.org/lax and see "Ground Transportation."
- **Public transportation:** Despite its reputation, LA does have public transportation, and the CSEC center is not far from rail and bus stops. There is also a free shuttle from LAX to the Aviation station on the Green Line, a rail line that is just two stops away from the El Segundo/Nash station. The Green Line runs every 7–15 minutes during rush hour. Get off at the El Segundo/Nash station, walk west on El Segundo Boulevard (0.5 miles/0.8 kM) toward the park on the south side of El Segundo, and make a right on North Sepulveda Boulevard. The hotels listed are also generally within walking distance of the stop. You can find more information and a Metro trip planner on the public transportation Web site, www.metro.net.

CSEC Center Location

The CSEC center is located on the west side of LA, only a few miles from LAX and about 20 miles/32.2 kM from downtown. It is situated at the corner of North Sepulveda and El Segundo Boulevards. You'll see a series of large office towers; turn in the first driveway marked "Pacific Corporate Towers." Follow the signs to get to visitors' parking ($9/day).

Where to Stay

The following hotels are situated around the test site. You can walk from most, although not all have great walking routes. Remember to ask hotels about their USMLE deals, listed on the AAMC Web site (marked with an asterisk below).

- ***Doubletree Hotel Los Angeles International Airport ($$):** 1985 East Grand Avenue (0.6 miles/1 kM away); 310-322-0999. The Doubletree is routinely recommended by guests for its comfortable beds and clean rooms.
- **Residence Inn by Marriott El Segundo ($$):** 2135 East El Segundo Boulevard (0.4 miles/0.6 kM away); 310-333-0888. Great quiet rooms and a good complimentary breakfast.
- ***Hacienda Hotel ($$):** 525 North Sepulveda Boulevard (0.4 miles/0.6 kM away); 310-615-0015. A convenient 10-minute walk to the CSEC center. An older but decent choice—just be ready for small elevators.
- ***Travelodge LAX South ($$):** 1804 East Sycamore Avenue (0.9 miles/1.4 kM away); 310-615-1073. An acceptable budget option, but service can be spotty.
- ***Hilton Garden Inn El Segundo ($$):** 2100 East Mariposa Avenue (0.9 miles/1.4 kM away); 310-726-0100.

- ***Sheraton Gateway Hotel Los Angeles Airport ($$):** 6101 West Century Boulevard (2.3 miles/3.7 kM away); 310-642-1111.
- **USA Hostels Hollywood ($):** 1624 Schrader Boulevard; 323-462-3777. This hostel is very cheap ($30–$80/night) and is about 30 minutes away from the center by car if traffic is normal. It's fun but loud, so if you plan on staying here, be sure to bring earplugs (24 miles/38.6 kM away).

Where to Eat and Play

LA is one of the most ethnically diverse cities in the world, so you can find food for almost every taste. Here are just a few of our favorites:

- **Beachcomber Café ($$):** 23000 Pacific Coast Highway, Malibu; 310-456-9800. Situated on the historic Pacific Coast Highway about 40 minutes from El Segundo. Enjoy an amazing dinner on the beach in Malibu.
- **WoodSpoon ($):** 107 West Ninth Street; 213-629-1765. Located in downtown LA, this unassuming restaurant serves up Brazilian fare. Grilled plates come with rice, beans, plantains, and collard greens. Simple and delicious.
- **Medusa Lounge ($$$):** 3211 Beverly Boulevard; 213-382-5723. An exciting place to get dinner and enjoy the nightly DJs. Offers great beers, sushi, duck, and bratwurst. You'll have to see it to believe it.

What to See

If your exam is over by early afternoon, you might have some extra time to see a bit of LA. As the locals say, LA is very "spread out," so the sights aren't always easy to reach without a car, but it's worth a try.

- **Hollywood:** Enjoy a stroll down Hollywood Boulevard and the Walk of Fame. If you don't have a car, you can ride the Metro Rail, but remember that this will take some time. From the test center, take the Green Line to the Blue Line and transfer to the Red Line. Exit at the Hollywood/Highland station.
- **Venice Beach:** Only 15 minutes away. Take in some of the uniqueness of LA with attractions like Muscle Beach and the area's renowned street performers!

For more information, check out:

- www.latourist.com
- www.laweekly.com

PHILADELPHIA ("THE CITY OF BROTHERLY LOVE")

Clinical Skills Evaluation Collaboration Center
3624 Market Street, 3rd Floor
Philadelphia, PA 19104

Philadelphia is a great city that is steeped in US history. It was a major hub of social and political activity during the American Revolution, and there is a wealth of places you can visit to soak it all up. Today, Philadelphia is thriving, boasting the fifth-largest metro area in the country. While you're in town, check out Independence Hall, where the Declaration of Independence was first signed on July 4, 1776. And be sure to eat a Philly cheesesteak!

Getting There

- **Air:** Philadelphia is served by one major airport, Philadelphia International Airport (PHL). It serves flights from all around the country and the world. PHL is located about 10 miles/16.1 kM from the CSEC center.
- **Ground:**
  - Greyhound, 1001 Filbert Street (www.greyhound.com): The Greyhound terminal is located near the downtown area. Plenty of taxis are available outside the station. A ride to your hotel should take about 5 minutes.
  - Peter Pan Trailways, 1001 Filbert Street (www.peterpanbus.com): This bus line is located at the same address as Greyhound.
  - Amtrak, 2955 Market Street (www.amtrak.com): Philadelphia is on multiple Amtrak lines, including the high-speed Acela line, which connects Boston, New York, Philadelphia, and Washington, DC. Other lines connect Philadelphia to the South and the Midwest.

Getting Around When You Arrive

- **Shuttles:** There is limited shuttle service from the airport, but one does cover the area: Lady Liberty Company (www.ladylibertyshuttle.com): 215-724-8888
- **Taxis:** A number of taxi companies operate in the city; below are just a few ($25 from the airport to the CSEC center):
  - Liberty Cab: 215-389-8000
  - Olde City Taxi Coach Association: 215-338-0838
  - PHL Taxi: 800-936-5111
  - Yellow Cab: 215-333-3333
  - Quaker City Cab: 215-728-8000
- **Rental cars:** Multiple rental car companies are available. The most popular companies are as follows:
  - Alamo (www.alamo.com): 800-462-5266
  - Avis (www.avis.com): 800-230-4898
  - Budget (www.budget.com): 800-527-0700
  - Dollar (www.dollar.com): 800-800-3665
  - Hertz (www.hertz.com): 800-654-3131
  - National (www.nationalcar.com): 800-227-7368
- **Public transportation:** Philadelphia has an extensive public transportation network, called SEPTA (www.septa.org). Buses and a high-speed rail line connect to the airport. Although the rail line is more expensive, it is easier to use. The Airport rail line (R1) connects all the terminals to the 30th Street station, which is six blocks from the testing center—or you can transfer to the Market-Frankford line and take it to 34th and Market Street, which is just two blocks from the testing center.

CSEC Center Location

The CSEC center is located downtown, near the University of Pennsylvania campus. It can be found near the intersection of Market and 36th Streets. There is a parking lot right across the street ($14/day).

Where to Stay

The following hotels are within walking distance of the test site. Since the CSEC center is downtown, these hotels are fairly expensive. Remember to ask hotels about their USMLE deals, listed on the AAMC Web site (marked below by an asterisk).

- ***Sheraton Philadelphia University City ($$):** 36th and Chestnut Streets (two blocks away); 800-596-0369. Well recommended and one of the only moderately priced hotels close by.
- **Hilton Inn at Penn ($$$):** 3600 Sansom Street (0.2 miles/0.3 kM away); 215-222-0200. Located on the University of Pennsylvania's campus, this hotel is close but expensive.
- ***Cornerstone Bed and Breakfast ($$):** 3300 Baring Street (0.6 miles/1 kM away); 215-387-6065. This B&B is a wonderful place to stay. The breakfasts are delicious.
- **Rodeway Inn Philadelphia ($$):** 1208 Walnut Street (2.1 miles/3.8 kM away); 215-546-7000. An acceptable budget option but not walkable. You can, however, ride the Market-Frankford line from City Hall to the 34th Street station.
- ***The Best Western Center City Hotel ($$):** 501 North 22nd Street (1.7 miles/2.7 kM away); 215-568-8300.
- **Apple Hostels of Philadelphia ($):** 32 South Bank Street (2.8 miles/4.5 kM away); 877-275-1971. This hostel offers both dorm-style and private rooms and is very well recommended. It is located just a block from the Market-Frankford line, so you can take the rail line to the 34th Street station and walk to the CSEC center.

Where to Eat and Play

Philadelphia is a great city with a variety of great restaurants. Here are a few of the best:

- **Geno's Steaks/Pat's King of Steaks ($):** 1219 South 9th Street; 215-389-0659/215-468-1547. The Philly cheesesteak (or "hoagie"), perhaps one of the best-known foods in the country, was born here. Just remember to drop the "Philly" while you're in town. Keys to a proper order: Cheese Whiz or provolone with or without fried onion rings.
- **Audrey Claire ($$):** 276 South 20th Street; 215-731-1222. One of the best restaurants in town, located in the heart of Rittenhouse Square.
- **Tangerine ($$$):** 232 Market Street; 215-627-5116. This is one of the tastiest experiences you'll ever have. There are too many great dishes to single out just one, but try the lobster risotto or the chicken tagine.

What to See

If your exam is over by early afternoon, you are likely to have some extra time to see the sights of Philadelphia. And since the CSEC center is downtown, you're already in the heart of it.

- **Independence Hall/Liberty Bell:** Located in the block between 5th and 6th Streets and Market and Chestnut Streets, Independence Hall and the Liberty Bell are two of the most iconic images in all of US history. You may want to make a reservation beforehand (www.nps.gov/inde).
- **Museum District:** Close by and home of the Philadelphia Museum of Art, the Franklin Institute of Science, the Philadelphia Zoo, Fairmont Park, and Eastern State Penitentiary.

For more information, check out:

- www.philly.com
- www.lonelyplanet.com/destinations/north_america/philadelphia

USEFUL WEB SITES

Here are a few other Web sites that you might find useful while you are planning your trip:

- **USMLE travel site:** www.usmle.org/Examinations/step2/cs/CSECAddresses.html
- **AAMC accommodations site:** www.aamc.org/meetings/153904/clinicalskills_mtgs_homepage_teaser.html
- **Travel and hotel sites:**
  - www.expedia.com
  - www.travelocity.com
  - www.orbitz.com
  - www.hotwire.com
  - www.hotels.com
  - www.priceline.com

► **NOTES**

The Patient Encounter

Introduction

Doorway Information

Taking the History

The Physical Exam

Closure

How to Interact with Special Patients

Challenging Questions and Situations

Counseling

The Patient Note

INTRODUCTION

As described in Section 1, the Step 2 Clinical Skills (CS) exam consists of 10–12 clinical encounters with trained "standardized patients" (SPs), with each encounter designed to replicate situations commonly seen in clinics, doctors' offices, and emergency departments.

Each encounter in the Step 2 CS lasts 15 minutes. You will be given a warning when 5 minutes remain in the session. The 15-minute period allotted for each of your interviews includes meeting the patient, taking the history, performing the physical exam, discussing your findings and plans, and answering any questions the patient might have. After that, you will have 10 minutes to summarize the patient history and physical exam and to formulate your differential diagnosis and workup plan. All this may seem overwhelming, but it doesn't need to be. This chapter will guide you through the process step by step.

Fifteen minutes should be adequate for each patient encounter as long as you budget your time wisely. The most common reasons for running out of time are as follows:

- Taking an overly detailed history
- Conducting an unnecessarily detailed physical exam
- Carrying out the encounter in a slow or disorganized fashion
- Allowing the patient to stray away from relevant topics
- Failing to adequately control challenging (eg, unresponsive, angry, crying) patients

To best manage your encounter, it is recommended that you distribute your time as follows:

- **Doorway information** (assessing preliminary information posted on the door of each room): 10–20 seconds
- **History:** 7–8 minutes
- **Physical exam:** 3–5 minutes
- **Closure:** 2–3 minutes

Of course, this is only an approximation. In reality, each encounter is different, so some will require more time for taking the history or doing the physical exam, whereas others will demand that more time be spent on closure and patient counseling. You should thus tailor your time to fit each case. Here are some additional time management tips:

- Do not waste valuable time looking at the clock on the wall. Use the official announcement that 5 minutes remain in the encounter as your only time indicator. If you have not begun to perform the physical exam by that point, you should do so.
- An organized and well-planned history is key. Stay focused on asking questions that are pertinent to the chief complaint.
- A brief and focused physical exam is also critical. There is no need to conduct a comprehensive physical exam during encounters.

- One of the major objectives of the Step CS is to evaluate your ability to communicate with patients. Make sure you leave time to discuss your management plan and never try to save time by ignoring the patient's questions, requests, or emotional status.
- Practice is the best way to improve your performance, efficiency, and sense of timing.

Figure 2-1 illustrates the key components and desired outcomes of the clinical encounter. The following sections will guide you through each of these components.

> *Any time saved from the patient encounter can be used to write the patient note.*

DOORWAY INFORMATION

As described, you will be given a chance to review preliminary patient information, known as "doorway information," at the outset of each encounter. This information, which is posted on the door of the examination room, includes the patient's name, age, and gender; the reason for the visit; the patient's vital signs (pulse, blood pressure, temperature in both degrees Celsius and Fahrenheit, and respiratory rate); and the task you will be called on to perform.

You should begin by reading the doorway information carefully, checking the chief complaint, and trying to organize in your mind the questions you will need to ask and the systems you will have to examine. Toward this goal, you should look for abnormalities in vital signs without trying to memorize actual numbers. Assume that these vital signs are accurate.

Remain calm and confident by reminding yourself that what you are about to encounter is a common medical case. You should also bear in mind that SPs are easier to deal with than real patients in that they are more predictable and already know what you are expected to do. Remember that a second copy of the doorway information sheet will be available on the other side of the door, so you can review that information at the end of each encounter. Note, however, that the time you spend reading the doorway information is included in the 15-minute time limitation.

Your entrance into the examination room is a critical part of the encounter. So before you enter the room, be sure to read and commit to memory the patient's last name, and then knock on the door. Once you have entered the examination room, ask the patient if he or she is the person identified on the door (eg, "Mr. Smith?"). You will receive credit for having done so and will not have to worry about remembering the patient's name for the remainder of the encounter. If the patient does not respond to your query, consider the possibility that there may be a change in mental status and that the SP might have been instructed not to respond to his or her name.

After your initial entrance, you should shake hands with the patient and introduce yourself in a confident yet friendly manner (eg, "Hi, I am Dr. Morton. Nice to meet you."). You may also add something like, "I would like to ask you some questions and

FIGURE 2-1. Overview of the Clinical Encounter

Doorway Information
Must get: Chief complaint, age, sex, and abnormal vital signs.
Leads to: Forming a hypothesis (broad differential, relevant points that should be elicited in the history, systems to examine).

History
Must get: Details of the chief complaint, associated symptoms, and any other relevant information that will help rule in or rule out each item in the differential.
Leads to: A more well-defined differential diagnosis, which will help narrow down the procedures that should be performed and the systems that should be examined in the physical exam.

Physical Exam
Must get: Evaluation of the appropriate systems to help rule in or rule out each item in the differential; any additional information on the patient's history if required.
Leads to: A final differential and an appropriate workup plan.

Closure
Explaining the findings, differential, and workup plan to the patient.
Answering the patient's questions and addressing his concerns.

Address the patient by his or her name when you enter the room. Always make eye contact with the patient.

do a physical exam." Again, make an effort to establish eye contact with the patient during this initial period.

The Patient-Centered Interview

Conducting a patient-centered interview (PCI) is an essential component of successfully completing the encounter in the Step 2 CS. The main goals of the PCI are to establish a trusting doctor–patient relationship and to ensure that the encounter is patient centered, not disease centered nor doctor centered.

Building a trusting relationship with the patient starts from the moment you enter the examination room. It includes the simple but essential components described previously: calling the patient by his/her name, introducing yourself, and shaking hands with the patient. Remember that these steps are not mere courtesies; they set a respectful and attentive tone to the entire encounter.

The next step in conducting a PCI involves **reflective listening.** Building trust with your patient requires you to be a good listener. Therefore, start the encounter by telling the patient what your role is and then asking about his or her concerns (eg, "I was asked to see you for your chest pain; what are your concerns?"). Once you have asked the patient to state his or her concerns, listen to what they are without interrupting or interjecting your own thoughts. Encourage the patient to express all the concerns by using phrases like, "Is there anything else?" or "Tell me more about that." When the patient has expressed all his or her concerns, summarize them using the patient's own words as much as possible. Doing this builds trust by showing the patient that you are actively listening.

The next step in the PCI involves setting a **joint agenda with the patient.** Once you have summarized the patient's concerns you need to prioritize these concerns and establish a joint agenda with the patient to address them. For example, you might say to the patient, "You are concerned about chest pain, cough, and smoking. I am concerned about all these things as well. Let's address first whichever of these things concerns you the most." By doing this, the patient will feel that he or she is an active part of the interview and that you are indeed conducting a *patient-centered* interview and not a *doctor-centered* interview.

Once this is established, you can begin gathering information and developing a diagnosis (discussed in the history-taking section, below).

Throughout the encounter, you should aim to **connect with the patient.** The patient is likely to express emotions such as anger, fear, sadness, and anxiety. Be alert to these emotions and be ready to respond with **"PEARLS"** (Partnership, Empathy, Apology, Respect, Legitimization, and Support). Look for opportunities to utilize the PEARLS in every patient encounter. Of course, you will not use all of them in each encounter; you will likely use only one or two, depending on the nature of the case. A brief description of each PEARLS is given below:

Partnership means that you and the patient are working together to identify the main concerns and to come up with solutions. Phrases that help facilitate partnership include "Let's deal with this together" and "We can do this."

Empathy is shown by acknowledging and showing understanding of the patient's feelings. For example, you might respond to a patient who expresses fear or anger with "That sounds hard" or "You look upset."

Apology refers to taking personal responsibility when it is appropriate to do so (eg, "I'm sorry I was late" or "I'm sorry this happened to you").

Respect means valuing the patient's choices, behaviors, and decisions (eg, "You have obviously worked hard on this.").

Legitimization validates the patient and shows understanding of his or her feelings and choices. For example, a legitimizing statement would be something like, "Anyone would be confused or sad or upset by this situation."

Support should be continually offered to the patient. You can offer support to the patient by saying something as simple as "I'll be here when you need me."

> The patient-centered interview is patient centered, not disease centered or doctor centered.

Again, the PCI is patient centered, not disease centered or doctor centered. Following these principles in the CS exam will help you establish a trusting doctor–patient relationship. From there, you can move on to making appropriate medical decisions and developing the differential diagnosis.

TAKING THE HISTORY

Your ability to take a detailed yet focused history is essential to the formulation of a differential diagnosis and workup plan. The discussion that follows will help guide you through this process in a manner that will maximize your chances of success.

Guidelines

You may take the history while standing in front of the patient or sitting on the stool that is usually located near the bed. You will find a sheet placed on this stool. Begin by removing the sheet and draping the patient. Do this before taking the history to make sure you get credit for doing so early on.

Don't cross your arms in front of your chest when talking to the patient, especially with the clipboard in your hands. It's best to sit down on the stool, relax, and keep the clipboard on your lap. If you decide to stand, maintain a distance of approximately two feet between yourself and the patient.

As noted, the interview as a whole should take no more than 7–8 minutes. You can start your interview by asking the patient an open-ended question such as, "So what brought you to the hospital/clinic today?" or "How can I help you today?" See Figure 2-2 to get an overview of the process.

Additional Tips

Once the interview has begun, be sure to maintain a professional yet friendly demeanor. You should speak clearly and slowly, and your questions should be short, well phrased, and simple. To that end, avoid the use of medical terms; instead, use simple words that a layperson can understand (eg, don't use the term *renal calculus*; use *kidney stone* instead). If you find yourself obliged to use a medical term that the patient may not understand, offer a quick explanation. Don't wait for the patient to ask you for the meaning of a term, or you may lose credit.

> *Use simple, nontechnical terminology when speaking to the patient.*

If you don't understand something the patient has said, you may ask him or her to explain or repeat it (eg, "Can you please explain what you mean by that?" or "Can you please repeat what you just said?"). At the same time, do not rush the patient. Instead, give the patient the time needed to respond. In interacting with the patient, you should always remember to ask questions in a neutral and nonjudgmental way.

FIGURE 2-2. History-Taking Overview

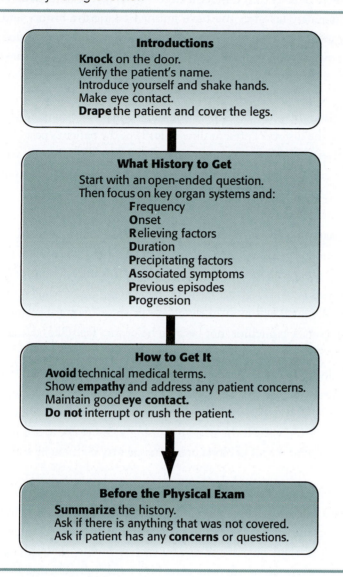

Introductions
Knock on the door.
Verify the patient's name.
Introduce yourself and shake hands.
Make eye contact.
Drape the patient and cover the legs.

What History to Get
Start with an open-ended question.
Then focus on key organ systems and:
       Frequency
       Onset
       Relieving factors
       Duration
       Precipitating factors
       Associated symptoms
       Previous episodes
       Progression

How to Get It
Avoid technical medical terms.
Show **empathy** and address any patient concerns.
Maintain good **eye contact**.
Do not interrupt or rush the patient.

Before the Physical Exam
Summarize the history.
Ask if there is anything that was not covered.
Ask if patient has any **concerns** or questions.

THE PATIENT ENCOUNTER

You should also remember not to interrupt the patient unless it is absolutely necessary. If the patient starts telling lengthy stories that are irrelevant to the chief complaint, you can interrupt politely but firmly by saying something like, "Excuse me, Mr. Johnson. I understand how important those issues are for you, but I'd like to ask you some additional questions about your current problem." You can also redirect the conversation by summarizing what the patient has told you thus far and then moving to the next step (eg, "So, as I understand it, your abdominal pains are infrequent, last a short time, and are always in the middle of your belly. Now tell me about . . . .").

It is critical to summarize what the patient has told you, not only to verify that you have understood him but also to ensure that you receive credit. You need to use this summary technique no more than once during the encounter to get credit, but you may use it more often if you consider it necessary. It is recommended, however, that you give a summary (1) after you have finished taking the history and before you start examining the patient, or (2) just after you have finished examining the patient and before you give him your medical opinion. In either case, your summary should include only the points that are relevant to the patient's chief complaint.

Minor transitions may also be used during the history. For example, when you want to move from the history of present illness (HPI) to the patient's past medical history or social and sexual history, you can say something like, "I need to ask you some questions about your health in the past" or "I'd like to ask you a few questions about your lifestyle and personal habits."

To ensure that you stay on track in gathering information, you will also need to watch the patient carefully, paying attention to his or her every word, move, or sign. Remember that clinical encounters are staged, so it is uncommon for something to occur for no reason. Although accidents do happen (eg, an SP once started to hiccup inadvertently), an SP will most likely cough in an encounter because he or she is intending to convey bronchitis, not because he or she "feels like" doing so.

By the same logic, you should address every sign you see in the patient (eg, "You look sad; do you know the reason?" or "You look concerned; is there anything that is making you worry?"). If your patient is coughing, ask about the cough even if it isn't cited as the reason for the visit. If the patient is using a tissue, ask to see it to check the color of the sputum. A spot of blood on the tissue may take you by surprise!

Look for nonverbal clues.

Finally, take brief notes throughout the interview, mainly to record relevant yet easy-to-forget pieces of information such as the duration of the chief complaint or the number of years the patient smoked. To facilitate this note taking, you will be given a clipboard with 12 blank blue sheets, one for each encounter. The extent of your note taking inside the encounter will depend on how much you trust your memory. Before you finish your interview and move to the physical exam, you may ask the patient something like, "Is there anything else you would like to tell me about?" or "Is there anything else you forgot to tell me about?"

Common Questions to Ask the Patient

In this section, we will cover a wide spectrum of questions that you may need to pose in the course of each of your patient interviews. This is not meant to be a complete list, nor do you have to use all of the questions outlined below. Instead, be selective in choosing the questions you ask in your efforts to obtain a concise, relevant history. You should also be sure to ask only one question at a time. If you ask complex questions (eg, "Is there any redness or swelling?"), the SP will likely answer only the last question you posed. Instead, you should slow down and ask about one symptom at a time.

Opening of the encounter:

- "Mr. Jones, hello; I am Dr. Singh. It's nice to meet you. I'd like to ask you some questions and examine you today."
- "How can I help you today?"
- "What brought you to the hospital/clinic today?"
- "What made you come in today?"

Pain:

- "Do you have pain?"
- "When did it start?"
- "How long have you had this pain?"
- "How long does it last?"
- "How often does it come on?"
- "Where do you feel the pain?"
- "Can you show me exactly where it is?"
- "Does the pain travel anywhere?"
- "What is the pain like?"
- "Can you describe it for me?"
- "Is it sharp, dull, burning, pulsating, cramping, or pressure-like?"
- "Is it constant, or does it come and go?"
- "On a scale of 1 to 10, with 10 being the worst pain of your life, how would you rate your pain?"
- "What brings the pain on?"
- "Do you know what causes the pain to start?"
- "Does anything make the pain better?"
- "Does anything make it worse?"
- "Have you had similar pain before?"

Nausea:

- "Do you feel nauseated?"
- "Do you feel sick to your stomach?"

Vomiting:

- "Did you vomit?"
- "Did you throw up?"
- "What color was the vomit?"
- "Did you see any blood in it?"

Cough:

- "Do you have a cough?"
- "When did it start?"
- "How often do you cough?"
- "Do you bring up any phlegm with your cough, or is it dry?"
- "Does anything come up when you cough?"
- "What color is it?"
- "Is there any blood in it?"

- "Can you estimate the amount of the phlegm? A teaspoon? A tablespoon? A cupful?"
- "Does anything make it better?"
- "Does anything make it worse?"

Headache:
- "Do you get headaches?"
- "Tell me about your headaches."
- "Tell me what happens before/during/after your headaches."
- "When do your headaches start?"
- "How often do you get them?"
- "When your headache starts, how long does it last?"
- "Can you show me exactly where you feel the headache?"
- "What causes the headache to start?"
- "Do you have headaches at certain times of the day?"
- "Do your headaches wake you up at night?"
- "What makes the headache worse?"
- "What makes it better?"
- "Can you describe the headache for me, please? Is it sharp, dull, pulsating, pounding, or pressure-like?"
- "Do you notice any change in your vision before/during/after the headaches?"
- "Do you notice any numbness or weakness before/during/after the headaches?"
- "Do you feel nauseated? Do you vomit?"
- "Do you notice any fever or stiff neck with your headaches?"

Fever:
- "Do you have a fever?"
- "Do you have chills?"
- "Do you have night sweats?"
- "Do you sweat during the night?"
- "How high is your fever?"

Shortness of breath:
- "Do you get short of breath?"
- "Do you get short of breath when you're climbing stairs?"
- "How many steps can you climb before you get short of breath?"
- "When did it start?"
- "When do you feel short of breath?"
- "What makes it worse?"
- "What makes it better?"
- "Do you wake up at night short of breath?"
- "Do you have to prop yourself up on pillows to sleep at night? How many pillows?"
- "Have you been wheezing?"
- "How far do you walk on level ground before you have shortness of breath?"
- "Have you noticed any fluid retention around your ankles?"

Urinary symptoms:

- "Has there been any change in your urinary habits?"
- "Do you have any pain or burning during urination?"
- "Have you noticed any change in the color of your urine?"
- "How often do you have to urinate?"
- "Do you have to wake up at night to urinate?"
- "Do you have any difficulty urinating?"
- "Do you feel that you haven't completely emptied your bladder after urination?"
- "Do you need to strain/push during urination?"
- "Have you noticed any weakness in your stream? Any dribbling of urine?"
- "Have you noticed any blood in your urine?"
- "Do you feel as though you need to urinate but then very little urine comes out?"
- "Do you feel as though you have to urinate all the time?"
- "Do you feel as though you have very little time to make it to the bathroom once you feel the urge to urinate?"

Bowel symptoms:

- "Has there been any change in your bowel movements?"
- "Do you have diarrhea?"
- "Are you constipated?"
- "How long have you had diarrhea/constipation?"
- "How many bowel movements do you have per day/week?"
- "What does your stool look like?"
- "What color is your stool?"
- "Is there any mucus or blood in it?"
- "Do you feel any pain when you have a bowel movement?"
- "Did you travel recently?"
- "Do you feel as though you strain to go to the bathroom and then very little feces or none at all comes out?"
- "Have you lost control of your bowels?"
- "Do you feel as though you have very little time to make it to the bathroom once you have the urge to have a bowel movement?"

Weight:

- "Have you noticed any change in your weight?"
- "How many pounds did you gain/lose?"
- "Over what period of time did it happen?"
- "Was the weight gain/loss intentional?"

Appetite:

- "How is your appetite?"
- "Has there been any change in your appetite?"

Diet:

- "Has there been any change in your eating habits?"
- "What do you usually eat?"

- "Did you eat anything unusual lately?"
- "What did you eat before the symptoms started?"
- "Is there any kind of special diet that you are following?"

Sleep:
- "Do you have any problems falling asleep?"
- "Do you have any problems staying asleep?"
- "Do you have any problems waking up?"
- "Do you feel refreshed when you wake up?"
- "Do you snore?"
- "Do you feel sleepy during the day?"
- "How many hours do you sleep?"
- "Do you take any pills to help you go to sleep?"

Dizziness:
- "Do you ever feel dizzy?"
- "Tell me exactly what you mean by dizziness."
- "Did you feel the room spinning around you, or did you feel light-headed as if you were going to pass out?"
- "Did you black out?"
- "Did you lose consciousness?"
- "Did you notice any change in your hearing?"
- "Do your ears ring?"
- "Do you feel nauseated? Do you vomit?"
- "What causes this dizziness to happen?"
- "What makes you feel better?"

Joint pain:
- "Do you have pain in any of your joints?"
- "Have you noticed any rash with your joint pain?"
- "Is there any redness or swelling of the joint?"

Travel history:
- "Have you traveled recently?"

Past medical history:
- "Have you had this problem or anything similar before?"
- "Have you had any other major illnesses before?"
- "Do you have any other medical problems?"
- "Have you been hospitalized before?"
- "Have you had any surgeries before?"
- "Have you had any accidents or injuries before?"
- "Are you taking any medications?"
- "Are you taking any over-the-counter drugs, vitamins, or herbs?"
- "Do you have any allergies?"

Family history:

- "Does anyone in your family have the same problem or anything similar?"
- "Are your parents alive?"
- "Are they in good health?"
- "What did your mother/father die of?"
- "Are your brothers or sisters alive?"
- "Are they in good health?"

Social history:

- "Do you smoke?"
- "How many packs a day?"
- "How long have you smoked?"
- "Do you drink alcohol?"
- "What do you drink?"
- "How much do you drink per week?"
- "Do you use any recreational drugs such as marijuana or cocaine?"
- "Which ones do you use?"
- "How often do you use them?"
- "Do you smoke or inject them?"
- "What type of work do you do?"
- "Where do you live? With whom?"
- "Tell me about your life at home."
- "Are you married?"
- "Do you have children?"
- "Do you have a lot of stressful situations on your job?"
- "Are you exposed to environmental hazards on your job?"

Alcohol history:

- "How much alcohol do you drink?"
- "Tell me about your use of alcohol."
- "Have you ever had a drinking problem?"
- "When was your last drink?"
- Administer the CAGE questionnaire:
    - "Have you ever felt a need to **cut down** on drinking?"
    - "Have you ever felt **annoyed** by criticism of your drinking?"
    - "Have you ever had **guilty** feelings about drinking?"
    - "Have you ever had a drink first thing in the morning (**'eye opener'**) to steady your nerves or get rid of a hangover?"

Sexual history:

- "I would like to ask you some questions about your sexual health and practice."
- "Are you sexually active?"
- "Do you use condoms? Always? Other contraceptives?"
- "Are you sexually active? With men, women, or both?"
- "Tell me about your sexual partner or partners."

- "How many sexual partners have you had in the past year?"
- "Do you currently have one partner or more than one?"
- "Have you ever had a sexually transmitted disease?"
- "Do you have any problems with sexual function?"
- "Do you have any problems with erections?"
- "Do you use any contraception?"
- "Have you ever been tested for HIV?"

Gynecologic/obstetric history:
- "At what age did you have your first menstrual period?"
- "How often do you get your menstrual period?"
- "How long does it last?"
- "When was the first day of your last menstrual period?"
- "Have you noticed any change in your periods?"
- "Do you have cramps?"
- "How many pads or tampons do you use per day?"
- "Have you noticed any spotting between periods?"
- "Have you ever been pregnant?"
- "How many times?"
- "How many children do you have?"
- "Have you ever had a miscarriage or an abortion?"
- "In what trimester?"
- "Do you have pain during intercourse?"
- "Do you have any vaginal discharge?"
- "Do you have any problems controlling your bladder?"
- "Have you had a Pap smear before?"

Pediatric history:
- "Was your pregnancy full term (40 weeks or 9 months)?"
- "Did you have routine checkups during your pregnancy? How often?"
- "Did you have any complications during your pregnancy/during your delivery/after delivery?"
- "Was an ultrasound performed during your pregnancy?"
- "Did you smoke, drink, or use drugs during your pregnancy?"
- "Was it a vaginal delivery or a C-section?"
- "Did your child have any medical problems after birth?"
- "When did your child have his first bowel movement?"

Growth and development:
- "When did your child first smile?"
- "When did your child first sit up?"
- "When did your child start crawling?"
- "When did your child start talking?"
- "When did your child start walking?"
- "When did your child learn to dress himself?"
- "When did your child learn to tie his shoes?"
- "When did your child start using short sentences?"
- "When did your child start putting things in his mouth?"

Feeding history:

- "Did you breast-feed your child?"
- "When did your child start eating solid food?"
- "How is your child's appetite?"
- "Does your child have any allergies?"
- "Is your child's formula fortified with iron?"
- "Are you giving your child pediatric multivitamins?"

Routine care:

- "Are your child's immunizations up to date?"
- "When was the date of your child's last routine checkup?"
- "Has your child had any serious illnesses?"
- "Is your child taking any medications?"
- "Has your child ever been hospitalized?"

Psychiatric history:

- "Tell me about yourself and your future goals."
- "How long have you been feeling unhappy/sad/anxious/confused?"
- "Do you have any idea what might be causing this?"
- "Would you like to share with me what made you feel this way?"
- "Do you have any friends or family members you can talk to?"
- "Has your appetite changed lately?"
- "Has your weight changed recently?"
- "Tell me how you spend your time/day."
- "Do you have any problems falling asleep/staying asleep/waking up?"
- "Has there been any change in your sleeping habits lately?"
- "What interests/hobbies do you have? Do you enjoy them?"
- "Do you take interest or pleasure in your daily activities?"
- "Do you have any memory problems?"
- "Do you have difficulty concentrating?"
- "Do you have hope for the future?"
- "Have you ever thought about hurting yourself or ending your life?"
- "Do you think of killing yourself/putting an end to your own life?"
- "Do you have a plan to end your life?"
- "Would you mind telling me about it?"
- "Do you feel that you want to hurt other people? Have you ever done so?"
- "Do you ever see or hear things that others can't see or hear?"
- "Do you hold beliefs about yourself or the world that other people would find odd?"
- "Do you feel as if other people are trying to harm or control you?"
- "Has anyone in your family ever experienced depression?"
- "Has anyone in your family ever been diagnosed with a mental illness?"
- "Would you like to meet with a counselor to help you with your problem?"
- "Would you like to join a support group?"
- "What do you think makes you feel this way?"
- "Can you tell me more about it?"
- "Have you lost any interest in your social activities and relationships?"

- "Do you feel hopeless?"
- "Do you feel guilty about anything?"
- "How is your energy level?"
- "Can you still perform your daily functions or activities?"
- "Do you have any thoughts of harming yourself?"
- "Do you have any thoughts of harming others?"
- "Whom do you live with?"
- "How do they react to your behavior?"
- "Do you have any problems in your job?"
- "How is your performance on your job?"
- "Have you had any recent emotional or financial problems?"
- "Have you had any recent traumatic event in your family?"
- "Does anyone support you?"

Daily activities (for dementia patients):
- "Tell me about your day yesterday."
- "Do you need any help bathing?"
- "Do you need any help getting dressed?"
- "What do you need help with when you are getting dressed?"
- "Do you need any help going to the toilet?"
- "Do you need any help transferring from your bed to the chair?"
- "Do you ever have accidents with your urine or bowel movements?"
- "Do you ever not make it to the toilet on time?"
- "Do you need any help feeding yourself?"
- "What do you need help with when you eat?"
- "Do you need any help taking your medications/using the telephone/shopping/preparing food/cleaning your house/doing laundry/getting from place to place/managing money?"

Abuse:
- "Are you safe at home?"
- "Is there any threat to your personal safety at home or anywhere else?"
- "Does anyone (your husband/wife/parents/boyfriend) treat you in a way that hurts you or threatens to hurt you?"
- "Can you tell me about the bruises on your arm?"

THE PHYSICAL EXAM

Guidelines

In this section, we recommend a systematic way to perform the physical exam. You can use this method or any other system with which you feel comfortable. Regardless of the method you choose, however, it is essential that you practice until you can perform the physical exam without mistakes or hesitation.

As described earlier, the physical exam can take up to five minutes. Given that the history portion of the encounter is estimated to take 7–8 minutes, you should already

> The key is a focused physical exam.

have started the physical exam by the time you hear the announcement that you have five minutes remaining in the encounter. Bear in mind that there is no time for a complete physical exam. Instead, you should aim at conducting a focused exam to look for physical findings that can support the differential diagnosis you made after taking the history. See Figure 2-3 for an overview of the process.

Before you begin, you should inform the patient of the need for the physical exam. Then, don't forget to wash your hands with soap and water and dry them carefully. (You can wear gloves instead if you so choose.) While you are washing your hands, use the time to think about what you should examine and whether there is anything you neglected to ask the patient. You should then drape the patient if you have not yet done so. The drape will be on the stool; unfold it and cover the patient from the waist down.

Before you touch the patient, make sure your hands are warm (rub your hands together if they are cold). In a similar manner, rub the diaphragm of your stethoscope to warm it up before you use it. Do not auscultate or palpate through the patient's gown.

As you proceed, be sure to ask the patient's permission before you uncover any part of his or her body (eg, "Is it okay if I untie your gown to examine your chest?" or "Can I move down the sheet to examine your belly?"). You may also ask the patient to uncover himself. You should expose only the area you need to examine. Do not expose large areas of the patient's body at once. After you have examined a given area, cover it immediately.

Ask permission before touching or uncovering the patient. Drape the patient appropriately.

During the physical exam, you will be scored both for performing a given procedure and for doing so correctly. You will not get credit for conducting an extra maneuver or for examining a nonrequired system, but failure to perform a required procedure will cost you a check mark on your list. You should also bear in mind that you are not allowed to perform a corneal reflex, breast, rectal, pelvic, or genital exam. If you think any of the above-mentioned exams is indicated, you should tell the patient that you will need to do the specific exam later and then remember to add the exam to your orders on your patient note (PN). When you have concluded a given procedure, remember to say "thank you." Then explain the next step, and ask the patient for permission to proceed. The patient should always be made to feel that he or she is in control of his or her body.

In the course of the physical exam, you may ask the patient any additional questions that you feel may be pertinent to the history. It is recommended, however, that you stop the physical exam while doing so to reestablish eye contact. After the patient has answered your questions, you may resume the exam.

Finally, you should remain alert to special situations that may not unfold as they would in an ordinary physical exam. When you enter the examination room, for example, the patient may hand you an insurance form requesting that only certain

FIGURE 2-3. Physical Exam Overview

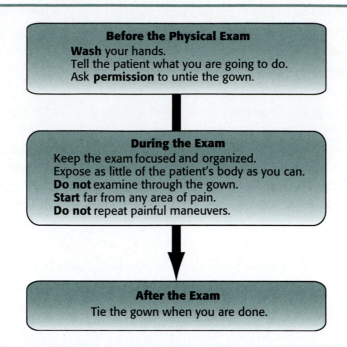

Before the Physical Exam
Wash your hands.
Tell the patient what you are going to do.
Ask **permission** to untie the gown.

During the Exam
Keep the exam focused and organized.
Expose as little of the patient's body as you can.
Do not examine through the gown.
Start far from any area of pain.
Do not repeat painful maneuvers.

After the Exam
Tie the gown when you are done.

THE PATIENT ENCOUNTER

systems be examined. In such cases, the patient will usually tell you that you do not need to take a history. Should this occur, simply introduce yourself, proceed to examine the systems listed, and then leave the room. No PN is required under such circumstances; instead, you are required only to fill out the form the patient gave you with the appropriate findings. In such encounters, the emphasis will be on the correct performance of the physical exam maneuvers and on professional and appropriate interaction with the patient.

> Not every patient will require an interview and physical exam.

Physical Exam Review

The following is a review of the steps involved in the examination of each of the body's main systems. Included are samples of statements that can be used during the physical exam. Remember that it is crucial to keep the patient informed of what is going on as well as to ask for consent before each step.

1. **HEENT exam:**
- **What to say to the patient before and during the exam:**
    - "I need to examine your sinuses, so I am going to press on your forehead and cheeks. Please tell me if you feel pain anywhere."
    - "I would like to examine your eyes now."
    - "I am going to shine this light in your eyes. Can you please look at the clock on the wall?"
    - "I need to examine your ears now."
    - "Can you please open your mouth? I need to check the inside of your mouth and your throat."

- **What to perform during the HEENT exam:**
  - Head:
    1. Inspect the head for signs of trauma and scars.
    2. Palpate the head for tenderness or abnormalities.
  - Eyes:
    1. Inspect the sclerae and conjunctivae for color and irritation.
    2. Check the pupils for symmetry and reactivity to light.
    3. Check the extraocular movements of the eyes.
    4. Check visual acuity with the Snellen eye chart.
    5. Perform a funduscopic exam. Remember the rule "right-right-right" (ophthalmoscope in examiner's right hand—patient's right eye—examiner's right eye) and the rule "left-left-left" (ophthalmoscope in examiner's left hand—patient's left eye—examiner's left eye).
  - Ears:
    1. Conduct an external ear inspection for discharge, skin changes, or masses.
    2. Palpate the external ear for pain (otitis externa); do the same for the mastoid.
    3. Examine the ear canal and the tympanic membrane using an otoscope. (Don't forget to use a new speculum for the patient.)
    4. Conduct the Rinne and Weber tests.
  - Nose:
    1. Inspect the nose.
    2. Palpate the nose and sinuses.
    3. Inspect the nasal turbinates and the nasal septum with a light source.
  - Mouth and throat:
    1. Inspect with a light.
    2. Tooth tapping may be performed if needed.

2. **Cardiovascular exam:**
- **What to say to the patient before and during the exam:**
  - "I need to listen to your heart."
  - "Can you hold your breath, please?"
  - "Can you sit, please?"
  - "Can you turn to your left side, please?"
  - "I am going to examine your legs to check for fluid retention. Is that okay with you?"
  - "I need to check the pulse in your arms and legs now."

- **What to perform during the cardiovascular exam:**
  - When examining the heart, do not lift up the patient's gown. Rather, pull the gown down the shoulder, exposing only the area to be examined.
  - Listen to the carotids for bruits (use the diaphragm of the stethoscope).

- Look for JVD. Remember to raise the head of the bed to 45 degrees.
- Palpate the chest for the PMI, retrosternal heave, and thrills.
- Listen to at least two of the four cardiac areas. (Listen to the mitral area with the patient on his left side.)
- Listen to the base of the heart with the patient leaning forward.
- Check for pedal edema.
- Check the peripheral pulses.

3. **Pulmonary exam:**
- **What to say to the patient before and during the exam:**
  - "I need to listen to your lungs now."
  - "Can you take a deep breath for me, please?"
  - "Can you say '99' for me, please?"
  - "I am going to tap on your back to check your lungs. Is that okay with you?"

- **What to perform during the pulmonary exam:**
  - Examine both the front and the back of the chest.
  - Don't percuss or auscultate through the patient's gown.
  - Don't percuss or auscultate over the scapula.
  - Allow a full inspiration and expiration in each area of the chest.
  - Inspect: The shape of the chest, respiratory pattern, deformities.
  - Palpate: Tenderness, tactile fremitus.
  - Percuss.
  - Auscultate, egophony.

4. **Abdominal exam:**
- **What to say to the patient before and during the exam:**
  - "I need to examine your belly/stomach now."
  - "I am going to listen to your belly now."
  - "I am going to press on your belly. Tell me if you feel any pain or discomfort."
  - "Now I need to tap on your belly."
  - "Do you feel any pain when I press in or when I let go? Which hurts more?"

- **What to perform during the abdominal exam:**
  - Inspect.
  - Auscultate (always auscultate before you palpate the abdomen).
  - Percuss.
  - Palpate: Start from the point that is farthest from the pain; be gentle on the painful area, and don't try to reelicit the pain. Check for rebound tenderness, CVA tenderness, obturator sign, psoas sign, and Murphy sign.
  - Check the liver span.

5. **Neurologic exam:**
- **What to say to the patient before and during the exam—mini-mental status exam questions:**
  - "I would like to ask you some questions to test your orientation."
  - "I would like to check your memory and concentration by asking you some questions."

- "Can you tell me your name and age?"
- "Do you know where you are now?"
- "Do you know the date today?"
- Show the patient your pen and ask, "Do you know what this is?"
- "Now I would like to ask you some questions to check your memory."
- "I will name three objects for you, and I want you to repeat them immediately, okay? Chair, bed, and pen." (Tests immediate memory.)
- "I will ask you to repeat the names of these three objects after a few minutes." (Tests short-term memory.)
- "Do you remember what you had for lunch yesterday?" (Tests recent memory.)
- "When did you get married?" (Tests distant memory.)
- "Now, can you repeat for me the names of the three objects that I mentioned to you?" (Tests short-term memory.)
- "Are you left-handed or right-handed?"
- "I will give you a piece of paper. I want you to take the paper in your right hand, fold the paper in half, and put it on the floor." (Three-step command.)
- "Now I want you to write your name on the paper."
- "I want you to count backward starting with the number 100," or
- "Take 7 away from 100 and tell me what number you get; then keep taking 7 away until I tell you to stop." (Tests concentration.)
- "Spell *world* forward and backward." (Tests concentration.)
- "What would you do if you saw a fire coming out of a paper basket?" (Tests judgment.)

- **What to say to the patient before and during the exam—neurologic exam questions:**
  - "I am going to check your reflexes now."
  - "I am going to test the strength of your muscles now."
  - "This is up, and this is down. Tell me which direction I am moving your big toe."
  - "Can you walk across the room for me, please?"

- **What to perform during the neurologic exam:**
  - Mental status examination: Orientation, memory, concentration.
  - Cranial nerves:
    1. II: Vision.
    2. III, IV, VI: Extraocular movements.
    3. V: Facial sensation, muscles of mastication.
    4. VII: "Smile, lift your brows, close your eyes and don't let me open them."
    5. IX, X: Symmetrical palate movement, gag reflex.
    6. XI: "Shrug your shoulders."
    7. XII: "Stick out your tongue."

- Motor system:
  1. Passive motion.
  2. Active motion: Arms—flexion ("pull in"), extension ("push out"); wrists—flexion ("push down"), extension ("pull up").
  3. Hands: "Spread your fingers apart; close your fist."
  4. Legs: Knee extension ("kick out"), knee flexion ("pull in").
  5. Ankles: "Push on the gas pedal."
- Reflexes: Biceps, triceps, brachioradialis, patellar, Achilles, Babinski.
- Sensory system: Sharp (pin)/dull (cotton swab), vibration, position sense.
- Cerebellum: Finger-to-nose, heel-to-shin, rapid alternating movements, Romberg sign, gait.
- Meningeal signs: Neck stiffness, Kernig, Brudzinski.

6. **Joint exam:**
- **What to say to the patient before and during the exam:**
  - "Tell me if you feel pain anywhere."
  - "I am going to examine your knee/ankle now."

- **What to perform during the joint exam:**
  - Inspect and compare joint with the opposite side.
  - Palpate.
  - Check for joint effusion.
  - Check for crepitus.
  - Check the joint range of motion.

- **Useful scales:**
  - Reflexes (0–4), with 0 being completely areflexic:
    - 1: Hyporeflexia
    - 2: Normal reflexes
    - 3: Hyperreflexia
    - 4: Hyperreflexia plus clonus (test the ankle and the knee)
  - Strength (0–5), with 0 representing an inability to move the limb:
    - 1: Can move limb (wiggle toes)
    - 2: Can lift limb against gravity
    - 3: Can lift limb with 1-finger resistance from the examiner
    - 4: Can lift limb with 2-finger resistance from the examiner
    - 5: Has full strength
  - Pulses (0–4), with 0 representing pulselessness:
    - 1: Weak pulse
    - 2: Regular pulse
    - 3: Increased pulse
    - 4: Pounding pulse

Special Challenges During the Physical Exam

During the course of the physical exam, you may encounter any number of special problems. The following are examples of such challenges along with potential responses to them.

- **Listening to the heart in a female patient:** You can place the stethoscope anywhere around the patient's bra and between the breasts. To auscultate or palpate the PMI, if necessary, ask the patient, "Can you please lift up your breast?"
- **Examining a patient who is in severe pain:** A patient in severe pain may initially seem unapproachable, refuse the physical exam, or insist that you give him something to stop his pain. In such cases, you should first ask the patient's permission to perform the physical exam. If he refuses, gently say, "I understand that you are in severe pain, and I want to help you. The physical exam that I want to do is very important to help determine what is causing your pain. I will be as quick and gentle as possible, and once I find the reason for your pain, I should be able to give you something to make you more comfortable."
- **Examining lesions:** If you see a scar, a mole (nevus), a psoriatic lesion, or any other skin lesion during the exam, you should mention it and ask the patient about it even if it is not related to the patient's complaint.
- **Examining bruising:** Inquire about any bruises you see on the patient's body, and think about abuse as a possible cause.
- **Running out of time:** If you don't have time for a full mini-mental status exam, at least ask patients if they know their name, where they are, and what day it is.

SP Simulation of Physical Exam Findings

It bears repeating that during the physical exam it is necessary to remain cautious and attentive, as the symptoms patients exhibit during the encounter are seldom accidental and are usually reproducible. So when you notice any positive sign, take it seriously. The following are some physical signs that may be simulated by the SP:

1. **Abdomen:**
    - Abdominal tenderness: The patient feels pain when you press on his abdomen. Remember that the patient is an actor. When you palpate the area, he will feel pain where he is supposed to feel pain regardless of the amount of pressure you exert. So don't try to palpate the same area again; instead, move on, and consider the pain on palpation a positive sign.
    - Abdominal rigidity: The patient will contract his abdominal muscles when you try to palpate the abdomen.
    - Rebound tenderness of the abdomen.
    - CVA tenderness.

2. **Chest:**
    - Shortness of breath.
    - Wheezing: This may often sound strange, as if the patient were whistling from his mouth.

- Decreased respiratory sounds: The patient will move his chest without really inhaling any air so that you do not hear any respiratory sounds.
- Increased fremitus: The patient will say "99" in a coarse voice, creating more fremitus than usual.

3. **Nervous system:**
   - Confusion.
   - Dementia.
   - Extensor plantar response (Babinski sign).
   - Absent or hyperactive tendon reflexes (stroke, diabetes mellitus): Eliciting the reflex in the SP is not like doing so in a real patient, where you must try more than once to ensure that you have not missed the tendon and that your strike is strong enough. In a clinical encounter, try the reflex only once; if you don't see it, it is not there. If the patient wants to show you hyperactive DTRs, he will make sure to respond with an exaggerated jerk even to the lightest and most awkward hammer hit.
   - Tremor (resting, intentional).
   - Facial paralysis.
   - Hemiparesis.
   - Gait abnormalities.
   - Ataxia.
   - Chorea.
   - Hearing loss.
   - Tinel sign.
   - Phalen sign.
   - Nuchal rigidity.
   - Kernig sign.
   - Brudzinski sign.

4. **Eyes:**
   - Visual loss (central, peripheral): In a young patient, this may be multiple sclerosis.
   - Photophobia: The patient will say, "I hate the light" or "I don't feel comfortable in bright light." Dim the light to make the patient feel more comfortable.
   - Lid lag.
   - Nystagmus.

5. **Muscles and joints:**
   - Muscle weakness.
   - Rigidity.
   - Spasticity.
   - Parkinsonism: Shuffling gait (difficulty initiating and stopping ambulation, small steps, no swinging of the arms), resting tremor, masked facies, rare blinking, and cogwheel rigidity.
   - Restricted range of motion of joints.

6. **Bruits and murmurs:**
   - Renal artery stenosis: A patient with hypertension who is not responding to multiple antihypertensive medications. Do not be surprised if you hear an abdominal bruit.
   - Thyroid bruit.
   - Carotid bruit: The patient says "Hush, hush" when you place the stethoscope over his neck.
   - Heart murmur: Once you place the stethoscope on the patient's heart, you will hear him saying "Hush, hush."

7. **Skin:**
   - Skin lesions: You may see artificial skin discoloration (eg, painful red spots on the shin for erythema nodosum in a patient with sarcoidosis; redness over an inflamed joint in a patient with arthritis).

8. **Real physical exam findings:**
   - You may see real C-section, appendectomy, cholecystectomy, or other scars. Don't overlook them. Always inquire about any scar you see.
   - You may see a real nevus (mole). Ask the patient about it and advise him to check it routinely and report any change in it.
   - You may see real skin lesions, such as pityriasis rosea in a Christmas tree pattern, seborrheic dermatitis of the scalp, or acne vulgaris.
   - When you listen to a patient's heart, don't be surprised to hear a real heart murmur.
   - A patient with a sore throat may present with enlarged tonsils.

CLOSURE

Finishing the history and the physical exam does not mean that the encounter is over. To the contrary, closure is a critical part of the encounter. See Figure 2-4 for an overview of the process. During closure, you are expected to do several things:

- Make a transition to mark the end of your encounter.
- Summarize the chief complaint and the HPI if you have not already done so before the physical exam.
- Summarize your findings from the physical exam.
- Give your impression of the patient's clinical condition and most likely diagnosis.
- Suggest a diagnostic workup.
- Answer any questions the patient might have.
- Address the patient's concerns.
- Check to see if the patient has any more questions.
- Leave the room.

> Leave a few minutes for closure to summarize key points to the patient.

To transition into the closure, you should begin by saying something like, "Thank you for letting me examine you, Mrs. Jones. Now I would like to sit down with you and give you my impression." You should then tell the patient about the possible differential diagnoses (keep to a maximum of three) and explain the meaning of any

FIGURE 2-4. Closure Overview

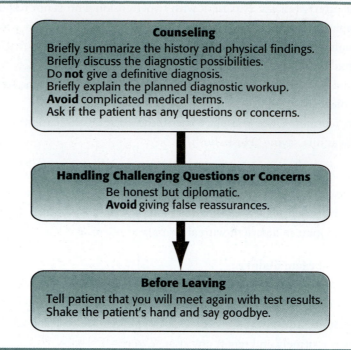

Counseling
Briefly summarize the history and physical findings.
Briefly discuss the diagnostic possibilities.
Do **not** give a definitive diagnosis.
Briefly explain the planned diagnostic workup.
Avoid complicated medical terms.
Ask if the patient has any questions or concerns.

Handling Challenging Questions or Concerns
Be honest but diplomatic.
Avoid giving false reassurances.

Before Leaving
Tell patient that you will meet again with test results.
Shake the patient's hand and say goodbye.

complicated medical terms you might use. You might also point out the organ or system that you think is involved and explain a simple mechanism of the disease. You should not, however, give the patient a definitive diagnosis at this time. Instead, tell her that you still need to run some tests to establish the final diagnosis. In some cases there will actually be no final diagnosis; instead, the case will be constructed in such a way as to be a mixture of signs and symptoms that can be construed to indicate any number of diseases.

During closure, almost every patient will have at least one challenging question to which you must respond (eg, "Do you think I have cancer, doctor?" or "Am I going to get better?"). In answering these questions, be honest yet diplomatic. Essentially, being honest with the patient means not giving false reassurances such as, "I am sure you will be cured after a week of antibiotics" or "Don't worry, I am sure that it is not cancer." What you might say instead is, "Well, I cannot exclude the possibility of cancer at this point. We need to do additional testing. Regardless of the final diagnosis, however, I want you to be assured that I will be available for any support you need."

If you do not know the answer to a patient's question, you should state as much. See the end of this section for examples of challenging questions patients might pose along with potential responses to them.

During closure, you should also explain to the patient the diagnostic tests you are planning to order. In doing so, you should again use nontechnical terms—for example, "We need to run some blood tests to check the function of your liver and kidneys" or "You need to have a chest x-ray and a CT scan of the head." You may further explain the latter by saying, "The CT scan is a type of x-ray imaging that gives us clear images of sections of the body." You should then add, "After we get the results of those tests, we will meet again to discuss them in detail, along with the final diagnosis and the treatment plan." Finally, you should conclude by asking the patient if he or she still has any questions.

If you find you are running out of time, do not compromise the closure. If time constraints dictate that you choose between a thorough physical exam and an appropriate closure, give priority to the execution of a proper closure.

Before you leave the room, you can finish your encounter by looking the patient in the eye and saying something like, "Okay, Mr. Jones, I'll contact you when I have your test results. It was nice meeting you." You may then shake the patient's hand and leave the room. You are allowed to leave the room as soon as you think you have completed the encounter. Once you have left the encounter room, you will not be allowed to go back inside.

> *You cannot reenter the examination room once you leave.*

HOW TO INTERACT WITH SPECIAL PATIENTS

The following guidelines can help you deal with atypical patients and uncommon encounters.

- **The anxious patient:** Encourage the patient to talk about his feelings. Ask about the things that are causing the anxiety. Give reasonable reassurance.
- **The angry patient:** Stay calm and don't be scared. Remember that the patient is not really angry; he is just acting angry to test your response. Let the patient express his feelings, and ask about the reason for his anger. You should also address the patient's anger in a reasonable way. For example, if the patient is complaining that he has been waiting for a long time, express that you understand. Explain that the clinic is crowded, and there were many patients who had appointments before his. Reassure the patient that now that it is his turn, you will focus on his case and take care of him.
- **The crying patient:** Allow the crying patient to express his feelings, and wait in silence for him to finish. Offer him a tissue, and show him empathy in your facial expressions. You may also place your hand lightly on the patient's shoulder or arm and say something like, "I know that you feel sad. Would you like to tell me about it?" Don't worry about time constraints in such cases. Remember that the patient is an actor and that his crying is timed. He will allow you to continue the encounter in peace if you respond correctly.
- **The patient who is in pain:** Show compassion for the patient's pain. Say something like, "I know that you are in pain." Offer help by asking, "Is there anything I can do for you to help you feel more comfortable?" Do not repeat painful maneuvers. If the patient does not allow you to touch his abdomen because of the

severe pain he is experiencing, tell him, "I know that you are in pain, and I want to help you. I need to examine you, though, to be able to locate the source of pain and give you the right treatment." Reassure the patient by saying, "I will be as quick and gentle as possible."

- **The patient who can't pay for the tests or for treatment:** Reassure the patient by saying, "Not having enough money doesn't mean you can't get treatment." You might also add, "We will refer you to a social worker who can help you find resources."

- **The patient who refuses to answer your question or let you examine him:** Explain to the patient why the question or the physical exam is important. Tell him that they are necessary to allow you to understand the problem and arrive at a diagnosis. If the patient still refuses to cooperate, skip the question or the maneuver and document his refusal and your counseling in the PN.

- **The hard-of-hearing patient:** Face the patient directly to allow him to read your lips. Speak slowly, and do not cover your mouth. Use gestures to reinforce your words. If the patient has unilateral hearing loss, sit close to the hearing side.

- **The patient who doesn't know the names of his medications or is taking medications whose names *you* don't recognize:** Ask the patient if he has a prescription or a written list of the medications he is currently taking.

- **The phone encounter:** The Step 2 CS may include a telephone encounter. As with other encounters, patient information will be posted on the door before you enter the examination room. Once you are inside, sit in front of the desk with the telephone, and push the speaker button by the yellow dot to be connected to the patient. Do not dial any numbers or touch any other buttons. You are permitted to call the SP only once. Treat this like a normal encounter and gather all the necessary information. To end the call, press the speaker button above the yellow dot. As in the pediatric encounter, there is no physical exam, so leave this portion of the PN blank.

CHALLENGING QUESTIONS AND SITUATIONS

During your encounters, every patient will ask you one or more challenging questions. Your reactions and answers to these questions will be scored. Such questions may be explicit ones that you are expected to answer directly, or they may take the form of indirect comments or statements that must be properly addressed to reveal an underlying concern. When answering the challenging questions, try to remember the following guidelines:

- Be honest and diplomatic.
- Before addressing the patient's issue, you might restate the issue back to the patient to let him know that you understand.
- Don't give the patient a final diagnosis. Instead, tell the patient about your initial impressions and about the workup you have in mind to reach a conclusive diagnosis.
- Do not give false reassurances.
- If you do not know the answer to the patient's question, just tell him so.

Do not give the patient a definitive diagnosis.

The following are examples of challenging questions:

Confidentiality/Ethical Issues

Challenging Question	Possible Response
A patient who needs emergent surgery says, "I can't afford the cost of staying in the hospital. I have no insurance. Just give me something to relieve the pain, and I will leave."	"I know that you are concerned about medical costs, but your life will be in danger if you don't have surgery. Let our social workers help you with the cost issues."
"Should I tell my sexual partner about my venereal disease?"	"Yes. There is a chance that you have already transmitted the disease to your partner, or he/she may be the source of your infection. The important step is to have you both evaluated and appropriately treated."
An anxious patient whom you suspect has been abused asks, "Why are you asking me these questions?"	"I am concerned that domestic abuse may be involved. My goal is to make sure that you are in a safe environment and that you are not a victim of abuse."
A patient recently diagnosed with HIV asks, "Do I have to tell my wife?"	"I know that it's difficult, but doing so will allow you and your wife to take the appropriate precautions to treat and prevent the transmission of the disease."

Patient Belief/Behavioral Issues

Challenging Question	Possible Response
An elderly patient says, "I think that it is normal at my age to have this problem" (impotence) or "I am just getting old."	"Age may play a role in the change you are experiencing in your sexual function, but your problem may have other causes that we should rule out, such as certain diseases (hypertension, diabetes) or certain medications. We also have medications that may improve your sexual function."
"I read in a journal that the treatment for this disease is herbal compounds."	"Herbal medicines have been suggested for many diseases. However, their safety and efficacy may not always be clear-cut. Let me know the name of the herbal medicine and I will check into its potential treatment role for this disease."

"I am afraid of surgery."	"I understand your feelings. It is normal and very common to have these feelings before surgery. Is there anything specific that you are concerned about?"
A patient who has a serious problem (unstable angina, colon cancer) asks, "I want to go on a trip with my wife. Can we do the tests after I come back?"	"I know that you don't want to put off your trip, but you may have a serious problem that may benefit from early diagnosis and management."
"I did not understand your question, doctor. Could you repeat it, please?"	Repeat the question again slowly. If the patient still doesn't comprehend the question, ask if there is any specific word he didn't understand and try to explain it or use a simpler one.
"What is a bronchoscopy?" (MRI, CT, x-ray, colonoscopy)	Explain the meaning using simple words. For example, "Bronchoscopy is using a thin tube connected to a camera to look into your respiratory airways and parts of your lungs," or "An MRI is a machine that uses a big magnet to obtain detailed pictures of your brain or body."
"What do you mean by *workup*?"	"It means all the tests that we are going to do to help us make the final diagnosis."
A patient who is late in seeking medical advice asks, "Do you think it is too late for recovery?"	"I am glad that you came for help. We will do our best and hope for the best."
A patient with pleuritic chest pain asks, "Is this a heart attack? Am I going to die?"	"Given your current presentation, my suspicion for a heart attack is low. It is more likely that inflammation of the membranes surrounding your lungs is causing your pain, and this is usually not a life-threatening condition. However, we still need to do some tests to confirm the diagnosis and rule out heart problems."
"Do you think I have colon cancer?" "Do you think I have a brain tumor?" "Do I have endometrial cancer?"	"That is one of the possibilities, but there are other explanations for your symptoms that we should rule out before making a diagnosis."

"My friend told me that you are a very fine doctor. That's why I came to you to refill my prescription."	"I am flattered, but since this is your first visit, I can't give you a refill without reviewing your history to better understand your need for this medication. I will also need to do a physical exam and perhaps order some tests."
"Will my insurance cover the expenses of this test?"	"I'm not sure, but I can refer you to a social worker who does have that information. If necessary, I can write a note to your insurance company indicating the importance of this test."
A person who wants to return to work at a job that can negatively affect his health asks, "Can I go back to work?"	"Unfortunately, work may actually worsen your condition. Therefore, I would prefer that you stay at home for now. I can write a letter to your employer explaining your situation."
"Do you think that this tumor I have could become malignant?"	"We really won't know until we remove the mass and get a pathology report on it."
"Since I stopped smoking, I have gained weight. I want to go back to smoking in order to lose weight."	"There are healthier ways to lose weight than smoking, such as exercise and diet. Smoking will increase your risk of cancer, heart problems, and lung disease."
A patient with a shoulder injury says, "I am afraid of losing my job if my shoulder doesn't get better."	"We will do our best to help you recover from your shoulder injury. With your permission, I will communicate the situation to your employer."
"Will I ever feel better, doctor?"	The answer differs depending on the prognosis of the disease and can vary from, "Yes, most people with this disease are completely cured" to, "Complete cure may be difficult at this advanced stage, but we have a lot to offer in terms of controlling the symptoms and improving your quality of life."
A person who has a broken arm asks, "Doctor, do you think I will be able to move my arm again like before?"	"It is hard to tell right now, but those fractures usually heal well, and with physical therapy you should regain the normal range of motion of your arm."

THE PATIENT ENCOUNTER

"I think that life is full of misery. Why do we have to live?"	"Life can be challenging. Is there something in particular that is bothering you? Have you thought of ending your life?" You can then continue screening for depression.
A young man with multiple sexual partners and a recent-onset skin rash says, "I am afraid that I might have AIDS."	"Having multiple sexual partners does put you at risk for HIV infection, but this rash may be due to many other causes. I agree that we should do an HIV test on you in addition to a few other tests."
A patient who needs hospitalization says, "My child is at home alone. I have to leave now."	"I understand your concern about your child, but right now staying in the hospital is in your best interest. One of our social workers can make some phone calls to arrange for child care."
"Do you have anything that will make me feel better? Please, doctor, I am in pain."	"I know that you're in pain, but I need to know what's causing your pain to give you the appropriate treatment. After I am done with my evaluation, we can decide on the best way to help manage your pain."
A patient you believe is pretending (malingering) says, "Please, doctor, I need a week off from work. The pain in my back is terrible."	"I know that you are uncomfortable, but after examining you, I don't find disability significant enough to keep you out of work. I plan to prescribe pain medication and exercises, but a big part of your recovery will be continuing your normal daily activities."
"Stop asking me all these stupid questions and just give me something for this pain."	"I know that you're in pain, but I need to determine the cause of the pain to give you the right treatment. After I am done with my evaluation, we will give you the appropriate treatment."
"So what's the plan, doctor?"	"After we get the results of your tests, we will meet again. At that time, I will try to answer any questions you may have."

"Do you think I will need surgery?"	"I will try to manage your problem medically, but if that doesn't work, you may need surgery. We can see how things go and then try to make that decision together in the future."
A female patient has only one sexual partner, and she is diagnosed with an STD. She asks you, "Could he possibly be cheating on me?"	"You most likely contracted this infection from your partner. It would be best to talk to your partner about this to clear things up. He needs to be tested and treated, or else you risk becoming reinfected."
A patient is shouting angrily, "Where have you been, doctor? I have been waiting here for the whole day."	"I am sorry you had to wait so long. We had some unexpected delays with a few of the earlier patients this morning. But I'm here now, and I will focus on you and your concerns."

Disease-Related Issues

Challenging Question	Possible Response
An educated 58-year-old woman asks, "I read in a scientific journal that hormonal replacement therapy causes breast cancer. What do you think of that, doctor?"	"It appears to be true. Studies show a slight increase in the risk of developing breast cancer after 4 years of combination estrogen and progesterone use for hormonal replacement therapy. The current recommendations are to use hormonal replacement therapy solely for the relief of hot flashes, and only for a limited period of time."
"Did I have a stroke?"	"We don't know yet. Your symptoms could be explained by a small stroke, but we need to wait for the results of your MRI."
"Do I have lung cancer?"	"We don't know at this point. It is a possibility, but we still need to do additional tests."
An African American man with sickle cell anemia presents with back and chest pain and says, "Please, doctor, I need some Demerol now or I will die from pain."	"I know that you are in pain, but I need to ask you a few questions first to better understand your pain. Then we will get you medicines for your pain."

A patient with symptoms of a common cold says, "I think I need antibiotics, doctor."	"It appears that you have a viral common cold. Antibiotics do not treat viruses, and they have adverse effects that could even make you feel worse. We should focus on treating your symptoms."
"My mother had breast cancer. What is the possibility that I will have breast cancer, too?"	"You are at increased risk, but it doesn't mean that you will get it. There are other risk factors that need to be considered, and regular screening tests will be very important."
A 55-year-old man says, "I had a colonoscopy six years ago, and they removed a polyp. Do you think that I have to repeat the colonoscopy?"	"Yes, it should be repeated. We need to screen for more polyps, and in this way we hope to prevent the development of colon cancer."
A patient with headache or confusion asks, "Do you think I have Alzheimer disease?"	"I don't know. Alzheimer disease is one of several possible causes that we will investigate."
"Can I get pregnant even though my tubes are tied?"	"There is no single contraceptive method that is 100% effective. The risk of pregnancy after tubal ligation is less than 1%, but it is a real risk."
A woman who is in her first trimester of pregnancy with vaginal bleeding asks, "Do you think I am losing my pregnancy?"	"Bleeding early in pregnancy increases your risk of losing the pregnancy, but at the same time, most women who have bleeding carry the pregnancy to term without problems."
"My brother has colon cancer. What are the chances that I will have colon cancer as well?"	"Some types of colon cancer are hereditary, and you may be at increased risk, but it doesn't mean that you will get colon cancer for sure. I need to get more information about your personal and family history to determine your level of risk."
A patient with palpitations says, "My mother had a thyroid problem; do you think it is my thyroid?"	"It's possible. We always check a thyroid blood test, but we will also consider many other possible causes of palpitations."

"Obesity runs in my family. Do you think that this is why I am overweight?"	"Genes play an important role in obesity, but lifestyle, diet, and daily habits are also major factors influencing weight. These factors can be used in a way that can help you lose weight."
A young man with dysuria asks, "Do you think I have an STD?"	"That is one of the possibilities. We will do some cultures to find out for sure, and we will also check a urine sample, since your symptoms may be due to a urinary tract infection."
"I am drinking a lot of water, doctor. What do you think the reason is?"	"This may simply be due to dehydration, or it may be a sign of a disease such as diabetes. We need to do some tests to determine the cause."
A patient with COPD asks, "Will I get better if I stop smoking?"	"Most patients with your condition who stop smoking will experience a gradual improvement in their symptoms, in addition to a significantly decreased risk of lung cancer in the future."
A patient with possible appendicitis is asking for a cup of water to drink.	"I am sorry, but I can't give you anything to eat or drink right now. You may need emergent surgery, and anesthesia is much safer if your stomach is completely empty."
A patient with infectious mononucleosis asks, "Can I go back to school, doctor?"	"Now that you have recovered from the acute stage of the disease, you can go back to school, but I want you to stay away from any strenuous exercise or contact sports, as you may rupture your spleen."

COUNSELING

During at least one of your encounters, you are likely to find a patient who smokes, drinks, or has another habit that may adversely affect his or her health. Although these behaviors may or may not be relevant to your primary diagnosis, it is important that they be addressed in a rapid yet caring manner. Here are some examples of conversations you might have with your patient. Try to practice saying some of these aloud, making sure to change them to fit your personality and style.

The **5 A's** are recommended guidelines to help patients quit smoking.
1. **A**sk the patient about tobacco use.
2. **A**dvise him or her to quit.
3. **A**ssess the patient's willingness to make an attempt to quit.
4. **A**ssist in the quit attempt.
5. **A**rrange for follow-up.

The Smoker

Examinee: Do you smoke cigarettes?

SP: Yes, I have smoked one pack a day for 20 years.

Examinee: Have you ever tried to quit?

SP: Of course, but it never works.

Examinee: Well, I strongly recommend that you quit smoking. Smoking is a major cause of cancer and heart disease. Are you interested in trying to quit now?

SP1: Yes. (If the answer is "no," see below.)

Examinee: I would be happy to help you quit smoking. We have many tools to help you do that, and I will be with you every step of the way. Let's set up an appointment for two weeks from today, and we can get started on it then. Is that okay with you?

SP2: No, I don't want to quit.

Examinee: I understand that you aren't ready to quit smoking yet, but I want to assure you that whenever you are ready, I will be here to help you.

The Alcoholic

Examinee: How many drinks do you have in a week?

SP: It is hard to say. Too many.

Examinee: How many drinks do you have per day?

SP: Oh, maybe five or so.

Examinee: Have you ever felt the need to **cut down** on your drinking? Have you ever felt **annoyed** by criticism of your drinking? Have you ever felt **guilty** about drinking? Have you ever had to take a morning **eye opener?** (A "yes" answer to any one of the questions in the CAGE questionnaire should raise suspicion and prompt further questioning.)

SP: All of these things apply.

Examinee: I am concerned about your drinking. It can lead to liver disease, cause problems with bleeding, or even predispose you to early dementia. Are you interested in cutting down or quitting?

SP1: Yes. (If the answer is "no," see below.)

Examinee: I am glad you want to quit. A variety of resources are available to help you quit drinking, and I would like to discuss them with you. Let's make an appointment later this week to talk about your options. In the meantime, I have printed up a list of resources, and my office assistant will bring it to you.

SP2: No, I am not ready to quit.

Examinee: I realize that you are not ready to quit drinking, but I want to assure you that if you do decide to try, I will be here for you. Okay?

The Patient With Uncontrolled Diabetes

Examinee: According to your blood glucose readings, your diabetes is not adequately controlled. How often do you forget to take your medication? (Check for noncompliance.)

SP1: Taking all these medications just gets so confusing. I can never remember when to take them.

Examinee: Diabetes can certainly be a challenge to manage. Do you have someone who could help you take your medications? If not, we have a social worker who might be able to arrange for a nurse to come to your home. Are you interested in that?

SP2: I have been taking my medications exactly as they were prescribed to me.

Examinee: Tell me about your diet. (Check for dietary management.)

SP2: I eat regular meals, but I really like to drink soda. Diet soda tastes awful!

Examinee: You must be very careful about your sugar consumption. It is prudent to keep your blood sugar within normal limits. Persistently high blood sugar can cause damage to your eyes, kidneys, and nerves. Also, you will be at higher risk for developing infections, heart attacks, and strokes. Fortunately, we have a diabetes educator who may be able to help you. Are you interested in meeting with her?

The Sexually Promiscuous Patient

Examinee: Are you currently in a sexual relationship?

SP: Yes.

Examinee: Can you tell me about your partner or partners?

SP: I have a girlfriend, but I also see a couple of other women on the side.

Examinee: Are you using any type of protection with these partners?

SP: My girlfriend is on the pill, but I don't use anything with the other women I see.

Examinee: Condoms reduce the risk of sexually transmitted infections. Do you think you could try to use condoms?

SP: I tried them, but I just don't like them.

Examinee: I understand that you may not like to use condoms, but I am concerned that you may be putting yourself at risk for STDs. You could contract HIV, herpes, chlamydia, or any of a number of other STDs. The complications of these diseases include infertility, painful infections, or even death. If anyone with whom you have sexual contact has an STD, you could share it among all of them, including your girlfriend. I hope you will consider using a condom in the future. Do you have any questions for me?

The Depressed Patient

Examinee: Do you have problems **sleeping?** Have you lost **interest** in things that used to interest you? Do you feel **guilty?** Do you lack your usual **energy?** Has it been difficult for you to **concentrate?** Has your **appetite** changed? Do you feel as though you want to hurt yourself or someone else or commit **suicide?** (If you suspect depression, ask the questions posed in the mnemonic **SIG E CAPS.**)

SP: (Answers affirmatively to many of these questions.)

Examinee: You answered "yes" to many of my questions. I believe that you might have the diagnosis of depression. Depression is a common disease; it is due to a chemical imbalance in the brain that causes many of the symptoms you have described to me. Fortunately, we have medications that can help; however, these medications work best when they are combined with counseling. I can write you a prescription and also give you a referral to see a therapist. Is this something you are interested in?

The Patient With an STD (Trichomoniasis)

Examinee: Your symptoms are due to an infection called trichomoniasis, a sexually transmitted infection that has been given to you by one of your sexual partners. This infection responds well to treatment with antibiotics and is curable. You will also need to be tested for all other STDs. Your sexual partner needs to be treated as well; otherwise, you will be at risk of contracting the infection again. You should avoid sexual intercourse (unless you use condoms) until you finish the course of antibiotics and your partner gets treated.

THE PATIENT NOTE

Once you have completed an encounter, your final task will be to compose a PN (see Figure 2-5 for a detailed overview of the clinical encounter and PN). Toward this goal, you will find a desk with a computer on it immediately outside the encounter room. Remember that all examinees taking the Step 2 CS will be now required to type, not handwrite, the PN. You will be given 10 minutes to type the PN and will be notified when two minutes remain. If you leave the encounter room before the end of the 15-minute period allotted for your patient encounter, you can devote the extra time you have to typing the PN. You are allowed to review the doorway information while you are typing the PN.

The PN screen located outside the encounter room will have your identification information and fields for History, Physical Exam, Differential Diagnosis, and Diagnostic Workup. Each field can only accommodate a certain number of characters: The character limits are 950 for History, 500 for Physical Exam, and 80 for each of the five fields in Differential Diagnosis and Diagnostic Workup. One benefit of the computer note is that it allows you to delete extraneous information in favor of more pertinent portions of your note if you run out of space, so use this to your advantage and use the space wisely.

Before you start typing the PN, take a few seconds to review the history, including the chief complaint, how it started, its progression, and the main symptoms. Then take a deep breath and try to relax. If you get nervous and try to rush, your thoughts may become garbled, and you will risk losing the point of your story.

Note that you will not be able to render diagrams such as the neurology stick figure for reflexes. You can simulate typing the PN online at the USMLE Web site.

> Starting in July 2011, all PNs must be typed. You may type your PN in either bullet style or regular style.

Writing the Patient Note

You will be required to fill out four main sections in your PN: the history, physical exam, differential diagnosis, and initial diagnostic workup.

Summarizing the history. In writing the history, be clear, direct, and concise, and avoid long and complex phrases. Make sure the history flows in a logical sequence. Also bear in mind that it is not necessary to write a detailed, all-inclusive history.

FIGURE 2-5. Summary Overview of the Patient Encounter

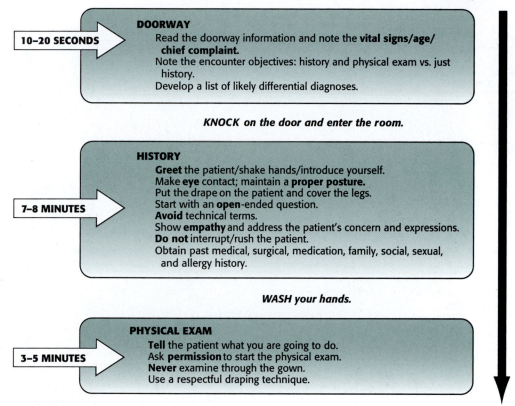

First announcement:
"Examinees, you may enter the room."

10–20 SECONDS

DOORWAY
Read the doorway information and note the **vital signs/age/ chief complaint.**
Note the encounter objectives: history and physical exam vs. just history.
Develop a list of likely differential diagnoses.

KNOCK on the door and enter the room.

7–8 MINUTES

HISTORY
Greet the patient/shake hands/introduce yourself.
Make **eye** contact; maintain a **proper posture.**
Put the drape on the patient and cover the legs.
Start with an **open**-ended question.
Avoid technical terms.
Show **empathy** and address the patient's concern and expressions.
Do not interrupt/rush the patient.
Obtain past medical, surgical, medication, family, social, sexual, and allergy history.

WASH your hands.

3–5 MINUTES

PHYSICAL EXAM
Tell the patient what you are going to do.
Ask **permission** to start the physical exam.
Never examine through the gown.
Use a respectful draping technique.

(continued)

The components that should be included are as follows:

- Chief complaint (CC)
- History of present illness (HPI)
- Review of systems (ROS)
- Past medical history (PMH)
- Past surgical history (PSH)
- Social history (SH)
- Family history (FH)

When you are summarizing the history, use the space assigned to you for that purpose prudently. One way to save time is to make ample use of abbreviations. Train yourself to use the abbreviations that are listed in the USMLE Step 2 CS orientation materials (also see the inside back inside cover of this text). You will find a copy of this list on each desk. You are allowed to use any abbreviations that are commonly used in US hospitals. If you are unsure of the correct abbreviation, it is better to spell out the word or phrase.

FIGURE 2-5. Summary Overview of the Patient Encounter *(continued)*

THE PATIENT ENCOUNTER

Second announcement:
*"Examinees, you have **five minutes left** for this encounter."*
By this time you should be **halfway** through your exam.

CLOSURE
2–3 MINUTES
Explain your diagnostic possibilities/workups.
Avoid complicated medical terms.
Ask if the patient has any concerns.
Be prepared to handle **challenging questions.**
Avoid giving false reassurances.
Do the **counseling.**
Say goodbye, thank the patient, and leave the encounter.

Third announcement:
*"This encounter is now **finished.**"*

TYPED PATIENT NOTE
10 MINUTES
Document **key** CC, HPI, PMH, meds, PSH, SH, ROS, FH.
Document **key** physical findings.
Include **pertinent positives** and **negatives.**
Give a maximum of **five** diagnostic possibilities.
Order maximum of **five** diagnostic tests.
Do **not** consult, hospitalize, or treat the patient.
Order **rectal, pelvic, genital,** or **breast** exams if needed.

Fourth announcement:
"You have two minutes left."

Fifth announcement:
"Your time is now finished."

In general, two styles of writing—narrative and "bullet"—are acceptable as long as your history is both comprehensive and coherent. Two examples can be found in the candidate orientation manual and multiple examples of both are included in this book's sample cases.

Outlining the physical exam. To summarize the physical exam, write a list of the systems that you examined, outlining all the relevant positive and negative findings. If you did not perform a maneuver that you think was necessary, it is better not to lie and pretend that you did. Be honest and list only the items you examined. For example, do not claim that you saw diabetic retinopathy in a patient with diabetes mellitus if you did not even get to see the eye fundus. See Figure 2-6 for some examples of how to document physical exam findings.

Developing a differential. In writing the differential, you should list a maximum of 5 diagnoses. You are not required to list that many if 3 or 4 diagnoses suffice. The diagnoses should be directly related to the history and physical exam, and it is preferable that they be listed in order of probability, from the most to the least probable.

Specifying the initial diagnostic workup. In summarizing your workup, list a maximum of 5 tests. It is best to start with the "forbidden physical exam maneuvers" (eg, rectal exam, pelvic exam) if you feel such procedures are indicated. Then state the required laboratory and radiologic tests, starting with the most simple and straightforward tests and ending with the most complex. Do not include referrals, treatments, hospitalizations, or consults, as these will not be scored.

Be specific in your orders. Instead of "chem 7," "thyroid panel," or "liver function tests," you should specify "Na, K," "TSH and total T_4," and "AST and ALT." You may, however, order electrolytes. Each group of related tests (blood tests, x-rays) should be listed together.

> *Tests in the diagnostic workup should be specific.*

Scoring the Patient Note

The PN will be scored by a physician on the basis of its organization, quality of information, interpretation of data, and legibility. The final score will represent the average PN score of all 10 scored encounters.

How to Prepare

The cardinal rule for preparing to write a PN is to practice, practice, and practice. Imagine that you are in the actual exam, and try to type the PN within 10 minutes. You should also practice writing the note so that it will fit in the allotted space. When using the cases presented in this book, try to write your PN and then compare your note with ours. Ask yourself the following questions:

- Is the history complete?
- Does it make sense?
- Are the physical exam results complete?
- Is the differential diagnosis correct?
- Are the tests correct and in the right order?

There are two styles you can use both to document the physical exam and to compose the PN. So choose a method, memorize it, and stick with it. In this book, we give you samples of bullet-style and traditional narrative-style formats so that you may familiarize yourself with both.

If you are running out of time, start from the bottom of the PN. Write down the differential diagnosis, the tests conducted, the physical exam, and then the history and the review of systems (listing only the positives first).

FIGURE 2-6. Examples of How to Document Physical Exam Findings

- **HEENT:**
  - Head: Atraumatic, normocephalic.
  - Eyes: EOMI, PERRLA, normal eye fundus.
  - Nose: No nasal congestion.
  - Throat: No tonsillar erythema, exudates, or enlargement.
  - Mouth: Moist mucous membranes, good dentition, no lesions.

- **Neck:** Supple, no JVD, normal thyroid, no cervical LAD.

- **Nervous System:**
  - Mental status: Alert and oriented x 3, good concentration.
  - Cranial nerves II–XII grossly intact.
  - Motor: Strength 5/5 in all muscle groups.
  - DTRs: 2+ intact and symmetric, Babinski ⊖.
  - Sensation: Intact to sharp and dull.
  - Cerebellum: ⊖ Romberg sign, intact finger to nose.

- **Chest/Lung:**
  - Clear to percussion bilaterally.
  - No rales, rhonchi, wheezing, or rubs.
  - No tenderness to palpation.
  - Tactile fremitus WNL.

- **Heart:**
  - PMI not displaced.
  - Regular rate and rhythm.
  - Normal S1, S2.
  - No murmurs, rubs, or gallops.

- **Abdomen:**
  - Soft, nontender, nondistended, BS ⊕, no hepatosplenomegaly.

- **Extremities:**
  - No clubbing, cyanosis, or edema.

- **Mental Status Exam:**
  - Patient speaks slowly.
  - No hostile behavior toward the interviewer.
  - Blunt affect with poor eye contact.
  - Inattentive to interviewer.
  - 3/3 registration, 3/3 recall at 3 times.
  - Distant memories are impaired.
  - Oriented to person, date, and place.
  - Completed three-step command.
  - Right-handed.
  - 1/5 on serial 7s.
  - Poor judgment.

Minicases

Headache / 81

Confusion/Memory Loss / 83

Depressed Mood / 85

Psychosis / 86

Dizziness / 87

Loss of Consciousness / 89

Numbness/Weakness / 90

Fatigue and Sleepiness / 91

Night Sweats / 93

Insomnia / 93

Sore Throat / 94

Cough/Shortness of Breath / 95

Chest Pain / 97

Palpitations / 99

Weight Loss / 100

Weight Gain / 101

Dysphagia / 101

Nausea/Vomiting / 102

Abdominal Pain / 103

Constipation/Diarrhea / 107

Upper GI Bleeding / 109

Blood in Stool / 110

Hematuria / 111

Other Urinary Symptoms / 112

Erectile Dysfunction / 113

Amenorrhea / 114

Vaginal Bleeding / 116

Vaginal Discharge / 117

Dyspareunia / 118

Abuse / 118

Joint/Limb Pain / 119

Low Back Pain / 122

Child with Fever / 123

Child with GI Symptoms / 124

Child with Red Eye / 126

Child with Short Stature / 126

Behavioral Problems in Childhood / 127

In this chapter, we will attempt to cover most of the clinical cases that you are likely to encounter on the Step 2 CS. The main title of each case represents a chief complaint that you may see on the doorway information sheet before you enter the examination room. After each chief complaint, key points pertinent to the history and physical exam are reviewed. Each clinical case consists of three components:

- **Presentation:** A brief clinical case with some pertinent positives and negatives.
- **Differential:** An appropriate differential diagnosis; the most likely diagnosis appears in boldface.
- **Workup:** The main diagnostic tests that should be considered for each disease. Note that the diagnostic tests in the third column are generally listed in order of priority. In clinical practice, many tests may be performed at the same time or not at all.

The sum of the **Differential** column will give you a wide differential diagnosis for the chief complaint, whereas the sum of the **Workup** column will give you a pool of tests from which to choose in the exam.

If you are studying by yourself, we suggest that you read the vignette and then try to figure out the diagnosis and workup. If you are studying with a partner or in a group, we suggest that you take turns reading the vignette aloud and allow each other to figure out the differential diagnosis and workup.

HEADACHE

Key History

Location (unilateral vs. bilateral), quality (dull vs. stabbing), intensity (is it the "worst headache of their life"?), duration, timing (does it disturb sleep?); presence of associated neurologic symptoms (paresthesias, visual stigmata, weakness, numbness, ataxia, photophobia, dizziness, auras, neck stiffness); nausea/vomiting, jaw claudication, recent trauma, dental surgery, sinusitis symptoms; exacerbating factors (stress, fatigue, menses, exercise, certain foods) and alleviating factors (rest, medications); patient and family history of headache.

Key Physical Exam

Vital signs; inspection and palpation of entire head; ENT inspection; complete neurologic exam, including funduscopic exam.

Presentation	Differential	Workup
21 yo F presents with several episodes of throbbing left temporal pain that lasts for 2–3 hours. Before onset, she sees flashes of light in her right visual field and feels weakness and numbness on the right side of her body for a few minutes. Headaches are often associated with nausea and vomiting. She has a family history of migraine.	**Migraine (complicated)** Tension headache Cluster headache Pseudotumor cerebri Trigeminal neuralgia CNS vasculitis Partial seizure Intracranial neoplasm	CBC ESR CT—head MRI—brain LP
26 yo M presents with severe right temporal headaches associated with ipsilateral rhinorrhea, eye tearing, and redness. Episodes have occurred at the same time every night for the past week and last for 45 minutes.	**Cluster headache** Migraine Tension headache Sinusitis Pseudotumor cerebri Trigeminal neuralgia Intracranial neoplasm	CBC CT—head MRI—brain LP ESR
65 yo F presents with severe, intermittent right temporal headache, fever, blurred vision in her right eye, and pain in her jaw when chewing.	**Temporal arteritis (giant cell arteritis)** Migraine Cluster headache Tension headache Meningitis Carotid artery dissection Pseudotumor cerebri Trigeminal neuralgia Intracranial neoplasm Temporomandibular joint disorder	CBC ESR CRP Temporal artery biopsy Doppler U/S—carotid MRI—brain LP

Presentation	Differential	Workup
▪ 30 yo F presents with frontal headache, fever, and nasal discharge. There is pain on palpation of the frontal and maxillary sinuses. She has a history of allergies.	**Sinusitis** Migraine Tension headache Meningitis Intracranial neoplasm	CBC XR—sinus CT—sinus LP
▪ 50 yo F presents with recurrent episodes of bilateral squeezing headaches that occur 3–4 times a week, typically toward the end of her work day. She is experiencing significant stress in her life.	**Tension headache** Migraine Depression Caffeine or analgesic withdrawal Hypertension Cluster headache Pseudotumor cerebri Intracranial neoplasm	CBC Electrolytes ESR CT—head LP

▪ 35 yo M presents with sudden severe headache, vomiting, confusion, left hemiplegia, and nuchal rigidity.	**Subarachnoid**
	  hemorrhage
	Migraine
	Meningitis/encephalitis
	Intracranial hemorrhage
	Vertebral artery dissection
	Intracranial venous
	  thrombosis
	Acute hypertension
	Intracranial neoplasm
		Noncontrast CT—head
		LP
		CBC
		PT/PTT/INR

▪ 25 yo M presents with high fever, severe headache, confusion, photophobia, and nuchal rigidity. Kernig and Brudzinski signs are positive.	**Meningitis (bacterial)**
	Meningitis (HSV)
	Migraine
	Subarachnoid hemorrhage
	Sinusitis/encephalitis
	Intracranial or epidural
	  abscess
		CBC
		CT—head
		MRI—brain
		LP—CSF analysis (cell
		  count, protein, glucose,
		  Gram stain, PCR for
		  antigens, culture)

▪ 18 yo obese F presents with a pulsatile headache, vomiting, and blurred vision for the past 2–3 weeks. She is taking OCPs.	**Pseudotumor cerebri**
	Tension headache
	Migraine
	Cluster headache
	Meningitis
	Intracranial venous
	  thrombosis
	Intracranial neoplasm
		Urine hCG
		CBC
		CT—head
		LP—opening pressure and
		  CSF analysis

MINICASES

Presentation	Differential	Workup
■ 57 yo M c/o daily pain in the right cheek for the past month. The pain is electric and stabbing in character and occurs while he is shaving. Each episode lasts 2–4 minutes.	**Trigeminal neuralgia** Tension headache Migraine Cluster headache TMJ dysfunction Intracranial neoplasm	CBC ESR MRI—brain

CONFUSION/MEMORY LOSS

Key History

Must include history from family members/caregivers. Detailed time course of cognitive deficits (acute vs. chronic/gradual onset), associated symptoms (constitutional, incontinence, ataxia, hypothyroid symptoms, depression); screen for delirium (waxing/waning level of alertness); falls, medications (and recent medication changes); history of stroke or other atherosclerotic vascular disease, syphilis, HIV risk factors, alcohol use, or vitamin B_{12} deficiency; family history of Alzheimer disease.

Key Physical Exam

Vital signs; complete neurologic exam, including mini-mental status exam and gait; general physical exam, including ENT, heart, lungs, abdomen, and extremities.

Presentation	Differential	Workup
■ 81 yo M presents with progressive confusion for the past several years accompanied by forgetfulness and clumsiness. He has a history of hypertension, diabetes mellitus, and 2 strokes with residual left hemiparesis. His mental status has worsened after each stroke (stepwise decline in cognitive function).	**Vascular ("multi-infarct") dementia** Alzheimer disease Normal pressure hydrocephalus Chronic subdural hematoma Intracranial tumor Depression B_{12} deficiency Neurosyphilis Hypothyroidism	CBC VDRL/RPR Serum B_{12} TSH MRI—brain CT—head LP—CSF analysis (rare)

MINICASES

Presentation	Differential	Workup
■ 84 yo F brought by her son c/o forgetfulness (eg, forgets phone numbers, loses her way back home) and difficulty performing some of her daily activities (eg, bathing, dressing, managing money, using the phone). The problem has progressed gradually in the past few years.	**Alzheimer disease** Vascular dementia Depression Hypothyroidism Chronic subdural hematoma Normal pressure hydrocephalus Intracranial neoplasm B_{12} deficiency Neurosyphilis	CBC VDRL/RPR Serum B_{12} TSH MRI—brain (preferred) CT—head LP—CSF analysis (rare)
■ 72 yo M presents with memory loss, gait disturbance, and urinary incontinence for the past 6 months.	**Normal pressure hydrocephalus** Alzheimer disease Vascular dementia Chronic subdural hematoma Intracranial neoplasm Depression B_{12} deficiency Neurosyphilis Hypothyroidism	CT—head LP—opening pressure and CSF analysis Serum B_{12} VDRL/RPR TSH
■ 55 yo M presents with a rapidly progressive change in mental status, inability to concentrate, and memory impairment for the past 2 months. His symptoms are associated with myoclonus and ataxia.	**Creutzfeldt-Jakob disease** Vascular dementia Lewy body dementia Wernicke encephalopathy Normal pressure hydrocephalus Chronic subdural hematoma Intracranial neoplasm Depression Delirium B_{12} deficiency Neurosyphilis	CBC, electrolytes, calcium Serum B_{12} VDRL/RPR MRI—brain (preferred) CT—head EEG LP—CSF analysis Brain biopsy

MINICASES

CONFUSION/MEMORY LOSS *(cont'd)*

Presentation	Differential	Workup
■ 70 yo insulin-dependent diabetic M presents with episodes of confusion, dizziness, palpitation, diaphoresis, and weakness.	**Hypoglycemia** Transient ischemic attack Arrhythmia Delirium Angina	Glucose CBC, electrolytes Echocardiography ECG MRI—brain Doppler U/S—carotid
■ 55 yo F presents with gradual altered mental status and headache. Two weeks ago she slipped, hit her head on the ground, and lost consciousness for 2 minutes.	**Subdural hematoma** SIADH (causing hyponatremia) Creutzfeldt-Jakob disease Intracranial neoplasm	Electrolytes CT—head MRI—brain LP

DEPRESSED MOOD

Key History

Onset, duration; sleep patterns; appetite and weight change; drug and alcohol use; life stresses, excessive guilt, suicidality, social function, decreased interest (anhedonia), decreased energy, decreased concentration, psychomotor agitation or retardation; family history of mood disorders; prior episodes; medications.

Key Physical Exam

Vital signs; head and neck exam; neurologic exam; mental status exam, including documentation of appearance, behavior, speech, mood, affect, thought process, thought content, cognition (measured by the 30-point mini-mental status exam), insight, and judgment.

Presentation	Differential	Workup
■ 68 yo M presents with a 2-month history of crying spells, excessive sleep, poor hygiene, and a 7-kg weight loss, all following his wife's death. He cannot enjoy time with his grandchildren and reluctantly admits to thinking he has seen his dead wife in line at the supermarket or standing in the kitchen making dinner.	**Normal bereavement** Adjustment disorder with depressed mood Major depressive disorder with psychotic features Schizoaffective disorder Depressive disorder not otherwise specified	Physical exam Mental status exam TSH CBC Urine toxicology

Presentation	Differential	Workup
▪ 42 yo F presents with a 4-week history of excessive fatigue, insomnia, and anhedonia. She states that she thinks constantly about death. She has suffered 5 similar episodes in the past, the first in her 20s, and has made 2 previous suicide attempts. She further admits to increased alcohol use in the past month.	**Major depressive disorder** Substance-induced mood disorder Dysthymic disorder	Physical exam Mental status exam Blood alcohol level TSH CBC Urine toxicology
▪ 26 yo F presents with a 3-kg weight loss in the past 2 months, accompanied by early-morning awakening, excessive guilt, and psychomotor retardation. She does not identify a trigger for the depressive episode but reports several weeks of increased energy, sexual promiscuity, irresponsible spending, and racing thoughts approximately 6 months before her presentation.	**Bipolar I disorder** Bipolar II disorder Cyclothymic disorder Major depressive disorder Schizoaffective disorder	Physical exam Mental status exam Urine toxicology

PSYCHOSIS

Key History

Positive symptoms (delusions, hallucinations, disorganized thoughts, disorganized or catatonic behavior), negative symptoms (blunted affect, social withdrawal, decreased motivation, decreased speech/thought), cognitive symptoms (disorganized speech or thought patterns, paranoia); age at first symptoms and/or hospitalization; previous psychiatric medications; alcohol and substance use.

Key Physical Exam

Vital signs; mental status exam.

Presentation	Differential	Workup
▪ 19 yo M c/o receiving messages from his television set. He reports that he did not have many friends in high school. In college, he started to suspect his roommate of bugging the phone. He stopped going to classes because he felt that his professors were saying horrible things about him that no one else noticed. He rarely showered or left his room and recently has been hearing a voice from his television set telling him to "guard against the evil empire."	**Schizophrenia** Schizoid or schizotypal personality disorder Schizophreniform disorder Psychotic disorder due to a general medical condition Substance-induced psychosis Depression with psychotic features	Mental status exam Urine toxicology TSH CBC Electrolytes

Presentation	Differential	Workup
■ 28 yo F c/o seeing bugs crawling on her bed for the past 2 days and hearing loud voices when she is alone in her room. She has never experienced anything similar in the past. She recently ingested an unknown substance.	**Substance-induced psychosis** Brief psychotic disorder Schizophreniform disorder Schizophrenia Psychotic disorder due to a general medical condition	Urine toxicology Mental status exam TSH CBC Electrolytes, BUN/Cr, AST/ALT
■ 48 yo F presents with a 1-week history of auditory hallucinations that state, "I am worthless" and "I should kill myself." She also reports a 2-week history of weight loss, early-morning awakening, decreased motivation, and overwhelming feelings of guilt.	**Schizoaffective disorder** Mood disorder with psychotic features Schizophrenia Schizophreniform disorder Psychotic disorder due to a general medical condition	Mental status exam Beck Depression Inventory TSH CBC Electrolytes

DIZZINESS

Key History

Lightheadedness vs. vertigo, ± auditory symptoms (hearing loss, tinnitus), duration of episodes, context (occurs with positioning, following head trauma), other associated symptoms (visual disturbance, URI, nausea); neck pain or injury; medications; history of atherosclerotic vascular disease.

Key Physical Exam

Vital signs; complete neurologic exam, including Romberg test, nystagmus, tilt test (eg, Dix-Hallpike maneuver), gait, hearing, and Weber and Rinne tests; ENT exam; cardiovascular exam.

Presentation	Differential	Workup
■ 35 yo F presents with intermittent episodes of vertigo, tinnitus, nausea, and hearing loss within the past week.	**Ménière disease** Vestibular neuronitis Labyrinthitis Benign positional vertigo Acoustic neuroma	CBC VDRL/RPR (syphilis is a cause of Ménière disease) MRI—brain

Presentation	Differential	Workup
■ 55 yo F c/o dizziness for the past day. She feels faint and has severe diarrhea that started 2 days ago. She takes furosemide for hypertension.	**Orthostatic hypotension due to dehydration** (diarrhea, diuretic use) Vestibular neuronitis Labyrinthitis Benign positional vertigo Vertebrobasilar insufficiency	Orthostatic vital signs CBC Electrolytes Stool exam (occult blood, fecal leukocytes)
■ 65 yo M presents with postural dizziness and unsteadiness. He has hypertension and was started on hydrochlorothiazide 2 days ago.	**Drug-induced orthostatic hypotension** Vestibular neuronitis Labyrinthitis Benign positional vertigo Brain stem or cerebellar tumor Acute renal failure	Orthostatic vital signs CBC Electrolytes MRI—brain
■ 44 yo F c/o dizziness on moving her head to the left. She feels that the room is spinning around her head. Tilt test results in nystagmus and nausea.	**Benign positional vertigo** Vestibular neuronitis Labyrinthitis Ménière disease	MRI—brain Audiogram Dix-Hallpike test
■ 55 yo F c/o dizziness that started this morning. She is nauseated and has vomited once in the past day. She had a URI 2 days ago and has experienced no hearing loss.	**Vestibular neuronitis** Labyrinthitis Ménière disease Benign positional vertigo Vertigo associated with cervical spine disease or injury Vertebrobasilar insufficiency	CBC Electrolytes Electronystagmography MRI/MRA—brain
■ 55 yo F c/o dizziness that started this morning and of "not hearing well." She feels nauseated and has vomited once in the past day. She had a URI 2 days ago.	**Labyrinthitis** Vestibular neuronitis Ménière disease Acoustic neuroma Vertebrobasilar insufficiency	Audiogram Electronystagmography MRI/MRA—brain

MINICASES

LOSS OF CONSCIOUSNESS (LOC)

Key History

Presence or absence of preceding symptoms (nausea, diaphoresis, palpitation, pallor, light-headedness), context (exertional, postural, traumatic; stressful, painful, or claustrophobic experience; dehydration); associated tongue biting or incontinence, tonic-clonic movements, prolonged confusion; dyspnea or pulmonary embolism risk factors; history of heart disease, arrhythmia, hypertension, or diabetes; alcohol and drug use.

Key Physical Exam

Vital signs, including orthostatics; complete neurologic exam; carotid and cardiac exam; lung exam; exam of the lower extremities.

Presentation	Differential	Workup
26 yo M presents after falling and losing consciousness at work. He had rhythmic movements of the limbs, bit his tongue, and lost control of his bladder. He was subsequently confused (as witnessed by his colleagues).	**Complex tonic-clonic seizure** Convulsive syncope Substance abuse/overdose Malingering Hypoglycemia	CBC, electrolytes, glucose Urine toxicology EEG MRI—brain CT—head LP—CSF analysis ECG
55 yo M c/o falling after feeling dizzy and unsteady. He experienced transient LOC. He has hypertension and is on numerous antihypertensive drugs.	**Drug-induced orthostatic hypotension (causing syncope)** Cardiac arrhythmia Syncope (vasovagal, other causes) Stroke MI Pulmonary embolism	Orthostatic vital signs CBC Electrolytes CT—head ECG V/Q scan CTA—chest with IV contrast
65 yo M presents after falling and losing consciousness for a few seconds. He had no warning before passing out but recently had palpitations. His past history includes coronary artery bypass grafting.	**Cardiac arrhythmia (causing syncope)** Severe aortic stenosis Syncope (other causes) Seizure Pulmonary embolism	ECG Holter monitoring CBC, electrolytes Glucose Echocardiography CT—head

NUMBNESS/WEAKNESS

Key History

Distribution (unilateral, bilateral, proximal, distal), duration, ± progression, pain (especially headache, neck or back pain); constitutional symptoms, other neurologic symptoms; history of diabetes, alcoholism, atherosclerotic vascular disease.

Key Physical Exam

Vital signs; neurologic and musculoskeletal exams; relevant vascular exam.

Presentation	Differential	Workup
■ 68 yo M presents following a 20-minute episode of slurred speech, right facial drooping and numbness, and right hand weakness. His symptoms had totally resolved by the time he got to the emergency department. He has a history of hypertension, diabetes mellitus, and heavy smoking.	**Transient ischemic attack (TIA)** Hypoglycemia Seizure Stroke Facial nerve palsy	CBC Glucose Electrolytes ECG CT—head MRI—brain Doppler U/S—carotid Echocardiography EEG
■ 68 yo M presents with slurred speech, right facial drooping and numbness, and right hand weakness. Babinski sign is present on the right. He has a history of hypertension, diabetes mellitus, and heavy smoking.	**Stroke** TIA Seizure Intracranial neoplasm Subdural or epidural hematoma	CBC, electrolytes PT/PTT/INR CT—head MRI—brain (preferred) Doppler U/S—carotid Echocardiography
■ 33 yo F presents with ascending loss of strength in her lower legs in the past 2 weeks. She had a recent URI.	**Guillain-Barré syndrome** Multiple sclerosis Polymyositis Myasthenia gravis Peripheral neuropathy Tumor in the vertebral canal	CBC, electrolytes CPK LP—CSF analysis MRI—spine EMG/nerve conduction study Tensilon test Serum B_{12}
■ 30 yo F presents with weakness, loss of sensation, and tingling in her left leg that started this morning. She is also experiencing right eye pain, decreased vision, and double vision. She reports feeling "electric shocks" down her spine upon flexing her head.	**Multiple sclerosis** Stroke Conversion disorder Malingering CNS tumor Neurosyphilis Syringomyelia CNS vasculitis	CBC, ESR VDRL/RPR MRI—brain, spine LP—CSF analysis Retinal evoked potentials

MINICASES

Presentation	Differential	Workup
■ 55 yo M presents with tingling and numbness in the hands and feet (glove-and-stocking distribution) for the past 2 months. He has a history of diabetes mellitus, hypertension, and alcoholism. There is decreased soft touch, vibratory, and position sense in the feet.	**Diabetic peripheral neuropathy** Alcoholic peripheral neuropathy B_{12} deficiency Hypocalcemia Hyperventilation Paraproteinemia/myeloma	HbA_{1c} ESR Calcium Serum B_{12} UA Serum and urine protein electrophoresis
■ 40 yo F presents with occasional double vision and droopy eyelids at night with normalization by morning.	**Myasthenia gravis** Horner syndrome Multiple sclerosis Intracranial tumor compressing CN III, IV, or VI Amyotrophic lateral sclerosis	Tensilon test ACh receptor antibodies (in serum) CXR CT—chest MRI—brain EMG
■ 25 yo M presents with hemiparesis after a tonic-clonic seizure that resolves within a few hours.	**Todd paralysis** TIA Stroke Complicated migraine Malingering	CBC, electrolytes EEG MRI—brain Doppler U/S—carotid

FATIGUE AND SLEEPINESS

Key History

Duration; sleep hygiene, snoring, waking up choking/gasping, witnessed apnea; overexertion; stress, depression, or other emotional problems; lifestyle changes, shift changes at work; diet, weight changes; other constitutional symptoms; symptoms of thyroid disease; history of bleeding or anemia; medications; alcohol and drug use.

Key Physical Exam

Vital signs; ENT exam (conjunctival pallor, oropharynx/palate, lymphadenopathy, thyroid exam); heart, lung, abdominal, neurologic, and extremity (pallor, coolness at distal extremities) exams; consider rectal exam and occult blood testing.

MINICASES

Presentation	Differential	Workup
■ 40 yo F c/o feeling tired, hopeless, and worthless and of having suicidal thoughts. She lost her job and has been having fights with her husband at home about money.	**Depression** Adjustment disorder Hypothyroidism Anemia	CBC TSH HIV/STD testing (given husband's possible risk factors)
■ 44 yo M presents with fatigue, insomnia, and night-mares about a murder that he witnessed in a mall 1 year ago. Since then, he has avoided that mall and has not gone out at night.	**Posttraumatic stress disorder** Depression Generalized anxiety disorder Psychotic or delusional disorder Hypothyroidism	CBC TSH Calcium Urine toxicology
■ 55 yo M presents with fatigue, weight loss, and constipation. He has a family history of colon cancer.	**Colon cancer** Hypothyroidism Renal failure Hypercalcemia Depression	Rectal exam, stool for occult blood CBC, electrolytes, calcium, BUN/Cr, AST/ALT, TSH Colonoscopy Barium enema
■ 40 yo F presents with fatigue, weight gain, sleepiness, cold intolerance, constipation, and dry skin.	**Hypothyroidism** Depression Diabetes Anemia	TSH, FT_3, FT_4 CBC Fasting glucose, HbA_{1c}
■ 50 yo obese F presents with fatigue and daytime sleepiness. She snores heavily and naps 3–4 times per day but never feels refreshed. She also has hypertension.	**Obstructive sleep apnea** Hypothyroidism Chronic fatigue syndrome Narcolepsy	CBC TSH Nocturnal pulse oximetry Polysomnography ECG
■ 20 yo M presents with fatigue, thirst, increased appetite, and polyuria.	**Diabetes mellitus** Atypical depression Primary polydipsia Diabetes insipidus	Glucose tolerance test, HbA_{1c} UA CBC, electrolytes, glucose BUN/Cr
■ 35 yo M policeman c/o feeling tired and sleepy during the day. He changed to the night shift last week.	**Sleep deprivation** Sleep apnea Depression Anemia	CBC Nocturnal pulse oximetry Polysomnography

MINICASES

NIGHT SWEATS

Key History

Onset, duration, severity, frequency, timing, patterns; recent URIs, associated cough, hemoptysis, pleuritic chest pain; lymphadenopathy, fever, rash, malaise, weight loss, itching; diarrhea, nausea/vomiting, early satiety, anorexia; alcohol history, sexual exposure, sick contacts, exposure to high-risk populations such as prisoners or homeless people; menstrual history, perimenopause.

Key Physical Exam

Vital signs; HEENT exam, including throat inspection for lymphadenopathy; heart and lung exam; abdominal exam for hepatosplenomegaly; skin exam; musculoskeletal exam for joint pain.

Presentation	Differential	Workup
■ 30 yo M presents with night sweats, cough, and swollen glands of 1 month's duration.	**Tuberculosis** Acute HIV infection Lymphoma Leukemia Hyperthyroidism	PPD CBC CXR Sputum Gram stain, acid- fast stain, and culture HIV antibody TSH, FT_4

INSOMNIA

Key History

Primary vs. secondary, duration, description (trouble falling asleep vs. multiple awakenings vs. early-morning awakening); daytime sleepiness; other medical problems keeping patient awake at night, such as arthritis (pain) or diabetes (polyuria); associated symptoms, including loud snoring, nightmares, and depression; caffeine use, recreational drug use; work or lifestyle (jet lag or shift work), stressors, sleep hygiene.

Key Physical Exam

Vital signs; mental status exam.

Presentation	Differential	Workup
■ 25 yo F presents with a 3-week history of difficulty falling asleep. She sleeps 7 hours per night without nightmares or snoring. She recently began college and is having trouble with her boyfriend. She drinks 3–4 cups of coffee a day.	**Stress-induced insomnia** Caffeine-induced insomnia Insomnia with circadian rhythm sleep disorder Insomnia related to major depressive disorder	Polysomnography Mental status exam Urine toxicology CBC TSH

Presentation	Differential	Workup
■ 55 yo obese M presents with several months of poor sleep and daytime fatigue. His wife reports that he snores loudly.	**Obstructive sleep apnea** Daytime fatigue in primary hypersomnia Insomnia with circadian rhythm sleep disorder Insomnia related to major depressive disorder	CBC TSH Polysomnography ECG
■ 33 yo F c/o 3 weeks of fatigue and trouble sleeping. She states that she falls asleep easily but wakes up at 3 A.M. and cannot return to sleep. She also reports an unintentional weight loss of 3.5 kg and an inability to enjoy the things she once liked to do.	**Insomnia related to major depressive disorder** Primary hypersomnia Insomnia with circadian rhythm sleep disorder	Mental status exam TSH CBC Polysomnography

SORE THROAT

Key History

Duration, fever, other ENT symptoms (ear pain, nasal or sinus congestion), odynophagia, swollen glands, ± cough, rash; sick contacts, HIV risk factors.

Key Physical Exam

Vital signs; ENT exam, including oral thrush, tonsillar exudate, and lymphadenopathy; lung, abdominal, and skin exams.

Presentation	Differential	Workup
■ 26 yo F presents with sore throat, fever, severe fatigue, and loss of appetite for the past week. She also reports epigastric and LUQ discomfort. She has cervical lymphadenopathy and a rash. Her boyfriend recently experienced similar symptoms.	**Infectious mononucleosis** Hepatitis Viral or bacterial pharyngitis Acute HIV infection Secondary syphilis	CBC with peripheral smear Monospot test Throat culture AST/ALT/bilirubin/ alkaline phosphatase HIV antibody and viral load Anti-EBV antibodies VDRL/RPR

Presentation	Differential	Workup
■ 26 yo M presents with sore throat, fever, rash, and weight loss. He has a history of IV drug abuse and sharing needles.	**HIV, acute retroviral syndrome** Infectious mononucleosis Hepatitis Viral pharyngitis Streptococcal tonsillitis/ scarlet fever Secondary syphilis	CBC Peripheral smear HIV antibody and viral load CD4 count Monospot test Throat culture VDRL/RPR AST/ALT/bilirubin/ alkaline phosphatase
■ 46 yo F presents with fever and sore throat.	Pharyngitis (bacterial or viral) *Mycoplasma* pneumonia Acute HIV infection Infectious mononucleosis	Throat swab for culture and rapid streptococcal antigen Monospot test CBC HIV antibody and viral load

COUGH/SHORTNESS OF BREATH

Key History

Acute vs. chronic, increased frequency of cough if chronic; presence/description of sputum; associated symptoms (constitutional, URI, postnasal drip, dyspnea, wheezing, chest pain, heartburn), exacerbating and alleviating factors, timing, exposures; smoking history; history of lung disease; allergies; medications (especially ACE inhibitors).

Key Physical Exam

Vital signs ± pulse oximetry; exam of nasal mucosa, oropharynx, heart, lungs, lymph nodes, and extremities (clubbing, cyanosis, edema).

Presentation	Differential	Workup
■ 30 yo M presents with shortness of breath, cough, and wheezing that worsen in cold air. He has had several such episodes in the past 4 months.	**Asthma** GERD Bronchitis Pneumonitis Foreign body	CBC CXR Peak flow measurement PFTs Methacholine challenge test

Presentation	Differential	Workup
■ 56 yo F presents with shortness of breath and productive cough that lasts for at least 3 months each year in the past 2 years. She is a heavy smoker.	**COPD—chronic bronchitis** Bronchiectasis Lung cancer Tuberculosis	CBC Sputum Gram stain and culture CXR PFTs CT—chest PPD
■ 58 yo M presents with 1 week of pleuritic chest pain, fever, chills, and cough with purulent yellow sputum. He is a heavy smoker with COPD.	**Pneumonia** COPD exacerbation (bronchitis) Lung abscess Lung cancer Tuberculosis Pericarditis	CBC Sputum Gram stain and culture CXR CT—chest ECG PPD
■ 25 yo F presents with 2 weeks of nonproductive cough. Three weeks ago she had a sore throat and runny nose.	**Atypical pneumonia** Reactive airway disease URI-associated cough ("postinfectious") Postnasal drip GERD	CBC Induced sputum Gram stain and culture CXR IgM detection for *Mycoplasma pneumoniae* Urine *Legionella* antigen
■ 65 yo M presents with worsening cough for the past 6 months accompanied by hemoptysis, dyspnea, weakness, and weight loss. He is a heavy smoker.	**Lung cancer** Tuberculosis Lung abscess COPD Vasculitis (ie, Wegener) Interstitial lung disease CHF	CBC Sputum Gram stain, culture, and cytology CXR CT—chest PPD Bronchoscopy
■ 55 yo M presents with increased dyspnea and sputum production for the past 3 days. He has COPD and stopped using his inhalers last week. He stopped smoking 2 days ago.	**COPD exacerbation (bronchitis)** Lung cancer Pneumonia URI CHF	CBC CXR PFTs Sputum Gram stain and culture CT—chest

Presentation	Differential	Workup
■ 34 yo F nurse presents with worsening cough of 6 weeks' duration accompanied by weight loss, fatigue, night sweats, and fever. She has a history of contact with tuberculosis patients at work.	**Tuberculosis** Pneumonia Lung abscess Vasculitis Lymphoma Metastatic cancer HIV/AIDS Sarcoidosis	CBC PPD Sputum Gram stain, acid- fast stain, and culture CXR CT—chest Bronchoscopy HIV antibody

■ 35 yo M presents with shortness of breath and cough. He has had unprotected sex with multiple sexual partners and was recently exposed to a patient with active tuberculosis.	**Tuberculosis**
	Pneumonia (including *Pneumocystis jiroveci*)
	Bronchitis
	CHF (cardiomyopathy)
	Asthma
	Acute HIV infection
		CBC
		PPD
		Sputum Gram stain, acid-
		   fast stain, silver stain,
		   and culture
		CXR
		HIV antibody

■ 50 yo M presents with a cough that is exacerbated by lying down at night and improved by propping up on 3 pillows. He also reports exertional dyspnea.	**CHF** Cardiac valvular disease GERD Pulmonary fibrosis COPD Postnasal drip	CBC CXR ECG Echocardiography PFTs BNP

CHEST PAIN

Key History

Location, quality, severity, radiation, duration, context (exertional, postprandial, positional, cocaine use, trauma), associated symptoms (sweating, nausea, dyspnea, palpitation, sense of doom), exacerbating and alleviating factors (especially medications); history of similar symptoms; known heart or lung disease or history of diagnostic testing; cardiac risk factors (hypertension, hyperlipidemia, smoking, family history of early MI); pulmonary embolism risk factors (history of DVT, coagulopathy, malignancy, recent immobilization).

Key Physical Exam

Vital signs ± BP in both arms; complete cardiovascular exam (JVD, PMI, chest wall tenderness, heart sounds, pulses, edema); lung and abdominal exams.

Presentation	Differential	Workup
■ 60 yo M presents with sudden onset of substernal heavy chest pain that has lasted for 30 minutes and radiates to the left arm. The pain is accompanied by dyspnea, diaphoresis, and nausea. He has a history of hypertension, hyperlipidemia, and smoking.	**Myocardial infarction (MI)** GERD Angina Costochondritis Aortic dissection Pericarditis Pulmonary embolism Pneumothorax	ECG CPK-MB, troponin × 3 CXR CBC, electrolytes Echocardiography Cardiac catheterization
■ 20 yo African American F presents with acute onset of severe chest pain for a few hours. She has a history of sickle cell disease and multiple previous hospitalizations for pain and anemia management.	**Sickle cell disease— pulmonary infarction** Pneumonia Pulmonary embolism MI Pneumothorax Aortic dissection	CBC, reticulocyte count, LDH, peripheral smear ABG CXR CPK-MB, troponin ECG CTA—chest with IV contrast
■ 45 yo F presents with a retrosternal burning sensation that occurs after heavy meals and when lying down. Her symptoms are relieved by antacids.	**GERD** Esophagitis Peptic ulcer disease Esophageal spasm MI Angina	ECG Barium swallow Upper endoscopy Esophageal pH monitoring
■ 55 yo M presents with retrosternal squeezing pain that lasts for 2 minutes and occurs with exercise. It is relieved by rest and is not related to food intake.	**Angina** Esophageal spasm Esophagitis	ECG CPK-MB, troponin CXR CBC, electrolytes Exercise stress test Upper endoscopy/pH monitor Cardiac catheterization
■ 34 yo F presents with retrosternal stabbing chest pain that improves when she leans forward and worsens with deep inspiration. She had a URI 1 week ago.	**Pericarditis** Aortic dissection MI Costochondritis GERD Esophageal rupture	ECG CPK-MB, troponin CXR Echocardiography CBC Upper endoscopy

MINICASES

Presentation	Differential	Workup
■ 34 yo F presents with stabbing chest pain that worsens with deep inspiration and is relieved by aspirin. She had a URI 1 week ago. Chest wall tenderness is noted.	**Costochondritis** Pneumonia MI Pulmonary embolism Pericarditis Muscle strain	ECG CPK-MB, troponin CXR CBC
■ 70 yo F presents with acute onset of shortness of breath at rest and pleuritic chest pain. She also presents with tachycardia, hypotension, tachypnea, and mild fever. She is recovering from hip replacement surgery.	**Pulmonary embolism** Pneumonia Costochondritis MI CHF Aortic dissection	ECG CXR ABG CPK-MB, troponin CBC, Chem 7 CTA—chest with IV contrast Doppler U/S—legs D-dimer
■ 55 yo M presents with sudden onset of severe chest pain that radiates to the back. He has a history of uncontrolled hypertension.	**Aortic dissection** MI Pericarditis Esophageal rupture Esophageal spasm GERD Pancreatitis Fat embolism	ECG, CPK-MB, troponin CXR CBC, amylase, lipase Transesophageal echocardiography (TEE), MRI/MRA—aorta Aortic angiography Upper endoscopy

PALPITATIONS

Key History

Gradual vs. acute onset/offset, context (exertion, caffeine, anxiety), associated symptoms (light-headedness, chest pain, dyspnea); hyperthyroid symptoms; history of bleeding or anemia; history of heart disease.

Key Physical Exam

Vital signs; endocrine/thyroid exam, including exophthalmos, lid retraction, lid lag, gland size, bruit, and tremor; complete cardiovascular exam.

MINICASES

Presentation	Differential	Workup
■ 70 yo diabetic M presents with episodes of palpitations and diaphoresis. He is on insulin.	**Hypoglycemia** Cardiac arrhythmias Angina Hyperthyroidism Hyperventilation episodes Panic attacks Pheochromocytoma Carcinoid syndrome	Glucose CBC, electrolytes TSH ECG Holter monitor
■ 35 yo M presents with several episodes of palpitations, sweating, and rapid breathing. Episodes occur unexpectedly and he does not recall any triggers. He has had 4–5 episodes per month for several months. Each episode lasts 2–3 minutes. He does not have any history of psychiatric illness except for separation anxiety as a child.	**Panic attack** Generalized anxiety disorder Acute stress disorder Specific phobia Hyperthyroidism Agoraphobia Substance abuse/ dependence Mitral valve prolapse Pheochromocytoma	CBC, electrolytes TSH, FT$_4$ ECG Echocardiography Urine toxicology
■ 19 yo F presents with episodic palpitations especially during presentations in front of her class. Episodes include heart pounding, facial blushing, and hand shaking. She also states she experiences excessive sweating and rapid breathing. She complains of intense worry and trouble sleeping for days or weeks before an upcoming social situation. Now she avoids all social events because she is always afraid of humiliating herself.	**Social phobia** Avoidant personality disorder Agoraphobia/specific phobia Panic attacks Generalized anxiety disorder Substance abuse/ dependence Hyperthyroidism	CBC, electrolytes ECG Echocardiography TSH, FT$_4$ Mental status exam

WEIGHT LOSS

Key History

Amount, duration, ± intention; diet history, body image, anxiety or depression; other constitutional symptoms; palpitation, tremor, diarrhea; family history of thyroid disease; HIV risk factors; tobacco, alcohol, and drug use; medications; history of cancer; blood in urine or stool.

Key Physical Exam

Vital signs; complete physical.

Presentation	Differential	Workup
■ 42 yo F presents with a 7-kg weight loss within the past 2 months. She has a fine tremor, and her pulse is 112.	**Hyperthyroidism** Cancer HIV infection Dieting/diet drugs Anorexia nervosa Malabsorption	TSH, FT$_4$ CBC, electrolytes HIV antibody Urine toxicology

WEIGHT GAIN

Key History

Amount, duration, timing (relation to medication changes, smoking cessation, depression); diet history; hypothyroid symptoms (fatigue, constipation, skin/hair/nail changes); menstrual irregularity; medical history; alcohol and drug use.

Key Physical Exam

Vital signs; complete exam, including signs of Cushing syndrome (hypertension, central obesity, moon face, buffalo hump, supraclavicular fat pads, purple abdominal striae).

Presentation	Differential	Workup
■ 44 yo F presents with a weight gain of > 11 kg within the past 2 months. She quit smoking 3 months ago and is on amitriptyline for depression. She also reports cold intolerance and constipation.	**Smoking cessation** Drug side effect Hypothyroidism Cushing syndrome Polycystic ovary syndrome Diabetes mellitus Atypical depression	CBC, electrolytes, glucose TSH 24-hour urine free cortisol Dexamethasone suppression test

DYSPHAGIA

Key History

Solids or liquids vs. both solids and liquids, ± progression, constitutional symptoms (especially weight loss), drooling, regurgitation, odynophagia, GERD symptoms; medications; HIV risk factors, history of smoking, history of Raynaud phenomenon.

DYSPHAGIA *(cont'd)*

Key Physical Exam

Vital signs; head and neck exam; heart, lung, and abdominal exams; skin exam (for signs of scleroderma/CREST).

Presentation	Differential	Workup
75 yo M presents with dysphagia that started with solids and progressed to liquids. He is an alcoholic and a heavy smoker. He has had an unintentional weight loss of 7 kg within the past 4 months.	**Esophageal cancer** Achalasia Esophagitis Systemic sclerosis Esophageal stricture Amyotrophic lateral sclerosis	CBC CXR Endoscopy with biopsy Barium swallow CT—chest
45 yo F presents with dysphagia for 2 weeks accompanied by mouth and throat pain, fatigue, and a craving for ice and clay.	**Plummer-Vinson syndrome** Esophageal cancer Esophagitis Achalasia Systemic sclerosis Mitral valve stenosis	CBC Serum iron, ferritin, TIBC Barium swallow Endoscopy
48 yo F presents with dysphagia for both solid and liquid foods that has slowly progressed in severity within the past year. It is associated with regurgitation of undigested food, especially at night.	**Achalasia** Plummer-Vinson syndrome Esophageal cancer Esophagitis Systemic sclerosis Mitral valve stenosis Esophageal stricture Zenker diverticulum	CXR XR—neck Endoscopy Barium swallow Esophageal manometry
38 yo M presents with dysphagia and pain on swallowing solids more than liquids. Exam reveals oral thrush.	**Esophagitis** (CMV, HSV, pill-induced) Systemic sclerosis GERD Esophageal stricture Zenker diverticulum	CBC Endoscopy Barium swallow HIV antibody and viral load CD4 count

NAUSEA/VOMITING

Key History

Acuity of onset, ± abdominal pain, relation to meals, sick contacts, possible food poisoning, possible pregnancy; neurologic symptoms (headache, stiff neck, vertigo, focal numbness or weakness), other associated symptoms (GI, chest pain), exacerbating and alleviating factors; medications.

Key Physical Exam

Vital signs; ENT; consider funduscopic exam (increased intracranial pressure); complete abdominal exam; consider heart, lung, and rectal exams.

Presentation	Differential	Workup
■ 20 yo F presents with nausea, vomiting (especially in the morning), fatigue, and polyuria. Her last menstrual period was 6 weeks ago, and her breasts are full and tender. She is sexually active with her boyfriend, and they use condoms for contraception.	**Pregnancy** Gastritis Hypercalcemia Diabetes mellitus UTI Depression	Urine hCG Pelvic exam U/S—pelvis CBC, electrolytes, calcium, glucose UA, urine culture Baseline Pap smear, cervical cultures, rubella antibody, HIV antibody, hepatitis B surface antigen, and VDRL/RPR

ABDOMINAL PAIN

Key History

Location, quality, intensity, duration, radiation, timing (relation to meals), associated symptoms (constitutional, GI, cardiac, pulmonary, renal, pelvic), exacerbating and alleviating factors; history of similar symptoms; history of abdominal surgeries, gallstones, renal stones, atherosclerotic vascular disease; medications; alcohol and drug use; domestic violence.

Key Physical Exam

Vital signs; heart and lung exams; abdominal exam, including guarding, rebound, Murphy sign, psoas and obturator signs, and CVA palpation; rectal exam; pelvic exam (women).

Presentation	Differential	Workup
■ 45 yo M presents with sudden onset of colicky right-sided flank pain that radiates to the testicles, accompanied by nausea, vomiting, hematuria, and CVA tenderness.	**Nephrolithiasis** Renal cell carcinoma Pyelonephritis GI etiology (eg, appendicitis)	Rectal exam UA Urine culture and sensitivity BUN/Cr CT—abdomen U/S—renal IVP

MINICASES

Presentation	Differential	Workup
■ 60 yo M presents with dull epigastric pain that radiates to the back, accompanied by weight loss, dark urine, and clay-colored stool. He is a heavy drinker and smoker.	**Pancreatic cancer** Acute viral hepatitis Chronic pancreatitis Cholecystitis/ choledocholithiasis Abdominal aortic aneurysm Peptic ulcer disease	Rectal exam CBC, electrolytes Amylase and lipase AST/ALT/bilirubin/ alkaline phosphatase U/S—abdomen CT—abdomen
■ 56 yo M presents with severe midepigastric abdominal pain that radiates to the back and improves when he leans forward. He also reports anorexia, nausea, and vomiting. He is an alcoholic and has spent the past 3 days binge drinking.	**Acute pancreatitis** Peptic ulcer disease Cholecystitis/ choledocholithiasis Gastritis Abdominal aortic aneurysm Mesenteric ischemia Alcoholic hepatitis Mallory-Weiss tear	Rectal exam CBC, electrolytes, BUN/ Cr, amylase, lipase, AST/ALT/bilirubin/ alkaline phosphatase U/S—abdomen CT—abdomen Upper endoscopy ECG
■ 41 yo obese F presents with RUQ abdominal pain that radiates to the right scapula and is associated with nausea, vomiting, and a fever of 101.5°F. The pain started after she ate fatty food. She has had similar but less intense episodes that lasted a few hours. Exam reveals a positive Murphy sign.	**Acute cholecystitis** Hepatitis Choledocholithiasis Ascending cholangitis Peptic ulcer disease Fitz-Hugh–Curtis syndrome	Rectal exam CBC AST/ALT/bilirubin/ alkaline phosphatase U/S—abdomen CT—abdomen HIDA scan
■ 43 yo obese F presents with RUQ abdominal pain, fever, and jaundice. She was diagnosed with asymptomatic gallstones 1 year ago.	**Ascending cholangitis** Acute cholecystitis Hepatitis Choledocholithiasis Sclerosing cholangitis Fitz-Hugh–Curtis syndrome	Rectal exam CBC AST/ALT/bilirubin/ alkaline phosphatase Viral hepatitis serologies U/S—abdomen MRCP ERCP

MINICASES

Presentation	Differential	Workup
25 yo M presents with RUQ pain, fever, anorexia, nausea, and vomiting. He has dark urine and clay-colored stool.	**Acute hepatitis** Acute cholecystitis Ascending cholangitis Choledocholithiasis Pancreatitis Acute glomerulonephritis	Rectal exam CBC, amylase, lipase AST/ALT/bilirubin/ alkaline phosphatase UA Viral hepatitis serologies U/S—abdomen

35 yo M presents with burning epigastric pain that starts 2–3 hours after meals. The pain is relieved by food and antacids.	**Peptic ulcer disease**
	Gastritis
	GERD
	Cholecystitis
	Chronic pancreatitis
	Mesenteric ischemia
		Rectal exam
		Amylase, lipase, lactate
		AST/ALT/bilirubin/
		    alkaline phosphatase
		Endoscopy (including
		    H. pylori testing)
		Upper GI series

37 yo M presents with severe epigastric pain, nausea, vomiting, and mild fever. He appears toxic. He has a history of intermittent epigastric pain that is relieved by food and antacids. He also smokes heavily and takes aspirin on a regular basis.	**Peptic ulcer perforation**
	Acute pancreatitis
	Hepatitis
	Cholecystitis
	Choledocholithiasis
	Mesenteric ischemia
		Rectal exam
		CBC, electrolytes,
		    amylase, lipase, lactate
		AST/ALT/bilirubin/
		    alkaline phosphatase
		KUB
		CT—abdomen
		Upright CXR
		Endoscopy (including
		    H. pylori testing)

18 yo M boxer presents with severe LUQ abdominal pain that radiates to the left scapula. He had infectious mononucleosis 3 weeks ago.	**Splenic rupture** Kidney stone Rib fracture Pneumonia Perforated peptic ulcer Splenic infarct	Rectal exam CBC, electrolytes CXR CT—abdomen U/S—abdomen
40 yo M presents with crampy abdominal pain, vomiting, abdominal distention, and inability to pass flatus or stool. He has a history of multiple abdominal surgeries.	**Intestinal obstruction** Small bowel or colon cancer Volvulus of the bowel Gastroenteritis Food poisoning Ileus Hernia	Rectal exam CBC, electrolytes AXR CT—abdomen/pelvis CXR

MINICASES

Presentation	Differential	Workup
■ 70 yo F presents with acute onset of severe, crampy abdominal pain. She recently vomited and had a massive dark bowel movement. She has a history of CHF and atrial fibrillation, for which she received digitalis. Her pain is out of proportion to the exam.	**Mesenteric ischemia/ infarction** Diverticulitis Peptic ulcer disease Gastroenteritis Acute pancreatitis Cholecystitis/ choledocholithiasis MI	Rectal exam CBC, amylase, lipase, lactate ECG, CPK-MB, troponin AXR CT—abdomen Mesenteric angiography Barium enema
■ 21 yo F presents with acute onset of severe RLQ pain, nausea, and vomiting. She has no fever, urinary symptoms, or vaginal bleeding and has never taken OCPs. Her last menstrual period was regular, and she has no history of STDs.	**Ovarian torsion** Appendicitis Nephrolithiasis Ectopic pregnancy Ruptured ovarian cyst Pelvic inflammatory disease Bowel infarction or perforation	Pelvic exam Rectal exam Urine hCG UA CBC Doppler U/S—pelvis CT—abdomen Laparoscopy
■ 68 yo M presents with LLQ abdominal pain, fever, and chills for the past 3 days. He also reports recent onset of alternating diarrhea and constipation. He consumes a low-fiber, high-fat diet.	**Diverticulitis** Crohn disease Ulcerative colitis Gastroenteritis Abscess	Rectal exam CBC, electrolytes CXR AXR CT—abdomen
■ 20 yo M presents with severe RLQ abdominal pain, nausea, and vomiting. His discomfort started yesterday as a vague pain around the umbilicus. As the pain worsened, it became sharp and migrated to the RLQ. McBurney and psoas signs are positive.	**Acute appendicitis** Gastroenteritis Diverticulitis Crohn disease Nephrolithiasis Volvulus or other intestinal obstruction/ perforation	Rectal exam CBC, electrolytes AXR CT—abdomen U/S—abdomen

Presentation	Differential	Workup
■ 30 yo F presents with periumbilical pain for 6 months. The pain never awakens her from sleep. It is relieved by defecation and worsens when she is upset. She has alternating constipation and diarrhea but no nausea, vomiting, weight loss, or anorexia.	**Irritable bowel syndrome** Crohn's disease Celiac disease Chronic pancreatitis GI parasitic infection (amebiasis, giardiasis) Endometriosis	Rectal exam, stool for occult blood Pelvic exam Urine hCG CBC/electrolytes Colonoscopy CT—abdomen/pelvis Stool for ova and parasitology, *Entamoeba histolytica* antigen
■ 24 yo F presents with bilateral lower abdominal pain that started with the first day of her menstrual period. The pain is associated with fever and a thick, green-yellow vaginal discharge. She has had unprotected sex with multiple sexual partners.	**Pelvic inflammatory disease** Endometriosis Dysmenorrhea Vaginitis Cystitis Spontaneous abortion Pyelonephritis	Pelvic exam Rectal exam Urine hCG Cervical cultures CBC/ESR UA, urine culture U/S—pelvis

CONSTIPATION/DIARRHEA

Key History

Frequency and volume of stools, duration of change in bowel habits, associated symptoms (constitutional, abdominal pain, bloating, sense of incomplete evacuation, melena or hematochezia); thyroid disease symptoms; diet (especially fiber and fluid intake); medications (including recent antibiotics); sick contacts, travel, camping, HIV risk factors; history of abdominal surgeries, diabetes, pancreatitis; alcohol and drug use; family history of colon cancer.

Key Physical Exam

Vital signs; relevant thyroid/endocrine exam; abdominal and rectal exams; ± female pelvic exam.

MINICASES

CONSTIPATION/DIARRHEA *(cont'd)*

Presentation	Differential	Workup
■ 67 yo M presents with alternating diarrhea and constipation, decreased stool caliber, and blood in the stool for the past 8 months. He also reports unintentional weight loss. He is on a low-fiber diet and has a family history of colon cancer.	**Colorectal cancer** Irritable bowel syndrome Diverticulosis GI parasitic infection (ascariasis, giardiasis) Inflammatory bowel disease Angiodysplasia	Rectal exam CBC, electrolytes AST/ALT/bilirubin/ alkaline phosphatase Colonoscopy Barium enema CT—abdomen/pelvis
■ 28 yo M presents with constipation (hard stool) for the past 3 weeks. Since his mother died 2 months ago, he and his father have eaten only junk food.	**Low-fiber diet** Irritable bowel syndrome Substance abuse (eg, heroin) Depression Hypothyroidism	Rectal exam TSH Electrolytes Urine toxicology
■ 30 yo F presents with alternating constipation and diarrhea and abdominal pain that is relieved by defecation. She has no nausea, vomiting, weight loss, or blood in her stool.	**Irritable bowel syndrome** Inflammatory bowel disease Celiac disease Chronic pancreatitis GI parasitic infection (ascariasis, giardiasis) Lactose intolerance	Rectal exam, stool for occult blood CBC, electrolytes Colonoscopy Stool for ova and parasitology KUB CT—abdomen/pelvis
■ 33 yo M presents with watery diarrhea, vomiting, and diffuse abdominal pain that began yesterday. He also reports feeling hot. Several of his coworkers are also ill.	**Infectious diarrhea (gastroenteritis)—** bacterial, viral, parasitic, protozoal Food poisoning Inflammatory bowel disease	Rectal exam, stool for occult blood Stool leukocytes and culture CBC Electrolytes CT—abdomen/pelvis
■ 40 yo F presents with watery diarrhea and abdominal cramps. Last week she was on antibiotics for a UTI.	**Pseudomembranous (*Clostridium difficile*) colitis** Gastroenteritis Cryptosporidiosis Food poisoning Inflammatory bowel disease	Rectal exam Stool leukocytes, culture, occult blood *C. difficile* toxin in stool CBC, electrolytes

CONSTIPATION/DIARRHEA *(cont'd)*

Presentation	Differential	Workup
▪ 25 yo M presents with watery diarrhea and abdominal cramps. He was recently in Mexico.	**Traveler's diarrhea** Giardiasis Amebiasis Food poisoning Hepatitis A	Rectal exam Stool leukocytes, culture, *Giardia* antigen, *Entamoeba histolytica* antigen CBC, electrolytes AST/ALT/bilirubin/ alkaline phosphatase Viral hepatitis serology
▪ 30 yo F presents with watery diarrhea, abdominal cramping, and bloating. Her symptoms are aggravated by milk ingestion and are relieved by fasting.	**Lactose intolerance** Gastroenteritis Inflammatory bowel disease Irritable bowel syndrome Hyperthyroidism	Rectal exam Stool exam Hydrogen breath test TSH
▪ 33 yo M presents with watery diarrhea, diffuse abdominal pain, and weight loss within the past 3 weeks. He has not responded to antibiotics.	**Crohn disease** Gastroenteritis Ulcerative colitis Celiac disease Pseudomembranous colitis Hyperthyroidism Small bowel lymphoma Carcinoid syndrome	Rectal exam Stool exam and culture CBC, electrolytes TSH CT—abdomen Colonoscopy Small bowel series Urinary 5-HIAA

UPPER GI BLEEDING

Key History

Amount, duration, context (after severe vomiting, alcohol ingestion, nosebleed), associated symptoms (constitutional, nausea, abdominal pain, dyspepsia); medications (especially warfarin, NSAIDs); history of peptic ulcer disease, liver disease, abdominal aortic aneurysm repair, easy bleeding.

Key Physical Exam

Vital signs, including orthostatics; ENT, heart, lung, abdominal, and rectal exams.

UPPER GI BLEEDING *(cont'd)*

Presentation	Differential	Workup

■ 45 yo F presents with coffee-ground emesis for the past 3 days. Her stool is dark and tarry. She has a history of intermittent epigastric pain that is relieved by food and antacids.	**Bleeding peptic ulcer**
	Gastritis
	Gastric cancer
	Esophageal varices
		Rectal exam
		CBC, electrolytes
		AST/ALT/bilirubin/
		    alkaline phosphatase
		Endoscopy (including
		    H. pylori testing if ulcer
		    is confirmed)

■ 40 yo F presents with epigastric pain and coffee-ground emesis. She has a history of rheumatoid arthritis that has been treated with aspirin. She is an alcoholic.	**Gastritis** Bleeding peptic ulcer Gastric cancer Esophageal varices Mallory-Weiss tear	Rectal exam CBC, electrolytes AST/ALT/bilirubin/ alkaline phosphatase Barium swallow Endoscopy

BLOOD IN STOOL

Key History

Melena vs. bright blood; amount, duration, associated symptoms (constitutional, abdominal or rectal pain, tenesmus, constipation/diarrhea); trauma; history of similar symptoms; prior colonoscopy; medications (especially warfarin); history of easy bleeding or atherosclerotic vascular disease.

Key Physical Exam

Vital signs ± orthostatics; abdominal and rectal exams.

Presentation	Differential	Workup

■ 67 yo M presents with blood in his stool, weight loss, and constipation. He has a family history of colon cancer.	**Colorectal cancer**
	Anal fissure
	Hemorrhoids
	Diverticulosis
	Ischemic bowel disease
	Angiodysplasia
	Upper GI bleeding
	Inflammatory bowel
	    disease
		Rectal exam
		CBC, PT/PTT
		AST/ALT/bilirubin/
		    alkaline phosphatase
		CEA
		Colonoscopy
		CT—abdomen/pelvis
		Barium enema

BLOOD IN STOOL *(cont'd)*

Presentation	Differential	Workup
■ 33 yo F presents with rectal bleeding and diarrhea for the past week. She has had lower abdominal pain and tenesmus for several months.	**Ulcerative colitis** Crohn disease Proctitis Anal fissure Hemorrhoids Diverticulosis Dysentery	Rectal exam CBC, PT/PTT AXR Colonoscopy CT—abdomen/pelvis Barium enema
■ 58 yo M presents with painless bright red blood per rectum and chronic constipation. He consumes a low-fiber diet.	**Diverticulosis** Anal fissure Hemorrhoids Angiodysplasia Colorectal cancer	Rectal exam CBC, PT/PTT Electrolytes Colonoscopy CT—abdomen/pelvis

HEMATURIA

Key History

Amount, duration, ± clots, associated symptoms (constitutional, renal colic, dysuria, irritative voiding symptoms); medications; history of vigorous exercise, trauma, smoking, stones, cancer, or easy bleeding.

Key Physical Exam

Vital signs; lymph nodes; abdominal exam; genitourinary and rectal exams; extremities.

Presentation	Differential	Workup
■ 65 yo M presents with painless hematuria. He is a heavy smoker and works as a painter.	**Bladder cancer** Renal cell carcinoma Nephrolithiasis Acute glomerulonephritis Prostate cancer Coagulation disorder (ie, factor VIII antibodies) Polycystic kidney disease	Genitourinary exam UA, urine cytology BUN/Cr, PSA, CBC, PT/PTT Cystoscopy U/S—renal/bladder CT—abdomen/pelvis IVP
■ 35 yo M presents with painless hematuria. He has a family history of kidney problems.	**Polycystic kidney disease** Nephrolithiasis Acute glomerulonephritis (eg, IgA nephropathy) UTI Coagulation disorder Bladder cancer	Genitourinary exam UA BUN/Cr, PSA, CBC, PT/PTT U/S—renal CT—abdomen/pelvis IVP

Presentation	Differential	Workup
■ 55 yo M presents with flank pain and blood in his urine without dysuria. He has experienced weight loss and fever in the past 2 months.	**Renal cell carcinoma** Bladder cancer Nephrolithiasis Acute glomerulonephritis Pyelonephritis Prostate cancer	Genitourinary, rectal exam UA, urine cytology, BUN/Cr, PSA, CBC, PT/PTT U/S—renal CT—abdomen/pelvis IVP

OTHER URINARY SYMPTOMS

Key History

Duration, obstructive symptoms (hesitancy, diminished stream, sense of incomplete bladder emptying, straining, postvoid dribbling), irritative symptoms (urgency, frequency, nocturia), constitutional symptoms; bone pain; medications; history of UTIs, urethral stricture, or urinary tract instrumentation; stones, diabetes, alcoholism.

Key Physical Exam

Vital signs; abdominal exam (including suprapubic percussion to assess for a distended bladder); genital and rectal exams; focused neurologic exam.

Presentation	Differential	Workup
■ 60 yo M presents with nocturia, urgency, weak stream, and terminal dribbling. He denies any weight loss, fatigue, or bone pain. He has had 2 episodes of urinary retention that required catheterization.	**Benign prostatic hyperplasia (BPH)** Prostate cancer UTI Bladder stones	Rectal exam UA CBC, BUN/Cr, PSA U/S—prostate (transrectal)
■ 71 yo M presents with nocturia, urgency, weak stream, terminal dribbling, hematuria, and lower back pain for the past 4 months. He has also experienced weight loss and fatigue.	**Prostate cancer** BPH Renal cell carcinoma UTI Bladder stones	Rectal exam UA CBC, BUN/Cr, PSA U/S—prostate (transrectal) CT—pelvis IVP

Presentation	Differential	Workup
■ 18 yo M presents with a burning sensation during urination and urethral discharge. He recently had unprotected sex with a new partner.	**Urethritis** Cystitis Prostatitis	Genital ± rectal exam UA Urine culture Gram stain and culture of urethral discharge Chlamydia and gonorrhea PCR
■ 45 yo diabetic F presents with dysuria, urinary frequency, fever, chills, and nausea for the past 3 days. There is left CVA tenderness on exam.	**Acute pyelonephritis** Nephrolithiasis Renal cell carcinoma Lower UTI (cystitis, urethritis)	UA Urine culture and sensitivity CBC, BUN/Cr U/S—renal CT—abdomen
■ 55 yo F presents with urinary leakage after exercise. She loses a small amount of urine when she coughs, laughs, or sneezes. She also complains of vague low back pain. She has a history of multiple C-sections and her mother had the same problem after the onset of menopause.	**Stress incontinence** Mixed incontinence Urge incontinence Overflow incontinence Functional incontinence UTI Diabetes mellitus	CBC, electrolytes, glucose UA, urine culture BUN/Cr Urodynamic testing IVP Cystourethroscopy
■ 33 yo F presents with urinary leakage. She is unable to suppress the urge to urinate. She loses large amounts of urine without warning. She has a history of UTIs and a family history of diabetes mellitus. She drinks 8 cups of coffee per day. She has been under a lot of stress since her sister passed away a few months ago.	**Urge incontinence** Mixed incontinence Stress incontinence Overflow incontinence Functional incontinence UTI Diabetes mellitus	CBC, electrolytes, glucose UA, urine culture BUN/Cr Urodynamic testing IVP Cystourethroscopy

ERECTILE DYSFUNCTION (ED)

Key History

Duration, severity, ± nocturnal erections, libido, stress or depression, trauma, associated incontinence; medications (and recent changes); medical history (hypertension, diabetes, high cholesterol, known atherosclerotic vascular disease, prior prostate surgery); smoking, alcohol, and drug use.

Key Physical Exam

Vital signs; cardiovascular exam; genital and rectal exams.

Presentation	Differential	Workup
■ 47 yo M presents with impotence that started 3 months ago. He has hypertension and was started on atenolol 4 months ago. He also has diabetes and is on insulin.	**Drug-related ED** ED caused by hypertension ED caused by diabetes mellitus Psychogenic ED Peyronie disease	Genital exam Rectal exam Glucose CBC

AMENORRHEA

Key History

Primary vs. secondary, duration, possible pregnancy, associated symptoms (headache, decreased peripheral vision, galactorrhea, hirsutism, virilization, hot flashes, vaginal dryness, symptoms of thyroid disease); history of anorexia nervosa, excessive dieting, vigorous exercise, pregnancies, D&Cs, uterine infections; drug use; medications.

Key Physical Exam

Vital signs; breast exam; complete pelvic exam.

Presentation	Differential	Workup
■ 40 yo F presents with amenorrhea, morning nausea and vomiting, fatigue, and polyuria. Her last menstrual period was 6 weeks ago, and her breasts are full and tender. She uses the rhythm method for contraception.	**Pregnancy** Anovulatory cycle Hyperprolactinemia UTI Thyroid disease	Pelvic exam Urine hCG U/S—pelvis CBC, electrolytes UA, urine culture Prolactin, TSH Baseline Pap smear, cervical cultures, rubella antibody, HIV antibody, hepatitis B surface antigen, and VDRL/RPR
■ 23 yo obese F presents with amenorrhea for 6 months, facial hair, and infertility for the past 3 years.	**Polycystic ovary syndrome** Thyroid disease Hyperprolactinemia Pregnancy Ovarian or adrenal malignancy Premature ovarian failure	Pelvic exam Urine hCG U/S—pelvis LH/FSH, TSH, prolactin Testosterone, DHEAS

MINICASES

Presentation	Differential	Workup
■ 35 yo F presents with amenorrhea, galactorrhea, visual field defects, and headaches for the past 6 months.	**Amenorrhea secondary to prolactinoma** Pregnancy Thyroid disease Premature ovarian failure Pituitary tumor	Pelvic and breast exam Urine hCG Prolactin LH/FSH, TSH MRI—brain
■ 48 yo F presents with amenorrhea for the past 6 months accompanied by hot flashes, night sweats, emotional lability, and dyspareunia.	**Menopause** Pregnancy Pituitary tumor Thyroid disease	Pelvic exam Urine hCG LH/FSH, TSH, prolactin, testosterone, DHEAS CBC MRI—brain
■ 35 yo F presents with amenorrhea, cold intolerance, coarse hair, weight loss, and fatigue. She has a history of abruptio placentae followed by hypovolemic shock and failure of lactation 2 years ago.	**Sheehan syndrome** Premature ovarian failure Pituitary tumor Thyroid disease Asherman syndrome	Pelvic exam Urine hCG CBC LH/FSH, prolactin TSH, FT_4 ACTH MRI—brain Hysteroscopy
■ 18 yo F presents with amenorrhea for the past 4 months. She is 5 feet, 6 inches (167.6 cm) tall and weighs 90 pounds (40.9 kg). She has a history of vigorous exercise and cold intolerance.	**Anorexia nervosa**	CBC TSH, FT_4 ACTH FSH LH
■ 29 yo F presents with amenorrhea for the past 6 months. She has a history of occasional palpitations and dizziness. She lost her fiancé in a car accident.	**Anxiety-induced amenorrhea**	CBC TSH, FT_4 ACTH Urine cortisol level Progesterone challenge test FSH/LH/estradiol levels

MINICASES

VAGINAL BLEEDING

Key History

Pre- vs. postmenopausal, duration, amount; menstrual history and relation to last menstrual period; associated discharge, pelvic or abdominal pain, or urinary symptoms; trauma; medications (especially warfarin, contraceptives); history of easy bleeding or bruising; history of abnormal Pap smears.

Key Physical Exam

Vital signs; abdominal exam; complete pelvic exam.

Presentation	Differential	Workup
■ 17 yo F presents with prolonged, excessive menstrual bleeding occurring irregularly within the past 6 months.	**Dysfunctional uterine bleeding** Coagulation disorders (eg, von Willebrand disease, hemophilia) Cervical cancer Molar pregnancy Hypothyroidism Diabetes mellitus	Pelvic exam Urine hCG Cervical cultures, Pap smear CBC, ESR, glucose PT/PTT Prolactin, LH/FSH TSH U/S—pelvis
■ 61 yo obese F presents with profuse vaginal bleeding for the past month. Her last menstrual period was 10 years ago. She has a history of hypertension and diabetes mellitus. She is nulliparous.	**Endometrial cancer** Cervical cancer Atrophic endometrium Endometrial hyperplasia Endometrial polyps Atrophic vaginitis	Pelvic exam Pap smear Endometrial biopsy U/S—pelvis Endometrial curettage Colposcopy Hysteroscopy
■ 45 yo G5P5 F presents with postcoital bleeding. She is a cigarette smoker and takes OCPs.	**Cervical cancer** Cervical polyp Cervicitis Trauma (eg, cervical laceration)	Pelvic exam Pap smear Colposcopy and biopsy
■ 28 yo F who is 8 weeks pregnant presents with lower abdominal pain and vaginal bleeding.	**Spontaneous abortion** Ectopic pregnancy Molar pregnancy	Pelvic exam Urine hCG U/S—pelvis CBC, PT/PTT Quantitative serum hCG

VAGINAL BLEEDING *(cont'd)*

Presentation	Differential	Workup
■ 32 yo F presents with sudden onset of left lower abdominal pain that radiates to the scapula and back and is associated with vaginal bleeding. Her last menstrual period was 5 weeks ago. She has a history of pelvic inflammatory disease and unprotected intercourse.	**Ectopic pregnancy** Ruptured ovarian cyst Ovarian torsion Pelvic inflammatory disease	Pelvic exam Urine hCG Cervical cultures U/S—pelvis Quantitative serum hCG

VAGINAL DISCHARGE

Key History

Amount, color, consistency, odor, duration; associated vaginal burning, pain, or pruritus; recent sexual activity; onset of last menstrual period; use of contraceptives, tampons, and douches; history of similar symptoms; history of STDs.

Key Physical Exam

Vital signs; abdominal exam; complete pelvic exam.

Presentation	Differential	Workup
■ 28 yo F presents with a thin, gray-white, foul-smelling vaginal discharge.	**Bacterial vaginosis** Vaginitis—candidal Vaginitis—trichomonal Cervicitis (chlamydia, gonorrhea)	Pelvic exam Wet mount Cervical cultures KOH prep ("whiff test") pH of vaginal fluid
■ 30 yo F presents with a thick, white, cottage cheese–like, odorless vaginal discharge and vaginal itching.	**Vaginitis—candidal** Bacterial vaginosis Vaginitis—trichomonal	Pelvic exam KOH prep ("whiff test") Wet mount Cervical cultures pH of vaginal fluid
■ 35 yo F presents with a malodorous, profuse, frothy, greenish vaginal discharge with intense vaginal itching and discomfort.	**Vaginitis—trichomonal** Vaginitis—candidal Bacterial vaginosis Cervicitis (chlamydia, gonorrhea)	Pelvic exam Wet mount Cervical cultures pH of the vaginal fluid KOH prep ("whiff test")

MINICASES

DYSPAREUNIA

Key History

Duration, timing, associated symptoms (vaginal discharge, rash, painful menses, GI symptoms, hot flashes), adequacy of lubrication; libido; sexual history; history of sexual trauma or domestic violence; history of endometriosis, pelvic inflammatory disease, or prior abdominal/pelvic surgeries.

Key Physical Exam

Vital signs; abdominal exam; complete pelvic exam.

Presentation	Differential	Workup
■ 54 yo F c/o painful intercourse. Her last menstrual period was 9 months ago. She has hot flashes.	**Atrophic vaginitis** Endometriosis Cervicitis Depression Domestic abuse	Pelvic exam Wet mount, KOH prep, cervical cultures U/S—pelvis

■ 37 yo F presents with dyspareunia, inability to conceive, and dysmenorrhea.	**Endometriosis**
	Cervicitis
	Vaginismus
	Vulvodynia
	Pelvic inflammatory
	   disease
	Depression
	Domestic violence
		Pelvic exam
		Wet mount, KOH prep,
		   cervical cultures
		U/S—pelvis
		Laparoscopy

ABUSE

Key History

Establish confidentiality; directly question about physical, sexual, or emotional abuse and about fear, safety, backup plan; history of frequent accidents/injuries, mental illness, drug use; firearms in the home.

Key Physical Exam

Vital signs; complete exam ± pelvic.

Presentation	Differential	Workup
■ 28 yo F c/o multiple facial and bodily injuries. She claims that she fell on the stairs. She was hospitalized for physical injuries 7 months ago. She presents with her husband.	**Domestic violence** Osteogenesis imperfecta Substance abuse Consensual violent sexual behavior	XR—skeletal survey CT—maxillofacial Urine toxicology CBC

ABUSE (cont'd)

Presentation	Differential	Workup
■ 30 yo F presents with multiple facial and physical injuries. She was attacked and raped by 2 men.	**Rape**	Pelvic exam Urine hCG Wet mount, KOH prep, cervical cultures XR—skeletal survey CBC HIV antibody Viral hepatitis serologies

JOINT/LIMB PAIN

Key History

Location, quality, intensity, duration, pattern (small vs. large joints; number involved; swelling, redness, warmth), associated symptoms (constitutional, red eye, oral or genital ulceration, diarrhea, dysuria, rash, focal numbness/weakness), exacerbating and alleviating factors; trauma (including vigorous exercise); medications; DVT risk factors; alcohol and drug use; family history of rheumatic disease.

Key Physical Exam

Vital signs; HEENT and musculoskeletal exams; relevant neurovascular exam.

Presentation	Differential	Workup
■ 30 yo F presents with wrist pain and a black eye after tripping, falling, and hitting her head on the edge of a table. She looks anxious and gives an inconsistent story.	**Domestic violence** Factitious disorder Substance abuse	XR—wrist CT—head Urine toxicology
■ 30 yo F secretary presents with wrist pain and a sensation of numbness and burning in her palm and the first, second, and third fingers of her right hand. The pain worsens at night and is relieved by loose shaking of the hand. There is sensory loss in the same fingers. Exam reveals a positive Tinel sign.	**Carpal tunnel syndrome** Median nerve compression in forearm or arm Radiculopathy of nerve roots C6 and C7 in cervical spine	Nerve conduction study EMG

Presentation	Differential	Workup
■ 28 yo F presents with pain in the interphalangeal joints of her hands accompanied by hair loss and a butterfly rash on her face.	**Systemic lupus erythematosus (SLE)** Rheumatoid arthritis Psoriatic arthritis Parvovirus B19 infection	ANA, anti-dsDNA, ESR, C3, C4, rheumatoid factor (RF), CBC XR—hands UA
■ 28 yo F presents with pain in the metacarpophalangeal joints of both hands. Her left knee is also painful and red. She has morning joint stiffness that lasts for an hour. Her mother had rheumatoid arthritis.	**Rheumatoid arthritis** SLE Disseminated gonorrhea Arthritis associated with inflammatory bowel disease Osteoarthritis	ANA, anti-dsDNA, CCP, ESR, RF, CBC XR—hands, left knee Cervical culture Arthrocentesis and synovial fluid analysis
■ 18 yo M presents with pain in the interphalangeal joints of both hands. He also has scaly, salmon-pink lesions on the extensor surface of his elbows and knees.	**Psoriatic arthritis** Rheumatoid arthritis SLE	RF, ANA, ESR CBC XR—hands XR—pelvis/sacroiliac joints Uric acid
■ 65 yo F presents with inability to use her left leg or bear weight on it after tripping on a carpet. Onset of menopause was 20 years ago, and she did not receive HRT or calcium supplements. Her left leg is externally rotated, shortened, and adducted, and there is tenderness in her left groin.	**Hip fracture** Hip dislocation Pelvic fracture	XR—hip/pelvis CT or MRI—hip CBC Serum calcium and vitamin D Bone density scan (DEXA)
■ 40 yo M presents with pain in the right groin after a motor vehicle accident. His right leg is flexed at the hip, adducted, and internally rotated.	**Hip dislocation—traumatic** Hip fracture	XR—hip CT or MRI—hip CBC PT/PTT Blood type and cross-match Urine toxicology and blood alcohol level

MINICASES

Presentation	Differential	Workup
■ 56 yo obese F presents with right knee stiffness and pain that increases with movement. Her symptoms have gradually worsened in the past 10 years. She has noticed swelling and deformity of the joint and is having difficulty walking.	**Osteoarthritis** Pseudogout Gout Meniscal or ligament damage	XR—knee CBC ESR Knee arthrocentesis and synovial fluid analysis (cell count, Gram stain, culture, crystals) MRI—knee
■ 45 yo M presents with fevers and right knee pain with swelling and redness.	**Septic arthritis** Gout Pseudogout Lyme arthritis Trauma Reiter arthritis	CBC Knee arthrocentesis and synovial fluid analysis (see above) Blood, urethral cultures XR—knee Uric acid Lyme antibody
■ 65 yo M presents with right foot pain. He has been training for a marathon.	**Stress fracture** Plantar fasciitis Foot sprain or strain	XR—foot Bone scan—foot MRI—foot
■ 65 yo M presents with pain in the heel of the right foot that is most notable with his first few steps and then improves as he continues walking. He has no known trauma.	**Plantar fasciitis** Heel fracture Splinter/foreign body	XR—heel Bone scan
■ 55 yo M presents with pain in the elbow when he plays tennis. His grip is impaired as a result of the pain. There is tenderness over the lateral epicondyle as well as pain on resisted wrist dorsiflexion (Cozen test) with the elbow in extension.	**Tennis elbow (lateral epicondylitis)** Stress fracture	XR—arm Bone scan MRI—elbow
■ 27 yo F presents with painful wrists and elbows, a swollen and hot knee joint that is painful on flexion, a rash on her limbs, and vaginal discharge. She is sexually active with multiple partners and occasionally uses condoms.	**Disseminated gonorrhea** Rheumatoid arthritis SLE Psoriatic arthritis Reiter arthritis	Knee arthrocentesis and synovial fluid analysis (cell count, Gram stain, culture) ANA, anti-dsDNA, ESR, RF, CBC Blood, cervical cultures XR—knee

MINICASES

121

Presentation	Differential	Workup
■ 60 yo F presents with pain in both legs that is induced by walking and is relieved by rest. She had cardiac bypass surgery 6 months ago and continues to smoke heavily.	**Peripheral vascular disease** (intermittent claudication) Leriche syndrome (aortoiliac occlusive disease) Lumbar spinal stenosis (pseudoclaudication) Osteoarthritis	Ankle-brachial index Doppler U/S—lower extremity Angiography MRI—lumbar spine
■ 45 yo F presents with right calf pain. Her calf is tender, warm, red, and swollen compared to the left side. She was started on OCPs 2 months ago for dysfunctional uterine bleeding.	**DVT** Baker cyst rupture Myositis Cellulitis Superficial venous thrombosis	Doppler U/S—right leg CBC CPK D-dimer PT, aPTT, fibrinogen XR—right leg
■ 60 yo F c/o left arm pain that started while she was swimming and was relieved by rest.	**Angina/MI** Tendonitis Osteoarthritis Shoulder dislocation	CPK-MB, troponin, ECG CBC ESR XR—shoulder CXR Echocardiography Stress test
■ 50 yo M presents with right shoulder pain after falling onto his outstretched hand while skiing. He noticed deformity of his shoulder and had to hold his right arm.	**Shoulder dislocation** Fracture of the humerus Rotator cuff injury	XR—shoulder XR—arm MRI—shoulder
■ 55 yo M presents with crampy bilateral thigh and calf pain, fatigue, and dark urine. He is on simvastatin and clofibrate for hyperlipidemia.	**Rhabdomyolysis due to simvastatin or clofibrate** Polymyositis Inclusion body myositis Thyroid disease	CBC, electrolytes CPK Aldolase UA Urine myoglobin TSH

LOW BACK PAIN

Key History

Location, quality, intensity, radiation, context (moving furniture, bending/twisting, trauma), timing (disturbs sleep), associated symptoms (especially constitutional, incontinence), exacerbating and alleviating factors; history of cancer, recurrent UTIs, diabetes, renal stones, IV drug use, smoking.

Key Physical Exam

Vital signs; neurologic exam (especially L4–S1 nerve roots); back palpation and range of motion (although rarely of diagnostic utility); hip exam (can refer pain to the back); consider rectal exam.

Presentation	Differential	Workup
■ 45 yo F presents with low back pain that radiates to the lateral aspect of her left foot. Straight leg raising is positive. The patient is unable to tiptoe.	**Disk herniation** Lumbar muscle strain Tumor in the vertebral canal	XR—L-spine MRI—L-spine
■ 45 yo F presents with low back pain that started after she cleaned her house. The pain does not radiate, and there is no sensory deficit or weakness in her legs. Paraspinal muscle tenderness and spasm are also noted.	**Lumbar muscle strain** Disk herniation Abdominal aortic aneurysm Vertebral compression fracture	XR—L-spine
■ 45 yo M presents with pain in the lower back and legs during prolonged standing and walking. The pain is relieved by sitting and leaning forward (eg, pushing a grocery cart).	**Lumbar spinal stenosis** Lumbar muscle strain Tumor in the vertebral canal Peripheral vascular disease	XR—L-spine MRI—L-spine (preferred) CT—L-spine Ankle-brachial index
■ 17 yo M presents with low back pain that radiates to the left leg and began after he fell on his knee during gym class. He also describes areas of loss of sensation in his left foot. The pain and sensory loss do not match any known distribution. He insists on requesting a week off from school because of his injury.	**Malingering** Lumbar muscle strain Disk herniation Knee or leg fracture Ankylosing spondylitis	XR—L-spine/knee MRI—L-spine

CHILD WITH FEVER

(No child will be present; only the mother will be present to tell the story.)

Key History

Severity, duration, associated localizing symptoms, appetite, rash, sick contacts, day care, immunizations, past history.

Key Physical Exam

Vital signs; HEENT; neck, heart, lung, abdominal, and skin exams.

MINICASES

Presentation	Differential	Workup
■ 20-day-old M presents with fever, decreased breast-feeding, and lethargy. He was born at 36 weeks as a result of premature rupture of membranes.	**Neonatal sepsis** Meningitis Pneumonia UTI	Physical exam CBC, electrolytes UA Urine culture Blood culture CXR LP—CSF analysis
■ 3 yo M presents with a 2-day history of fever and pulling on his right ear. He is otherwise healthy, and his immunizations are up to date. His older sister recently had a cold. The child attends a day care center.	**Acute otitis media** URI Meningitis UTI	Physical exam (including pneumatic otoscopy) CBC UA
■ 12-month-old M presents with fever for the past 2 days accompanied by a maculopapular rash on his face and body. He has not yet received the MMR vaccine.	**Measles (or other viral exanthem)** Rubella Roseola Fifth disease Varicella Scarlet fever Meningitis	Physical exam CBC Viral antibodies/titers Throat swab for culture LP
■ 4 yo M presents with diarrhea, vomiting, lethargy, weakness, and fever. The child attends a day care center where several children have had similar symptoms.	**Gastroenteritis** (viral, bacterial, parasitic) Food poisoning UTI URI Volvulus Intussusception	Physical exam Stool exam and culture CBC Electrolytes UA, urine culture AXR

CHILD WITH GI SYMPTOMS

(No child will be present; only the mother will be present to tell the story.)

Key History

Onset, location, quality, intensity, duration, radiation, timing (relation to meals), associated symptoms (constitutional, GI, cardiac, pulmonary, renal, pelvic), exacerbating and alleviating factors; history of similar symptoms; history of abdominal surgeries; medications; sick contacts, day care, immunizations, changes in weight.

Key Physical Exam

Vital signs; heart and lung exams; abdominal exam, rectal exam; pelvic exam (women).

Presentation	Differential	Workup
■ 1-month-old F is brought in because she has been spitting up her milk for the last 10 days. The vomiting episodes have increased in frequency and forcefulness. Emesis is nonbloody and nonbilious. The episodes usually occur immediately after breast-feeding. She has stopped gaining weight.	**Pyloric stenosis** Partial duodenal atresia GERD Gastroenteritis Hepatitis UTI	Physical exam CBC, electrolytes U/S—abdomen Barium swallow pH probe AST/ALT/bilirubin/ alkaline phosphatase UA, urine culture Endoscopy
■ 3 yo M presents with constipation. The child has had 1 bowel movement per week since birth despite use of stool softeners. At birth, he did not pass meconium for 48 hours. He has poor weight gain. There is a family history of this problem.	**Hirschsprung disease** Low-fiber diet Anal stenosis Hypothyroidism Lead poisoning	Physical exam Rectal exam Stool exam and culture TSH, FT_4 CBC, electrolytes Barium enema Anal biopsy
■ 8-month-old F presents with sudden-onset colicky abdominal pain with vomiting. The episodes are 20 minutes apart and the child is completely well between episodes. She had loose stools several hours before the pain but her stools are now bloody.	**Intussusception** Appendicitis Meckel diverticulum Volvulus Gastroenteritis Blunt abdominal trauma	Physical exam Rectal exam, stool for occult blood CBC, electrolytes Contrast enema U/S—abdomen CT—abdomen Blood culture
■ 7 yo M presents with abdominal pain that is generalized, crampy, worse in the morning, and seemingly less prominent during weekends and holidays. He has missed many school days because of the pain. Growth and development are normal. His parents recently divorced.	**Somatoform disorder** Malingering Irritable bowel syndrome Lactose intolerance Child abuse	Physical exam CBC, electrolytes U/S—abdomen CT—abdomen Amylase, lipase Stool exam and culture
■ 2-month-old M presents with persistent crying for 2 weeks. The episodes subside after passing flatus or eructation. There is no change in appetite, weight, or growth. There is no vomiting, constipation, or fever.	**Colic** Formula allergy GERD Lactose intolerance Strangulated hernia Testicular torsion Sepsis Aseptic meningitis Gastroenteritis	Physical exam Rectal exam Fecal occult blood test Lumbar puncture U/S—abdomen Blood culture

MINICASES

CHILD WITH RED EYE

(No child will be present; only the mother will be present to tell the story.)

Key History

Onset, location, duration, exacerbating and alleviating factors; eye discharge, medications; sick contacts, day care, immunizations, associated symptoms (constitutional, GI, cardiac, pulmonary, renal, pelvic), history of similar symptoms.

Key Physical Exam

Vital signs, HEENT exam.

Presentation	Differential	Workup
■ 3 yo F presents with a 3-day history of "pink eye." It began in the right eye but now involves both eyes. She has mucoid discharge, itching, and difficulty opening her eyes in the morning. Her mother had the flu last week. She has a history of asthma and atopic dermatitis.	**Bacterial conjunctivitis** Viral conjunctivitis Keratitis Seasonal allergies Uveitis	Physical exam Ophthalmoscopic eye exam CBC, electrolytes Discharge cultures Slit lamp exam

CHILD WITH SHORT STATURE

(No child will be present; only the mother will be present to tell the story.)

Key History

Prenatal and birth history, growth history, past medical history, medications, family history, any associated symptoms (constitutional, GI, cardiac, pulmonary, renal, pelvic).

Key Physical Exam

Vital signs, height, weight, HEENT exam; heart and lung exams; abdominal exam, neurologic exam.

Presentation	Differential	Workup
■ 14 yo M presents with short stature and lack of sexual development. His birth weight and length were normal but he is the shortest child in his class. His father and uncles had the same problem when they were young.	**Familial short stature** Growth hormone deficiency Hypothyroidism Chronic renal insufficiency Genetic causes	Physical exam CBC, electrolytes TSH, FT_4, GH XR—hand U/S—renal and cardiac Karyotype

BEHAVIORAL PROBLEMS IN CHILDHOOD

(No child will be present; only the mother will be present to tell the story.)

Key History

Onset, severity, duration, triggers; physical violence or use of weapons; substance use, developmental history, changes in environment, school performance.

Key Physical Exam

Vital signs; neurologic exam.

Presentation	Differential	Workup
9 yo M presents with a 2-year history of angry outbursts both in school and at home. His mother complains that he runs around "as if driven by a motor." His teacher reports that he cannot sit still in class, regularly interrupts his classmates, and has trouble making friends.	**Attention-deficit hyperactivity disorder (ADHD)** Oppositional defiant disorder Manic episode Conduct disorder	Physical exam Mental status exam
12 yo F presents with a 2-month history of fighting in school, truancy, and breaking curfew. Her parents recently divorced, and she just started school in a new district. Before her parents divorced, she was an average student with no behavioral problems.	**Adjustment disorder** Substance intoxication, abuse, or dependence Manic episode Oppositional defiant disorder Conduct disorder	Physical exam Mental status exam Urine toxicology
15 yo M presents with a 1-year history of failing grades, school absenteeism, and legal problems, including shoplifting. His parents report that he spends most of his time alone in his room, adding that when he does go out, it is with a new set of friends.	**Substance abuse** Conduct disorder Oppositional defiant disorder Adjustment disorder	Urine toxicology Mental status exam Physical exam
5 yo M presents with a 6-month history of temper tantrums that last 5–10 minutes and immediately follow a disappointment or a discipline. He has no trouble sleeping, has had no change in appetite, and does not display these behaviors when he is at day care.	**Age-appropriate behavior** ADHD Oppositional defiant disorder	Physical exam Mental status exam

Practice Cases

Case 1   48-year-old woman with abdominal pain / 132

Case 2   21-year-old woman with abdominal pain / 139

Case 3   74-year-old man with right arm pain / 147

Case 4   21-year-old man with sore throat / 154

Case 5   55-year-old man with bloody stool / 161

Case 6   46-year-old man with chest pain / 168

Case 7   7-month-old boy with fever / 175

Case 8   18-month-old girl with fever / 181

Case 9   26-year-old man with cough / 187

Case 10   54-year-old woman with cough / 194

Case 11   52-year-old woman with jaundice / 202

Case 12   65-year-old woman with forgetfulness and confusion / 209

Case 13   56-year-old man presents for diabetes follow-up / 216

Case 14   53-year-old man with dizziness / 223

Case 15   46-year-old man with fatigue / 230

Case 16   32-year-old woman with fatigue / 237

Case 17   61-year-old man with fatigue / 244

Case 18   35-year-old woman with headaches / 251

Case 19   57-year-old man with bloody urine / 258

Case 20   54-year-old man presents for hypertension follow-up / 265

Case 21   33-year-old woman with knee pain / 272

Case 22   66-year-old man with tremor / 280

Case 23   49-year-old man with loss of consciousness / 288

Case 24   30-year-old woman with weight gain / 295

Case 25   36-year-old woman with menstrual problems / 302

Case 26   28-year-old woman with pain during sex / 309

Case 27   51-year-old man with back pain / 316

Case 28   6-month-old girl with diarrhea / 322

Case 29   75-year-old man with hearing loss / 328

Case 30   8-year-old boy with bed-wetting / 335

Case 31   25-year-old man presents following motor vehicle accident / 341

Case 32   25-year-old woman presents following sexual assault / 349

Case 33   28-year-old woman presents with positive pregnancy test / 356

Case 34   20-year-old woman with sleeping problems / 363

Case 35   27-year-old man with visual hallucinations / 370

Case 36   10-year-old girl with new-onset diabetes / 377

Case 37   35-year-old woman with calf pain / 384

Case 38   31-year-old man with heel pain / 391

Case 39   5-day-old boy with jaundice / 399

Case 40   2-year-old girl with noisy breathing / 405

Case 41   32-year-old man presents for preemployment physical / 411

Case 42   62-year-old man with hoarseness / 418

Case 43   67-year-old woman with neck pain / 425

Case 44   11-month-old girl with seizures / 431

This chapter consists of 44 commonly encountered cases that approximate those on the actual USMLE Step 2 CS exam. Each case consists of four parts:

1. **Doorway information sheet:** Designed to simulate the actual information that you will find on the doorway of each examination room, this sheet contains the opening scenario, vital signs, and the tasks you are required to perform during the exam. You should read this sheet just before starting the 15-minute encounter.

2. **Checklist/SP sheet:** This sheet outlines information that standardized patients (SPs) will use to guide them during the interview and lists questions SPs might ask you, along with potential responses to these questions. It also includes a sample checklist that SPs will use to evaluate your performance in the areas of entrance, history taking, diagnosis, closure, and follow-up recommendations, as well as your ability to conduct a patient-centered interview overall.

3. **Blank patient note:** A blank form on which you can write your own note after the patient encounter.

4. **Sample patient note and discussion:** This sheet includes a sample patient note for you to review after you have written your own, as well as a discussion of reasonable differential diagnoses and diagnostic tests to consider in each case.

Because the cases in this section are designed to simulate the actual exam, you will derive the most benefit by practicing them with a friend who can act as an SP. To maximize the effectiveness of these practice cases, you should also time each encounter in accordance with the guidelines provided in Sections 1 and 2 and compare each of your patient notes with those provided in the text.

For a quicker self-review, you can try to formulate a patient note after reviewing the doorway sheet and the SP checklist, and then compare your note with the sample note provided.

Opening Scenario

Sharon Smith, a 48-year-old female, comes to the clinic complaining of abdominal pain.

Vital Signs

BP: 135/70 mm Hg

Temp: 98.5°F (36.9°C)

RR: 16/minute

HR: 76/minute, regular

Examinee Tasks

1. Take a focused history.

2. Perform a focused physical exam (do not perform rectal, genitourinary, or female breast exam).

3. Explain your clinical impression and workup plan to the patient.

4. Write the patient note after leaving the room.

Checklist/SP Sheet

Patient Description

Patient is a 48 yo F, married with four children.

Notes for the SP

- Sit up on the bed.
- Show pain on palpation of the right upper abdomen that is exacerbated during inspiration.
- Exhibit epigastric tenderness on palpation.
- If ultrasound is mentioned by the examinee, ask, "What is the meaning of this word?"

Challenging Questions to Ask

"My father had pancreatic cancer. Could I have it, too?"

Sample Examinee Response

"It's highly unlikely, as your symptoms are very unusual for pancreatic cancer. Regardless, some routine blood and x-ray tests should help us exclude that as a possibility."

Examinee Checklist

Building the Doctor-Patient Relationship

Entrance

☐ Examinee knocked on the door before entering.

☐ Examinee introduced self by name.

☐ Examinee identified his/her role or position.

☐ Examinee correctly used patient's name.

☐ Examinee made eye contact with the SP.

Reflective Listening

☐ Examinee asked an open-ended question and actively listened to the response.

☐ Examinee asked the SP to list his/her concerns and listened to the response without interrupting.

☐ Examinee summarized the SP's concerns, often using the SP's own words.

Information Gathering

☐ Examinee elicited data efficiently and accurately.

☑ Question	Patient Response
☐ Chief complaint	Abdominal pain.
☐ Onset	Two weeks ago.
☐ Constant/intermittent	Well, I don't have the pain all the time. It comes and goes.
☐ Frequency	At least once every day.
☐ Progression	It is getting worse.
☐ Severity on a scale	When I have the pain, it is 7/10, and then it may go down to 0.
☐ Location	It is here (points to the epigastrium).
☐ Radiation	No.
☐ Quality	Burning.
☐ Alleviating factors	Food, antacids, and milk.
☐ Exacerbating factors	Heavy meals and hunger.
☐ Types of food that exacerbate pain	Heavy, fatty meals, like pizza.
☐ Relationship of food to pain	Well, usually the pain will decrease or stop completely when I eat, but it comes back after 2–3 hours.
☐ Previous episodes of similar pain	No.
☐ Nausea/vomiting	Sometimes I feel nauseated when I am in pain. Yesterday I vomited for the first time.
☐ Description of vomitus	It was a sour, yellowish fluid.
☐ Blood in vomitus	No.
☐ Diarrhea/constipation	No.
☐ Weight changes	No.
☐ Appetite changes	No.
☐ Change in stool color	No.
☐ Current medications	Maalox, ibuprofen (two pills 2–3 times a day if asked).
☐ Past medical history	I had a urinary tract infection 1 year ago, treated with amoxicillin, and arthritis in both knees treated with ibuprofen.

☑ Question	Patient Response
☐ Past surgical history	I had two C-sections.
☐ Family history	My father died at 55 of pancreatic cancer. My mother is alive and healthy.
☐ Occupation	Housewife.
☐ Alcohol use	No.
☐ Illicit drug use	No.
☐ Tobacco	No.
☐ Sexual activity	With my husband (laughs).
☐ Drug allergies	No.

Connecting with the Patient

☐ Examinee recognized the SP's emotions and responded with PEARLS.

Physical Examination

☐ Examinee washed his/her hands.

☐ Examinee asked permission to start the exam.

☐ Examinee used respectful draping.

☐ Examinee did not repeat painful maneuvers.

☑ Exam Component	Maneuver
☐ CV exam	Auscultation
☐ Pulmonary exam	Auscultation
☐ Abdominal exam	Inspection, auscultation, palpation (including Murphy sign), percussion

Closure

☐ Examinee discussed initial diagnostic impressions.

☐ Examinee discussed initial management plans:

    ☐ Follow-up tests: Examinee mentioned the need for a rectal exam.

☐ Examinee asked if the SP had any other questions or concerns.

Sample Closure

Mrs. Smith, there are a number of disorders that can cause pain similar to what you have described. Pain of this type is most commonly due to an ulcer, an abdominal infection, or a gallstone. We will have to run some tests to confirm the diagnosis and to rule out more serious illness. These tests will include a rectal exam; an ultrasound of your abdomen; blood tests; and possibly an upper endoscopy, which examines your stomach by means of an optical instrument passed through your mouth. Once we have made the diagnosis, we will be able to treat your condition and help alleviate your pain. Do you have any questions for me?

Patient Note

History

_____

_____

_____

_____

_____

_____

_____

_____

Physical Examination

_____

_____

_____

_____

_____

_____

_____

_____

_____

Differential Diagnosis

1. _____

2. _____

3. _____

4. _____

5. _____

Diagnostic Workup

1. _____

2. _____

3. _____

4. _____

5. _____

History

HPI: *48 yo F c/o intermittent, burning, nonradiating epigastric pain that started for the first time 2 weeks ago. The pain occurs at least once a day, usually 2–3 hours after meals. It is exacerbated by hunger and heavy, fatty food and is alleviated by milk, antacids, and other food. It reaches 7/10 in severity and then diminishes to 0/10. It is sometimes accompanied by nausea. The patient vomited once yesterday: an acidic, yellowish, nonbloody fluid. No diarrhea or constipation. No changes in weight or appetite. No changes in the color of the stool.*

ROS: *Negative except as above.*

Allergies: *NKDA.*

Medications: *Maalox, ibuprofen.*

PMH: *Arthritis in the knees, treated with ibuprofen. UTI last year, treated with amoxicillin.*

PSH: *2 C-sections.*

SH: *No smoking, no EtOH, no illicit drugs. Sexually active with husband only.*

FH: *Father died of pancreatic cancer at age 55.*

Physical Examination

Patient is in no acute distress.

VS: *WNL.*

Chest: *No tenderness, clear breath sounds bilaterally.*

Heart: *RRR; normal S1/S2; no murmurs, rubs, or gallops.*

Abdomen: *Soft, nondistended, C-section scar, epigastric tenderness without rebound, ⊕ Murphy sign, ⊕ BS, no hepatosplenomegaly.*

Differential Diagnosis

1. *Peptic ulcer disease*
2. *Cholecystitis*
3. *Gastritis*
4. *Functional or nonulcer dyspepsia*
5. *Perforated ulcer*
6. *Gastric cancer*

Diagnostic Workup

1. *Rectal exam, stool for occult blood*
2. *AST/ALT/bilirubin/alkaline phosphatase, lipase*
3. *U/S—abdomen*
4. *Upper endoscopy*
5. *HIDA scan*
6. *H. pylori antibody testing*

CASE DISCUSSION

Differential Diagnosis

Although the causes of abdominal pain are many, this presentation should prompt you to ponder the common etiologies.

- **Peptic ulcer disease:** The history of NSAID use and burning epigastric pain alleviated by antacids and food are consistent with this diagnosis (although the clinical history cannot accurately distinguish duodenal from gastric ulcers).

- **Cholecystitis:** Several features suggest this diagnosis, but the pain in acute cholecystitis is usually unremitting and is not alleviated by milk or antacids. This patient's intermittent pain may be due to "biliary colic," representing transient obstruction of the cystic duct, usually due to gallstones.

- **Gastritis:** This can easily explain epigastric pain, nausea, and vomiting in patients taking NSAIDs.

- **Functional or nonulcer dyspepsia:** This is the most common cause of chronic dyspepsia. After thorough evaluation, no obvious organic etiology is discovered.

- **Perforated ulcer:** These patients appear toxic and have severe diffuse abdominal pain with rebound tenderness and involuntary guarding.

- **Gastric cancer:** Although this patient does not have early satiety, anorexia, weight loss, or a left supraclavicular mass (Virchow node), it should be noted that signs and symptoms are minimal until late in the course of this rare disease.

- **Other etiologies:** Less likely possibilities include pancreatitis, atypical GERD, choledocholithiasis, mesenteric ischemia, and extra-abdominal causes.

Diagnostic Workup

- **Rectal exam, stool for occult blood:** May document occult blood loss due to peptic ulcer, gastritis, cancer, or other causes.

- **AST/ALT/bilirubin/alkaline phosphatase, lipase:** To look for evidence of hepatocellular injury, biliary obstruction, or pancreatitis.

- **U/S—abdomen:** A quick, inexpensive imaging technique with which to examine a patient with suspected acute cholecystitis (it may show stones, pericholecystic fluid, a thickened gallbladder wall, and a sonographic Murphy sign).

- **Upper endoscopy:** Peptic ulcer, gastritis, and gastric cancer have lesions that can be visualized (biopsy is required for gastric cancer diagnosis and sometimes for *H. pylori* diagnosis).

- **HIDA (hepatobiliary) scan:** Can document obstruction of the cystic duct in acute cholecystitis; a positive scan shows absence of filling of the gallbladder. HIDA is usually ordered after U/S (ie, when the easier but less sensitive U/S does not establish the diagnosis of acute cholecystitis).

- **Noninvasive *H. pylori* testing:** Serologic tests for antibodies to *H. pylori* are adequate for diagnosis but not to document cure, as antibody levels often remain detectable after treatment (indicating exposure, not necessarily active infection). The urease breath test is a useful test with which to confirm *H. pylori* eradication in peptic ulcer disease.

CASE 2
DOORWAY INFORMATION

Opening Scenario

Jessica Anderson, a 21-year-old female, comes to the ED complaining of abdominal pain.

Vital Signs

BP: 120/80 mm Hg

Temp: 100.5°F (38.1°C)

RR: 20/minute

HR: 88/minute, regular

Examinee Tasks

1. Take a focused history.

2. Perform a focused physical exam (do not perform rectal, genitourinary, or female breast exam).

3. Explain your clinical impression and workup plan to the patient.

4. Write the patient note after leaving the room.

Checklist/SP Sheet

Patient Description

Patient is a 21 yo F, single with one child.

Notes for the SP

- Exhibit right lower abdominal tenderness on palpation.
- Show rebound tenderness (pain when the examinee removes his palpating hand).
- Demonstrate guarding (contraction of the abdominal muscles when palpating the RLQ).
- Experience pain in the RLQ when the examinee presses on the LLQ (Rovsing sign).
- Manifest pain when the examinee extends your right hip (psoas sign).

Challenging Questions to Ask

- "My child is in the house alone. I must leave now."
- "I can't afford to stay in the hospital. Please give me a prescription for antibiotics so that I can leave."

Sample Examinee Response

"First we have to make sure that your illness isn't life threatening. Our social worker would be happy to work with you to ensure that your child is taken care of, as well as to address any financial concerns you may have."

Examinee Checklist

Building the Doctor-Patient Relationship

Entrance

☐ Examinee knocked on the door before entering.

☐ Examinee introduced self by name.

☐ Examinee identified his/her role or position.

☐ Examinee correctly used patient's name.

☐ Examinee made eye contact with the SP.

Reflective Listening

☐ Examinee asked an open-ended question and actively listened to the response.

☐ Examinee asked the SP to list his/her concerns and listened to the response without interrupting.

☐ Examinee summarized the SP's concerns, often using the SP's own words.

Information Gathering

☐ Examinee elicited data efficiently and accurately.

☑ Question	Patient Response
☐ Chief complaint	Abdominal pain.
☐ Onset	This morning.
☐ Frequency	Strong, steady pain.
☐ Progression	It is getting worse.
☐ Severity on a scale	7/10.
☐ Location	It is here (points to the right lower abdomen).
☐ Radiation	No.
☐ Quality	Cramping.
☐ Alleviating factors	None.
☐ Exacerbating factors	Movement.
☐ Pain with ride to hospital	Yes.
☐ Precipitating events	None.
☐ Fever/chills	I've been a little hot since this morning, but no chills.
☐ Nausea/vomiting	I feel nauseated and vomited once two hours ago.
☐ Description of vomitus	It was a sour, yellowish fluid.
☐ Blood in vomitus	No.
☐ Diarrhea/constipation	Loose bowel movements this morning.
☐ Description of stool	Brown.

☑ Question	Patient Response
☐ Blood in stool	No.
☐ Urinary frequency/burning	No.
☐ Last menstrual period	Five weeks ago.
☐ Vaginal spotting	Yes, today is the first day of my menstrual period.
☐ Color of the spotting	Brownish.
☐ Vaginal discharge	No.
☐ Frequency of menstrual periods	Every four weeks; lasts for seven days.
☐ Starting menses	Age 13.
☐ Pads/tampons changed this day	Only one; usually 2–3 a day.
☐ Pregnancies	Three years ago.
☐ Problems during pregnancy/delivery	No, it was a normal delivery, and my child is healthy.
☐ Miscarriages/abortions	None.
☐ Current medications	Ibuprofen.
☐ Sexual activity	Yes.
☐ Contraceptives	Oral contraceptive pills. My boyfriend refuses to use condoms.
☐ Sexual partners	One partner; I met him two months ago.
☐ Over the past year	I had three sexual partners.
☐ History of STDs	Yes, I had some kind of infection a month ago, but I can't remember the name of it. The doctor gave me a shot and some pills for 1 week, and then it was over.
☐ Treatment of the partner	He refused the treatment.
☐ HIV test	No.
☐ Past medical history	None except for what I've mentioned.
☐ Past surgical history	None.
☐ Occupation	Waitress.
☐ Alcohol use	Two or three beers a week.
☐ Illicit drug use	No.
☐ Tobacco	One pack a day for the past six years.
☐ Drug allergies	No.

Connecting with the Patient

☐ Examinee recognized the SP's emotions and responded with PEARLS.

Physical Examination

☐ Examinee washed his/her hands.

☐ Examinee asked permission to start the exam.

☐ Examinee used respectful draping.

☐ Examinee did not repeat painful maneuvers.

☑ Exam Component	Maneuver
☐ CV exam	Auscultation
☐ Pulmonary exam	Auscultation
☐ Abdominal exam	Inspection, auscultation, palpation, percussion, psoas sign, obturator sign, Rovsing sign, CVA tenderness

Closure

☐ Examinee discussed initial diagnostic impressions.

☐ Examinee discussed initial management plans:

    ☐ Follow-up tests: Examinee mentioned the need for rectal and pelvic exams.

    ☐ Safe sex practices.

    ☐ Help with smoking cessation.

    ☐ Assistance of social workers to help the patient identify available financial resources.

☐ Examinee asked if the SP had any other questions or concerns.

Sample Closure

Ms. Anderson, your symptoms may be due to a problem with your reproductive organs, such as an infection in your fallopian tube or a cyst on your ovary. They might also result from a complicated pregnancy, which could be indicated if your pregnancy test comes back positive. Another possibility is an infection in your appendix, which could require surgery. To ensure an accurate diagnosis, we will need to run some tests, including a blood test, a urinalysis, a pregnancy test, and possibly a CT scan of your abdomen and pelvis. I will also need to perform rectal and pelvic exams. Since cigarette smoking is associated with a variety of diseases, I advise you to quit smoking; we have many ways to help you if you are interested. I also recommend that you use a condom every time you have intercourse to prevent STDs, including HIV, and to avoid pregnancy. Our social worker can meet you to discuss your social situation, and she can offer you a variety of resources. Do you have any questions for me?

Patient Note

History

_____
_____
_____
_____
_____
_____
_____
_____

Physical Examination

_____
_____
_____
_____
_____
_____
_____
_____
_____
_____

Differential Diagnosis

1. _____
2. _____
3. _____
4. _____
5. _____

Diagnostic Workup

1. _____
2. _____
3. _____
4. _____
5. _____

Patient Note

History

HPI: *21 yo G1P1 F c/o right lower abdominal pain that started this morning. The pain is 7/10, crampy, nonradiating, and constant. It is exacerbated by movement and accompanied by fever, nausea, vomiting, and loose stools. The patient noticed some brownish spotting this morning. No urinary symptoms; no abnormal vaginal discharge.*

OB/GYN: *LMP 5 weeks ago. Regular periods every 4 weeks lasting 7 days. Menarche at age 13. Uncomplicated NSVD at full term 3 years ago.*

Allergies: *NKDA.*

Medications: *Ibuprofen.*

PMH: *STD 1 month ago, possibly treated with ceftriaxone and doxycycline.*

PSH: *None.*

SH: *1 PPD for 6 years, 2–3 beers/week, no illicit drugs. Unprotected sex with multiple partners.*

Physical Examination

Patient is in pain.

VS: *WNL except for temperature of 100.5°F.*

Chest: *No tenderness, clear breath sounds bilaterally.*

Heart: *RRR; normal S1/S2; no murmurs, rubs, or gallops.*

Abdomen: *Soft, nondistended, hypoactive BS, no hepatosplenomegaly. Direct and rebound RLQ tenderness, RLQ guarding, ⊕ psoas sign, ⊕ Rovsing sign, ⊖ obturator sign, no CVA tenderness.*

Differential Diagnosis

1. *Pelvic inflammatory disease (PID)*
2. *Appendicitis*
3. *Ruptured ectopic pregnancy*
4. *Ruptured ovarian cyst*
5. *Adnexal torsion*
6. *Gastroenteritis*
7. *Abortion*
8. *Endometriosis*

Diagnostic Workup

1. *Rectal exam*
2. *Pelvic exam*
3. *Urine hCG*
4. *Cervical cultures*
5. *UA*
6. *CBC*
7. *U/S—abdomen/pelvis*
8. *CT—abdomen/pelvis*
9. *Laparoscopy*

CASE DISCUSSION

Differential Diagnosis

- **PID:** Suspicion is high for this diagnosis in a patient with multiple sexual partners and a history of STDs who presents with lower abdominal pain and fever. Other findings suggestive of PID include cervical motion tenderness, purulent cervical discharge, adnexal tenderness (usually bilateral), and fever > 101°F (38.3°C).

- **Appendicitis:** Acute right lower abdominal pain that is exacerbated by movement is compatible with this diagnosis. If peritoneal signs are present, patients will usually complain of pain with activity that jostles their abdomen (eg, the ride to the hospital). Patients may also present with low-grade fever, nausea, vomiting, direct and rebound RLQ tenderness, RLQ guarding, a positive psoas sign, and a positive Rovsing sign.

- **Ruptured ectopic pregnancy:** Even though this patient does not have previously documented PID (or previous tubal pregnancy), the crampy lower abdominal pain, nausea and vomiting, and vaginal spotting occurring after a 5-week period of amenorrhea suggest this diagnosis. However, positive psoas and Rovsing signs are not typical of ectopic pregnancy.

- **Ruptured ovarian cyst:** The sudden-onset unilateral lower abdominal pain, rebound tenderness, and guarding are consistent with this diagnosis. Rupture may occur at any time during the menstrual cycle, and symptoms may resemble a ruptured ectopic pregnancy as described above.

- **Adnexal torsion:** This presentation may be due to adnexal torsion, an uncommon complication that is most often associated with ovarian enlargement due to a benign mass.

- **Gastroenteritis:** Viral gastroenteritis presents with crampy abdominal pain, nausea and vomiting, low-grade fever, and diarrhea. It can be difficult to distinguish from appendicitis and gynecologic etiologies but is less likely in this case given the presence of rebound tenderness.

- **Abortion:** The fact that the patient's last menstrual period was only 5 weeks ago makes this less likely, but the crampy abdominal pain and vaginal spotting may signal an abortion. Furthermore, the presence of fever suggests possible septic abortion.

- **Endometriosis:** This is an unlikely diagnosis, in part because the patient has no history of chronic pelvic pain, dysmenorrhea, dyspareunia, or infertility, which are often associated. In a patient with established endometriosis, this presentation with acute severe pain, including rebound tenderness, could be due to rupture of an endometrioma ("chocolate cyst").

Diagnostic Workup

- **Rectal exam:** Elicits pain on the right side of the abdomen in acute appendicitis (not very specific).

- **Pelvic exam:** Look for cervical motion tenderness and discharge, uterine size, and adnexal masses or tenderness.

- **Urine hCG:** Positive in pregnancy. Urine and serum tests are equally sensitive, but obtaining quantitative hCG levels (available only via serum test) may help diagnose and treat ectopic pregnancy.

- **Cervical cultures:** *Neisseria gonorrhoeae* and *Chlamydia trachomatis*, the main causes of PID, are detected via DNA probes.

- **UA:** To rule out UTI.

- **CBC:** Findings are nonspecific, but leukocytosis may be seen in infection or appendicitis.

- **U/S—abdomen/pelvis:** Can help diagnose appendiceal or ovarian pathology. Transvaginal U/S can identify an intrauterine gestational sac when the time elapsed since the last menstrual period is 35 days (this corresponds to a β-hCG of approximately 1500); fluid in the cul-de-sac is nonspecific and may suggest ectopic pregnancy or a ruptured ovarian cyst.

- **CT—abdomen/pelvis:** Can detect the presence of appendiceal inflammation, abscess in appendicitis, or signs of other GI or gynecologic pathology.

- **Laparoscopy:** Can diagnose ectopic pregnancy (gold standard), ruptured ovarian cyst, ovarian torsion, PID ± tubo-ovarian abscess, appendicitis, etc.

Opening Scenario

Richard Green, a 74-year-old male, comes to the ED complaining of pain in his right arm.

Vital Signs

BP: 135/85 mm Hg

Temp: 98.0°F (36.7°C)

RR: 12/minute

HR: 76/minute, regular

Examinee Tasks

1. Take a focused history.

2. Perform a focused physical exam (do not perform rectal, genitourinary, or female breast exam).

3. Explain your clinical impression and workup plan to the patient.

4. Write the patient note after leaving the room.

Checklist/SP Sheet

Patient Description

Patient is a 74 yo M.

Notes for the SP

- Sit up on the bed.
- Hold your right arm close to your body with your left hand and keep it internally rotated.
- Show pain when the examinee tries to move your right shoulder in any direction.
- Do not allow the examinee to bring your shoulder to its full range of motion in flexion, extension, abduction, or external rotation.

Challenging Questions to Ask

"Doctor, do you think I will be able to move my arm again like before?"

Sample Examinee Response

"I hope so, but first we need to find out exactly what is causing your problem."

Examinee Checklist

Building the Doctor-Patient Relationship

Entrance

☐ Examinee knocked on the door before entering.

☐ Examinee introduced self by name.

☐ Examinee identified his/her role or position.

☐ Examinee correctly used patient's name.

☐ Examinee made eye contact with the SP.

Reflective Listening

☐ Examinee asked an open-ended question and actively listened to the response.

☐ Examinee asked the SP to list his/her concerns and listened to the response without interrupting.

☐ Examinee summarized the SP's concerns, often using the SP's own words.

Information Gathering

☐ Examinee elicited data efficiently and accurately.

☑ Question	Patient Response
☐ Chief complaint	Pain in the right arm.
☐ Onset	Three days ago.
☐ Precipitating events	I was playing with my grandchildren in the garden when I tripped and fell.
☐ Description of the fall	I tripped over a toy on the ground and fell on my hand. My arm was outstretched.
☐ Loss of consciousness	No.
☐ Location	The upper and middle parts of the arm.
☐ Weakness/paralysis	None.
☐ Numbness/loss of sensation	None.
☐ Progression of pain	I didn't feel any pain at the time, and then the pain started gradually. It is stable now, but it is still there.
☐ Pain anywhere else	No.
☐ Seen by a doctor since then	No.
☐ Any treatments	I used a sling and took some Tylenol, but the pain didn't get better.
☐ Alleviating factors	Not moving my arm and Tylenol.
☐ Exacerbating factors	Moving my arm.
☐ Reason for not seeking medical attention	Well, it wasn't that bad, and I thought it would get better on its own (looks anxious). Also, my son didn't have time to bring me to the hospital; he was busy.
☐ Living conditions	I live with my son. He is married and has three children. Life has been hard on him lately. He lost his job and is looking for a new one.
☐ Social history	I am a widower; my wife died three years ago, and since then I've lived with my son.
☐ Bad treatment in his son's house	No (looks anxious). They are all nice.
☐ Do you feel safe at home?	Yes (looks anxious).

☑ Question	Patient Response
☐ Current medications	Tylenol, albuterol inhaler.
☐ Allergies	Yes, I am allergic to aspirin.
☐ Past medical history	Asthma.
☐ Past surgical history	They removed my prostate two years ago. It was very difficult for me to urinate, but that has gotten much better. They said there was no evidence of cancer.
☐ Occupation	Retired schoolteacher.
☐ Alcohol use	No.
☐ Tobacco	No.
☐ Exercise	Every day I walk for 20 minutes to the grocery store and back.

Connecting with the Patient

☐ Examinee recognized the SP's emotions and responded with PEARLS.

Physical Examination

☐ Examinee washed his/her hands.

☐ Examinee asked permission to start the exam.

☐ Examinee used respectful draping.

☐ Examinee did not repeat painful maneuvers.

☑ Exam Component	Maneuver
☐ Head and neck exam	Checked for bruises, neck movements
☐ CV exam	Auscultation
☐ Pulmonary exam	Auscultation
☐ Exam of the arms	Compared both arms in terms of strength, range of motion (shoulder, elbow, wrist), sensation, DTRs, pulses

Closure

☐ Examinee discussed initial diagnostic impressions.

☐ Examinee discussed initial management plans:

    ☐ Follow-up tests.

    ☐ Alternative living options such as assisted living.

    ☐ Social work assistance.

☐ Examinee offered a statement of support: "Your safety is my primary concern, and I am here for help and support when you need it."

☐ Examinee asked if the SP had any other questions or concerns.

Sample Closure

Mr. Green, you may have a fractured bone, a simple sprain, or a dislocation of the shoulder joint. We will need to obtain an x-ray of your shoulder to make a diagnosis, and more precise imaging studies may be necessary as well. Your safety is my primary concern, and I am here to offer you help and support whenever you need it. Sometimes living with a family can be stressful for the whole household. Have you ever considered moving to an assisted-living community or to an apartment complex for seniors? If you are interested, I can arrange a meeting with our social worker, who can assess your social situation and help you find the resources you need. Do you have any questions for me?

Patient Note

History

_____
_____
_____
_____
_____
_____
_____
_____
_____

Physical Examination

_____
_____
_____
_____
_____
_____
_____
_____
_____
_____
_____

Differential Diagnosis

1. _____

2. _____

3. _____

4. _____

5. _____

Diagnostic Workup

1. _____

2. _____

3. _____

4. _____

5. _____

History

HPI: 74 yo M c/o right arm pain for the past 3 days. The pain started after he fell on his outstretched right hand and persisted although he used Tylenol and a sling at home. No loss of consciousness before or after the fall. No paralysis or loss of sensation. The pain is in the upper and middle part of the arm, increases with any movement of the arm, and is alleviated by rest. When asked why he delayed in seeking medical assistance, the patient looked anxious and stated that his son didn't have time to take him to the hospital.

ROS: Negative except as above.
Allergies: Aspirin.
Medications: Tylenol, albuterol inhaler.
PMH: Asthma, probable BPH s/p prostate surgery.
SH: No smoking, no EtOH. Widower for the past 3 years; lives with his son, who recently lost his job. Walks 20 minutes every morning.

Physical Examination

Patient is in no acute distress.
VS: WNL.
HEENT: Normocephalic, atraumatic, no bruises.
Neck: Supple, full range of motion in all directions, no bruises.
Chest: Clear breath sounds bilaterally.
Heart: RRR; normal S1/S2; no murmurs, rubs, or gallops.
Extremities: Nonlocalized tenderness over middle and upper right arm and right shoulder; pain and restricted range of motion on flexion, extension, abduction, and external rotation of right shoulder. Right elbow and wrist are normal. Pulses normal and symmetric in brachial and radial arteries. Unable to assess muscle strength due to pain. DTRs intact and symmetric. Sensation intact to pinprick and soft touch.

Differential Diagnosis

1. Humeral fracture
2. Osteoporosis
3. Shoulder dislocation
4. Elder abuse
5. Rotator cuff tear

Diagnostic Workup

1. XR—right shoulder and arm
2. MRI—shoulder
3. Bone density scan (DEXA)

CASE DISCUSSION

Differential Diagnosis

- **Humeral fracture:** Most commonly occurs in elderly persons, usually after a fall. The axillary nerve can be injured in a proximal humerus fracture, causing sensory loss along the lateral aspect of the deltoid region. The radial nerve can be injured in a fracture of the midshaft/distal third of the humerus, causing wrist drop.

- **Osteoporosis:** Suspect underlying osteoporosis in elderly patients (especially women) presenting with fractures following minimal trauma. The most common sites of osteoporotic fractures are the thoracic and lumbar vertebral bodies, the neck of the femur, and the distal radius.

- **Shoulder dislocation:** The glenohumeral joint is the most commonly dislocated joint in the human body. It most often dislocates anteriorly and usually results from a fall on an outstretched hand with forceful abduction, extension, and external rotation of the shoulder. On exam the arm is held in the neutral position, and movement is avoided owing to pain.

- **Elder abuse:** The history contains red flags (bruises, anxious behavior) that may indicate elder abuse. The American Medical Association has defined elder abuse as "an act or omission which results in harm or threatened harm to the health or welfare of an elderly person." The diagnosis of elder abuse is not readily made because often both the abuser and the victim deny abuse. Thus, diagnosis is inferential in many cases, and supporting evidence must be sought.

- **Rotator cuff tear:** Patients usually present with nonspecific pain localized to the shoulder, but pain is often referred down the proximal lateral arm owing to shared innervation. There may be an inability to abduct or flex the shoulder. Patients may also demonstrate significant weakness in internal or external rotation strength.

Diagnostic Workup

- **XR—right shoulder and arm:** AP and lateral views that include the joints above and below the injury can show fracture or dislocation. An axillary view is useful to help diagnose proximal humeral fracture or dislocation.

- **MRI—shoulder:** Required to diagnose rotator cuff tears, labral disease, and other disorders.

- **Bone density scan (DEXA):** To diagnose and quantify osteoporosis.

Opening Scenario

Brian Davis, a 21-year-old male, comes to the office complaining of a sore throat.

Vital Signs

BP: 120/80 mm Hg

Temp: 99.5°F (37.5°C)

RR: 15/minute

HR: 75/minute, regular

Examinee Tasks

1. Take a focused history.

2. Perform a focused physical exam (do not perform rectal, genitourinary, or female breast exam).

3. Explain your clinical impression and workup plan to the patient.

4. Write the patient note after leaving the room.

Checklist/SP Sheet

Patient Description

Patient is a 21 yo M.

Notes for the SP

- Be rude and defensive.
- Make most of your answers a curt "yes" or "no."
- Pretend that you have LUQ tenderness on abdominal palpation.

Challenging Questions to Ask

"Do you think I have AIDS?"

Sample Examinee Response

"That's a difficult question. Do you believe you have been exposed to HIV?"

Examinee Checklist

Building the Doctor-Patient Relationship

Entrance

☐ Examinee knocked on the door before entering.

☐ Examinee introduced self by name.

☐ Examinee identified his/her role or position.

☐ Examinee correctly used patient's name.

☐ Examinee made eye contact with the SP.

Reflective Listening

☐ Examinee asked an open-ended question and actively listened to the response.

☐ Examinee asked the SP to list his/her concerns and listened to the response without interrupting.

☐ Examinee summarized the SP's concerns, often using the SP's own words.

Information Gathering

☐ Examinee elicited data efficiently and accurately.

☑ Question	Patient Response
☐ Chief complaint	Sore throat.
☐ Onset	Two weeks ago.
☐ Runny nose	No.
☐ Fever/chills	Mild fever over the past two weeks, but I didn't take my temperature. No chills.
☐ Night sweats	No.
☐ Cough	No.
☐ Swollen glands and lymph nodes	Yes, in my neck (if asked); a little painful (if asked).
☐ Jaundice	No.
☐ Chest pain	No.
☐ Shortness of breath	No.
☐ Abdominal pain	I've had some discomfort here (points to LUQ) constantly since yesterday.
☐ Radiation	No.
☐ Severity on a scale	4/10.
☐ Relationship of food to pain	No.
☐ Alleviating/exacerbating factors	None.
☐ Nausea/vomiting	No.
☐ Change in bowel habits	No.
☐ Change in urinary habits	No.
☐ Headache	No.
☐ Fatigue	I have been feeling tired for the past two weeks.
☐ Ill contacts	My ex-girlfriend had the same thing two months ago. I don't know what happened to her because we broke up around that time.
☐ Weight changes	Yes, I feel that I am losing weight, but I don't know how much.
☐ Appetite changes	I don't feel like eating anything at all.
☐ Current medications	Tylenol.
☐ Past medical history	I had gonorrhea four months ago. I took some antibiotics.

☑ Question	Patient Response
☐ Past surgical history	None.
☐ Family history	My father and mother are alive and in good health.
☐ Occupation	Last year in college.
☐ Alcohol use	Yes, on the weekends.
☐ Illicit drug use	No.
☐ Tobacco	Yes, I smoke one pack a day. I started when I was 15 years old.
☐ Sexual activity	I have a new girlfriend.
☐ Use of condoms	Yes.
☐ Active with men, women, or both	Men and women.
☐ Number of sexual partners during the past year	Two.
☐ History of STDs	I told you, I had gonorrhea four months ago, and I was cured after a course of antibiotics.
☐ Drug allergies	No.

Connecting with the Patient

☐ Examinee recognized the SP's emotions and responded with PEARLS.

Physical Examination

☐ Examinee washed his/her hands.

☐ Examinee asked permission to start the exam.

☐ Examinee used respectful draping.

☐ Examinee did not repeat painful maneuvers.

☑ Exam Component	Maneuver
☐ Head and neck exam	Examined nose, mouth, throat, lymph nodes; checked for sinus tenderness
☐ CV exam	Auscultation
☐ Pulmonary exam	Auscultation
☐ Abdominal exam	Auscultation, palpation, percussion
☐ Skin/lymph node exam	Inspected for rashes, lesions, lymphadenopathy

Closure

☐ Examinee discussed initial diagnostic impressions.

☐ Examinee discussed initial management plans:

☐ Follow-up tests (including consent for HIV testing).

☐ Safe sex practices.

☐ Help with smoking cessation.

☐ Recommendation to avoid contact sports because of the possible increased risk of traumatic splenic rupture.

☐ Examinee asked if the SP had any other questions or concerns.

Sample Closure

Mr. Davis, it is likely that you have acquired the same infection your girlfriend had. This may be no more than a transient viral infection, or it may represent a more serious illness such as HIV. We will need to run a few tests to help us make the diagnosis. I recommend that we obtain an HIV test. In any case, I strongly recommend using condoms to avoid an unwanted pregnancy and to prevent STDs. Since infectious mononucleosis is one of the diseases that might account for your symptoms, I also recommend that you avoid contact sports because of the possible risk of traumatic rupture of your spleen, which could be fatal. Also, since cigarette smoking is associated with a variety of diseases, I advise you to quit smoking; we have many ways to help you if you are interested. Do you have any questions for me?

Patient Note

History

_____
_____
_____
_____
_____
_____
_____
_____
_____
_____

Physical Examination

_____
_____
_____
_____
_____
_____
_____
_____
_____
_____
_____
_____

Differential Diagnosis

1. _____
2. _____
3. _____
4. _____
5. _____

Diagnostic Workup

1. _____
2. _____
3. _____
4. _____
5. _____

History

HPI: *21 yo M c/o sore throat for the past 2 weeks. Two weeks ago he had a mild fever and fatigue, but he denies any chills, runny nose, cough, night sweats, shortness of breath, or wheezing. The patient also notes LUQ abdominal pain since yesterday. The pain is 4/10 and constant with no radiation, no relation to food, and no alleviating or exacerbating factors. He has poor appetite and subjective weight loss. His ex-girlfriend had the same symptoms 2 months ago.*

ROS: *Negative except as above.*

Allergies: *NKDA.*

Medications: *Tylenol.*

PMH: *Gonorrhea 4 months ago, treated with antibiotics.*

SH: *1 PPD since age 15; drinks heavily on weekends. Multiple female and male partners; uses condoms.*

FH: *Noncontributory.*

Physical Examination

Patient is in no acute distress.

VS: *WNL.*

HEENT: *Nose, mouth, and pharynx WNL.*

Neck: *Supple, no lymphadenopathy.*

Chest: *Clear breath sounds bilaterally.*

Heart: *RRR; normal S1/S2; no murmurs, rubs, or gallops.*

Abdomen: *Soft, nondistended, ⊕ BS, no hepatosplenomegaly, mild LUQ tenderness on palpation.*

Skin: *No rash or lymphadenopathy.*

Differential Diagnosis

1. Infectious mononucleosis
2. Acute HIV infection
3. Viral pharyngitis
4. Bacterial pharyngitis

Diagnostic Workup

1. CBC
2. Peripheral smear
3. Monospot
4. Rapid streptococcal antigen
5. Throat culture
6. Anti-EBV antibodies
7. HIV antibody and viral load

CASE DISCUSSION

Differential Diagnosis

- **Infectious mononucleosis:** The differential diagnosis for "sore throat" includes many pathogens. This patient's LUQ pain suggests splenomegaly, which could limit the differential (for a unifying diagnosis) to an infectious mononucleosis caused by EBV or, less commonly, by CMV infection. The physical exam is notoriously insensitive for detecting splenomegaly and may be misleading, as in this case. However, this patient does not have other typical features of infectious mononucleosis, such as lymphadenopathy or exudative pharyngitis.

- **Group A streptococcal pharyngitis:** Clinical features in patients with sore throat that predict group A streptococcal pharyngitis include tonsillar exudates, tender anterior cervical lymphadenopathy, a history of fever (temperature > 100.4°F/38°C), and absence of cough. "Strep throat" must be recognized and treated to prevent acute rheumatic fever.

- **Other common etiologies:** Include viruses (including acute HIV infection, which is often associated with a generalized maculopapular rash), *Neisseria gonorrhoeae*, *Mycoplasma* (although lower respiratory symptoms usually predominate), rubella, and *Chlamydia trachomatis*.

Diagnostic Workup

- **CBC:** Findings are nonspecific, but leukocytosis may be seen in infection.

- **Peripheral smear:** Can reveal atypical lymphocytes in infectious mononucleosis.

- **Monospot (heterophil agglutination test):** Usually becomes positive in EBV-associated mononucleosis within 4 weeks of onset of illness.

- **Rapid streptococcal antigen:** Has high negative predictive value (ie, it can accurately confirm the absence of group A streptococcal pharyngitis).

- **Throat culture:** The gold standard for diagnosing bacterial pharyngitis.

- **Anti-EBV antibodies:** Antibodies to various EBV antigens can be detected, such as IgM antibody to virus capsid antigen (VCA) and to nuclear antigen (EBNA). There is also a PCR to detect EBV in serum.

- **HIV antibody and viral load:** Check antibody to exclude preexisting HIV infection, and check viral load to help document acute infection.

Opening Scenario

Kenneth Klein, a 55-year-old male, comes to the clinic complaining of blood in his stool.

Vital Signs

BP: 130/80 mm Hg

Temp: 98.5°F (36.9°C)

RR: 16/minute

HR: 76/minute, regular

Examinee Tasks

1. Take a focused history.

2. Perform a focused physical exam (do not perform rectal, genitourinary, or female breast exam).

3. Explain your clinical impression and workup plan to the patient.

4. Write the patient note after leaving the room.

Checklist/SP Sheet

Patient Description

Patient is a 55 yo M, married with two children.

Notes for the SP

If colonoscopy is mentioned by the examinee, ask, "What is the meaning of this word?"

Challenging Questions to Ask

"My father had colon cancer. Could I have it, too?"

Sample Examinee Response

"It is a possibility. Tell me more about the symptoms you're having that concern you with regard to cancer."

Examinee Checklist

Building the Doctor-Patient Relationship

Entrance

☐ Examinee knocked on the door before entering.

☐ Examinee introduced self by name.

☐ Examinee identified his/her role or position.

☐ Examinee correctly used patient's name.

☐ Examinee made eye contact with the SP.

Reflective Listening

☐ Examinee asked an open-ended question and actively listened to the response.

☐ Examinee asked the SP to list his/her concerns and listened to the response without interrupting.

☐ Examinee summarized the SP's concerns, often using the SP's own words.

Information Gathering

☐ Examinee elicited data efficiently and accurately.

☑ Question	Patient Response
☐ Chief complaint	Blood in stool.
☐ Onset	One month ago.
☐ Frequency	Every time I move my bowels, I see some blood mixed in with the stool.
☐ Description (blood before, during, or after defecation)	The blood is mixed in with the brown stool.
☐ Bright red or dark blood	Bright red.
☐ Pain during defecation	No.
☐ Constipation	Well, I have had constipation for a long time, and I keep taking laxatives. At first I used to get some relief, but now there is no benefit from them.
☐ Frequency of bowel movements	I have had two bowel movements a week for the past six months.
☐ Diarrhea	I have had diarrhea for the past two days.
☐ Urgency	No.
☐ Tenesmus (ineffectual spasms of the rectum, accompanied by the desire to empty the bowel)	A little.
☐ Frequency of diarrhea	Three times a day.
☐ Description of the diarrhea	Watery, brown, mixed with blood.
☐ Mucus in stool	No.
☐ Melena	No.
☐ Fever/chills	No.
☐ Abdominal pain	No.
☐ Nausea/vomiting	No.
☐ Diet	I eat a lot of junk food. I don't eat vegetables at all.
☐ Weight changes	I have lost about 10 pounds over the past six months.
☐ Appetite changes	My appetite has been the same.
☐ Recent travel	No, but I am thinking of going on a trip with my family next week. Do you think I should stay home?

☑ Question	Patient Response
☐ Contact with people with diarrhea	No.
☐ Exercise	I walk for half an hour every day.
☐ Urinary problems	No.
☐ Current medications	No. I used to take many laxatives, such as bisacodyl and phenolphthalein, but I stopped all of them when the diarrhea started.
☐ Past medical history (recent antibiotic use)	I had bronchitis three weeks ago; it was treated with amoxicillin.
☐ Past surgical history	Hemorrhoids resected four years ago.
☐ Family history	My father died at 55 of colon cancer. My mother is alive and healthy.
☐ Occupation	Lawyer.
☐ Alcohol use	No.
☐ Illicit drug use	No.
☐ Tobacco	No.
☐ Sexual activity	With my wife.
☐ Drug allergies	None.

Connecting with the Patient

☐ Examinee recognized the SP's emotions and responded with PEARLS.

Physical Examination

☐ Examinee washed his/her hands.

☐ Examinee asked permission to start the exam.

☐ Examinee used respectful draping.

☐ Examinee did not repeat painful maneuvers.

☑ Exam Component	Maneuver
☐ CV exam	Auscultation
☐ Pulmonary exam	Auscultation
☐ Abdominal exam	Auscultation, palpation, percussion

Closure

☐ Examinee discussed initial diagnostic impressions.

☐ Examinee discussed initial management plans:

    ☐ Follow-up tests: Examinee mentioned the need for a rectal exam.

☐ Examinee asked if the SP had any other questions or concerns.

Sample Closure

Mr. Klein, the symptoms you describe may be due to readily treatable problems, such as hemorrhoids, an infection in your colon, or diverticulosis, or they may be a sign of more serious disease, such as colorectal cancer. It is crucial that we run some blood tests; a stool exam; and probably a colonoscopy, which involves looking at your colon through a thin tube that contains a camera. I will also need to perform a rectal exam today. Once we make a diagnosis, we should be able to treat your problem. Do you have any questions for me?

Patient Note

History

_____

_____

_____

_____

_____

_____

_____

_____

_____

Physical Examination

_____

_____

_____

_____

_____

_____

_____

_____

_____

_____

_____

Differential Diagnosis

1. _____

2. _____

3. _____

4. _____

5. _____

Diagnostic Workup

1. _____

2. _____

3. _____

4. _____

5. _____

History

HPI: 55 yo M c/o bright red blood in stool. He has a history of constipation that started 6 months ago, consisting of 2 bowel movements a week. One month ago he noticed blood mixed with stool at every bowel movement. During the past 2 days he started to have tenesmus and watery brown diarrhea (3 times a day) mixed with blood. He has no urgency, no mucus in stool, and no pain during defecation. He denies any fever, chills, nausea, vomiting, abdominal pain, recent history of travel, or contact with ill persons. He recalls a 10-lb weight loss during the past 6 months despite a good appetite. His diet consists of a lot of junk food with no vegetables.

ROS: Negative except as above.

Allergies: NKDA.

Medications: Used to take many laxatives (bisacodyl, phenolphthalein) but stopped after the onset of diarrhea 2 days ago.

PMH: Bronchitis 3 weeks ago, treated with amoxicillin.

PSH: Hemorrhoids resected 4 years ago.

SH: No smoking, no EtOH, no illicit drugs. Sexually active with wife only.

FH: Father died of colon cancer at age 55.

Physical Examination

Patient is in no acute distress.

VS: WNL.

Chest: Clear breath sounds bilaterally.

Heart: RRR; normal S1/S2; no murmurs, rubs, or gallops.

Abdomen: Soft, nondistended, nontender, ⊕ BS, no hepatosplenomegaly.

Differential Diagnosis

1. Colorectal cancer
2. Hemorrhoids
3. Diverticulosis
4. Angiodysplasia
5. Pseudomembranous (C. difficile) colitis
6. Other infectious colitis
7. Ulcerative colitis

Diagnostic Workup

1. Rectal exam, stool for occult blood
2. Stool for C. difficile toxin
3. Fecal leukocytes
4. CBC
5. Anoscopy
6. Flexible proctosigmoidoscopy
7. Colonoscopy
8. Double-contrast (air contrast) barium enema
9. CT—abdomen/pelvis

CASE DISCUSSION

Differential Diagnosis

Bright red blood that is mixed with brown stool suggests a distal colonic or anorectal source. Otherwise, this patient's presentation is complex, and the differential remains broad. His chronic constipation may simply be due to a low-fiber diet or to irritable bowel syndrome, but neither of these entities explains hematochezia and weight loss.

- **Colorectal cancer:** A positive family history coupled with the presence of blood in the stool, a change in bowel habits, and weight loss makes colorectal cancer a plausible diagnosis. Screening colonoscopy should have been offered to the patient at age 45 (10 years before the age when a first-degree family member was diagnosed).

- **Hemorrhoids:** Recurrent hemorrhoids may explain the patient's hematochezia, although more typical findings in hemorrhoids are fresh blood on the paper or dripped into the toilet bowl.

- **Diverticulosis:** This is the most common cause of major lower GI bleeding, but it usually presents with larger-volume bleeds occurring in discrete, self-limited episodes.

- **Angiodysplasia:** This is another common cause of lower GI tract bleeding, but as with diverticular disease, it cannot explain the other features of this patient's presentation.

- **Pseudomembranous (*C. difficile*) colitis:** It is important to ask all patients with acute diarrhea about recent antibiotic exposure, as symptoms of antibiotic-associated colitis may be delayed for up to 6–8 weeks. Stools rarely contain gross blood, however. The absence of fever and lower abdominal cramping also makes this diagnosis (and other forms of infectious colitis) less likely.

- **Ulcerative colitis:** The absence of abdominal pain and the recent onset of diarrhea and tenesmus make inflammatory bowel disease a less likely etiology for this patient's month-long hematochezia.

Diagnostic Workup

- **Rectal exam, stool for occult blood:** Useful to detect masses and hemorrhoids. Always test for occult blood in stool.

- **Stool for *C. difficile* toxin:** Recall that 1 negative test does not exclude the diagnosis, as the assays are positive in only 80% of patients on the first stool sample and in 90% of patients after two stool samples.

- **Fecal leukocytes:** Usually present in invasive bacterial infection and in inflammatory bowel disease. Variably present in C. *difficile* colitis.

- **CBC:** To investigate anemia. Also, leukocytosis could suggest infection or inflammatory bowel disease.

- **Anoscopy:** Can identify bleeding internal hemorrhoids, rectal ulcers, and traumatic lesions.

- **Flexible proctosigmoidoscopy:** If nondiagnostic, follow up with a barium enema or a colonoscopy.

- **Colonoscopy:** Should be the initial test performed in patients older than 40 years of age presenting with hematochezia.

- **Double-contrast (air contrast) barium enema:** Not as accurate as colonoscopy for the diagnosis of polyps and cancer (and cannot diagnose angiodysplasia). Used mainly when colonoscopy is unavailable or contraindicated.

- **CT—abdomen/pelvis:** Contrast-enhanced exams can detect diverticulosis or masses but generally are not useful in the evaluation of GI bleeding.

CASE 6
DOORWAY INFORMATION

Opening Scenario

Joseph Short, a 46-year-old male, comes to the ED complaining of chest pain.

Vital Signs

BP: 165/85 mm Hg

Temp: 98.6°F (37°C)

RR: 22/minute

HR: 90/minute, regular

Examinee Tasks

1. Take a focused history.

2. Perform a focused physical exam (do not perform rectal, genitourinary, or female breast exam).

3. Explain your clinical impression and workup plan to the patient.

4. Write the patient note after leaving the room.

Checklist/SP Sheet

Patient Description

Patient is a 46 yo M.

Notes for the SP

- Lie on the bed and exhibit pain.
- Place your hands in the middle of your chest.
- Exhibit difficulty breathing.
- If ECG is mentioned by the examinee, ask, "What is an ECG?"

Challenging Questions to Ask

"Is this a heart attack? Am I going to die?"

Sample Examinee Response

"As you suspect, your symptoms are of significant concern. We need to learn more about what's going on to know if your pain is life threatening."

Examinee Checklist

Building the Doctor-Patient Relationship

Entrance

☐ Examinee knocked on the door before entering.

☐ Examinee introduced self by name.

☐ Examinee identified his/her role or position.

☐ Examinee correctly used patient's name.

☐ Examinee made eye contact with the SP.

Reflective Listening

☐ Examinee asked an open-ended question and actively listened to the response.

☐ Examinee asked the SP to list his/her concerns and listened to the response without interrupting.

☐ Examinee summarized the SP's concerns, often using the SP's own words.

Information Gathering

☐ Examinee elicited data efficiently and accurately.

☑ Question	Patient Response
☐ Chief complaint	Chest pain.
☐ Onset	Forty minutes ago.
☐ Precipitating events	Nothing; I was asleep and I woke up at 5:00 in the morning having this pain.
☐ Progression	Constant severity.
☐ Severity on a scale	7/10.
☐ Location	Middle of the chest.
☐ Radiation	To my neck and left arm.
☐ Quality	Pressure.
☐ Alleviating/exacerbating factors	Nothing.
☐ Shortness of breath	Yes.
☐ Nausea/vomiting	I feel nauseated, but I didn't vomit.
☐ Sweating	Yes.
☐ Associated symptoms (cough, wheezing, abdominal pain, diarrhea/constipation)	None.
☐ Previous episodes of similar pain	Yes, but not exactly the same.
☐ Onset	The past three months.
☐ Severity	Less severe.
☐ Frequency	Two to three episodes a week for 5–10 minutes.
☐ Precipitating events	Walking up the stairs, strenuous work, and heavy meals.
☐ Alleviating factors	Antacids.
☐ Associated symptoms	None.
☐ Current medications	Maalox, diuretic.

☑ Question	Patient Response
☐ Past medical history	Hypertension for five years, treated with a diuretic. High cholesterol, managed with diet; I have not been very compliant with the diet. GERD 10 years ago, treated with antacids.
☐ Past surgical history	None.
☐ Family history	My father died of lung cancer at age 72. My mother is alive and has a peptic ulcer. No early heart attacks.
☐ Occupation	Accountant.
☐ Alcohol use	Once in a while.
☐ Illicit drug use	Cocaine, once a week.
☐ Last time of cocaine use	Yesterday afternoon.
☐ Tobacco	Stopped three months ago.
☐ Duration	Twenty-five years.
☐ Amount	One pack a day.
☐ Sexual activity	Well, doctor, to be honest, I haven't had sex with my wife for the past three months because I get this pain in my chest during sex.
☐ Exercise	No.
☐ Diet	My doctor gave me a strict diet last year to lower my cholesterol, but I always cheat.
☐ Drug allergies	No.

Connecting with the Patient

☐ Examinee recognized the SP's emotions and responded with PEARLS.

Physical Examination

☐ Examinee washed his/her hands.

☐ Examinee asked permission to start the exam.

☐ Examinee used respectful draping.

☐ Examinee did not repeat painful maneuvers.

☑ Exam Component	Maneuver
☐ Neck exam	Looked for JVD, carotid auscultation
☐ CV exam	Inspection, auscultation, palpation
☐ Pulmonary exam	Auscultation, palpation, percussion
☐ Abdominal exam	Auscultation, palpation, percussion
☐ Extremities	Checked peripheral pulses, checked blood pressure in both arms, looked for edema and cyanosis

Closure

☐ Examinee discussed initial diagnostic impressions.

☐ Examinee discussed initial management plans:

　☐ Follow-up tests.

　☐ Lifestyle modification (diet, exercise).

☐ Examinee asked if the SP had any other questions or concerns.

Sample Closure

Mr. Short, the source of your pain can be a cardiac problem, such as a heart attack or angina, or it may be due to acid reflux, lung problems, or disorders related to the large blood vessels in your chest. It is crucial that we perform some tests to identify the source of your problem. We will start with an ECG and some blood work, but more complex tests may be needed as well. In the meantime, I strongly recommend that you stop using cocaine, since use of this drug can lead to a variety of medical problems, including heart attacks. Do you have any questions for me?

Patient Note

History

_____
_____
_____
_____
_____
_____
_____
_____
_____
_____

Physical Examination

_____
_____
_____
_____
_____
_____
_____
_____
_____
_____
_____
_____

Differential Diagnosis

1. _____
2. _____
3. _____
4. _____
5. _____

Diagnostic Workup

1. _____
2. _____
3. _____
4. _____
5. _____

Patient Note

History

HPI: *46 yo M c/o chest pain. Chest pain started 40 minutes before the patient presented to the ED. The pain woke the patient from sleep at 5:00 AM with a steady 7/10 pressure sensation in the middle of his chest that radiated to the left arm and the neck. Nothing makes it worse or better. Nausea, sweating, and dyspnea are also present. Similar episodes have occurred during the past 3 months, 2–3 times/week. These episodes were precipitated by walking up the stairs, strenuous work, sexual intercourse, and heavy meals. Pain during these episodes was less severe, lasted for 5–10 minutes, and disappeared spontaneously or after taking antacids.*

ROS: *Negative except as above.*

Allergies: *NKDA.*

Medications: *Maalox, diuretic.*

PMH: *Hypertension for 5 years, treated with a diuretic. High cholesterol, managed with diet. GERD 10 years ago, treated with antacids.*

SH: *1 PPD for 25 years; stopped 3 months ago. Occasional EtOH, occasional cocaine (last used yesterday afternoon). No regular exercise; poorly adherent to diet.*

FH: *Father died of lung cancer at age 72. Mother has peptic ulcers. No early coronary disease.*

Physical Examination

Patient is in severe pain.

BP: *165/85 mm Hg (both arms).*

RR: *22/minute.*

Neck: *No JVD, no bruits.*

Chest: *No tenderness, clear symmetric breath sounds bilaterally.*

Heart: *Apical impulse not displaced; RRR; normal S1/S2; no murmurs, rubs, or gallops.*

Abdomen: *Soft, nondistended, nontender, ⊕ BS, no hepatosplenomegaly.*

Extremities: *No edema, peripheral pulses 2+ and symmetric.*

Differential Diagnosis

1. *Myocardial ischemia or infarction*
2. *Cocaine-induced myocardial ischemia*
3. *GERD*
4. *Aortic dissection*
5. *Pericarditis*
6. *Pneumothorax*
7. *Pulmonary embolism*
8. *Costochondritis*

Diagnostic Workup

1. *ECG*
2. *Cardiac enzymes (CPK, CPK-MB, troponin)*
3. *CXR*
4. *Transthoracic echocardiogram*
5. *Cardiac catheterization*
6. *Transesophageal echocardiogram*
7. *CT—chest with IV contrast*
8. *Upper endoscopy*
9. *Cholesterol panel*

CASE DISCUSSION

Differential Diagnosis

- **Myocardial ischemia or infarction:** The patient has multiple cardiac risk factors (including smoking, hypertension, and hyperlipidemia), and his symptoms are classic for cardiac ischemia.

- **Cocaine-induced:** Cocaine can predispose to premature atherosclerosis or can induce myocardial ischemia and infarction by causing coronary artery vasoconstriction or by increasing myocardial energy requirements.

- **GERD:** Severe chest pain is atypical but not uncommon for GERD and may worsen with recumbency overnight. Other atypical symptoms may include chronic cough, wheezing, or dysphagia. The classic symptom of GERD is heartburn, which may be exacerbated by meals.

- **Aortic dissection:** With the sudden onset of severe chest pain, aortic dissection should be suspected given the high potential for death if missed (and the potential for harm if mistaken for acute MI and treated with thrombolytic therapy). However, the patient's pain is not the classic sudden tearing chest pain that radiates to the back. In addition, his peripheral pulses and blood pressures are not diminished or unequal, and there is no aortic regurgitant murmur (although physical exam findings have poor sensitivity and specificity to diagnose aortic dissection).

- **Pericarditis:** The absence of pain that changes with position or respiration and the absence of a pericardial friction rub make pericarditis less likely.

- **Pneumothorax:** This diagnosis should be considered in a patient with acute chest pain and difficulty breathing, but it is less likely in this case given that breath sounds are symmetric.

- **Pulmonary embolism:** As above, this is on the differential for acute chest pain and difficulty breathing, but this patient has no apparent risk factors for pulmonary embolism.

- **Costochondritis (or other musculoskeletal chest pain):** This is more typically associated with pain on palpation or pleuritic pain.

Diagnostic Workup

- **ECG:** Acute myocardial ischemia, infarction, and pericarditis have characteristic changes on ECG.

- **Cardiac enzymes (CPK, CPK-MB, troponin):** Specific tests for myocardial tissue necrosis that can turn positive as early as 4–6 hours after onset of pain.

- **CXR:** A widened mediastinum suggests aortic dissection and may reveal other causes of chest pain, including pneumothorax and pneumonia.

- **Transthoracic echocardiogram (TTE):** Can demonstrate segmental wall motion abnormalities in suspected acute MIs (infarction is unlikely in the absence of wall motion abnormalities).

- **Cardiac catheterization:** Can diagnose and treat coronary artery disease.

- **Transesophageal echocardiogram (TEE):** Highly specific and sensitive for aortic dissection, and can be done rapidly at the bedside.

- **CT—chest with IV contrast:** Another rapidly available diagnostic study that can rule out aortic dissection or pulmonary embolism.

- **Upper endoscopy:** Can be used to document tissue damage characteristic of GERD. However, it can be normal in up to one-half of symptomatic patients; esophageal probe (pH and manometry measurements) together with endoscopic visualization constitutes an effective diagnostic technique.

- **Cholesterol panel:** Can identify a critical risk factor for cardiovascular disease.

Opening Scenario

The mother of Josh White, a 7-month-old male child, comes to the office complaining that her child has a fever.

Examinee Tasks

1. Take a focused history.

2. Explain your clinical impression and workup plan to the mother.

3. Write the patient note after leaving the room.

Checklist/SP Sheet

Patient Description

The patient's mother offers the history; she is a fair historian.

Notes for the SP

Show concern regarding your child's situation.

Challenging Questions to Ask

- "Is my baby going to be okay?"
- "Do I need to bring my baby to the hospital?"

Sample Examinee Response

"I understand your concern and want answers, but I will need to examine your child first. Although I suspect that he has a viral infection, I need to make sure he does not have anything else."

Examinee Checklist

Building the Doctor-Patient Relationship

Entrance

☐ Examinee knocked on the door before entering.

☐ Examinee introduced self by name.

☐ Examinee identified his/her role or position.

☐ Examinee correctly used patient's name.

☐ Examinee made eye contact with the SP.

Reflective Listening

☐ Examinee asked an open-ended question and actively listened to the response.

☐ Examinee asked the SP to list his/her concerns and listened to the response without interrupting.

☐ Examinee summarized the SP's concerns, often using the SP's own words.

Information Gathering

☐ Examinee elicited data efficiently and accurately.

☑ Question	Patient Response
☐ Chief complaint	My child has a fever.
☐ Onset	Yesterday.
☐ Temperature	I measured it rectally, and it was 101.
☐ Runny nose	Yes.
☐ Ear pulling/ear discharge	No.
☐ Cough	No.
☐ Shortness of breath	I think so; breathing seems to be more difficult recently and he is breathing quickly.
☐ Difficulty swallowing	I don't know, but he hasn't eaten anything since yesterday and is refusing to drink from his bottle or my breast.
☐ Rash	No.
☐ Nausea/vomiting	No.
☐ Change in bowel habits or in stool color or consistency	No.
☐ Change in urinary habits, urine smell, or color (change in normal number of wet diapers)	No.
☐ Shaking (seizures)	No.
☐ How has the baby looked (lethargic, irritated, playful, etc)?	He has looked tired and irritated since yesterday.
☐ Appetite changes	He is not eating anything at all.
☐ Ill contacts	His 3-year-old brother had an upper respiratory tract infection 1 week ago, and he is fine now.
☐ Day care center	Yes.
☐ Ill contacts in day care center	I don't know.
☐ Vaccinations	Up to date.
☐ Last checkup	Two weeks ago, and everything was perfect with him.
☐ Birth history	It was a 40-week vaginal delivery with no complications.
☐ Child weight, height, and language development	Normal.
☐ Eating habits	I am breast-feeding him, and I give him all the vitamins that his pediatrician prescribes. He has refused my breast since yesterday. He also gets baby food three times a day.
☐ Sleeping habits	Last night he did not sleep well and cried when I laid him down.
☐ Current medications	Tylenol.
☐ Past medical history	Jaundice in the first week of life.

☑ Question	Patient Response
☐ Past surgical history	None.
☐ Drug allergies	No.

Connecting with the Patient

☐ Examinee recognized the SP's emotions and responded with PEARLS.

Physical Examination

None.

Closure

☐ Examinee discussed initial diagnostic impressions.

☐ Examinee discussed initial management plans:

   ☐ Follow-up tests.

☐ Examinee asked if the SP had any other questions or concerns.

Sample Closure

Mrs. White, your child's fever may be due to a simple upper respiratory tract infection or to an ear infection caused by a virus or certain types of bacteria. I would like to examine your baby so that I can better determine the cause of his fever and exclude more serious causes, such as meningitis. In addition to a detailed physical exam, your baby may need some blood tests, a urinalysis, and possibly a chest x-ray. Do you have any questions for me?

Patient Note

History

_____
_____
_____
_____
_____
_____
_____
_____
_____

Physical Examination

_____
_____
_____
_____
_____
_____
_____
_____
_____

Differential Diagnosis

1. _____
2. _____
3. _____
4. _____
5. _____

Diagnostic Workup

1. _____
2. _____
3. _____
4. _____
5. _____

Patient Note

History

HPI: *History obtained from mother. Patient is a 7-month-old M with fever × 1 day. Temperature recorded rectally 101°F yesterday. Child has been tired, irritated, breathing rapidly for past day. Mother also notes rhinorrhea and refusal of breast and baby food. History of sick contact with 3 yo brother who had URI 1 week ago, since resolved. Child attends day care. No cough, ear pulling, ear discharge, or rash.*

ROS: *Negative except as above.*

Allergies: *NKDA.*

Medications: *Tylenol.*

PMH: *Jaundice in the first week of life.*

Birth history: *40-week vaginal delivery with no complications.*

Dietary history: *Breast-feeding and supplemental vitamins.*

Immunization history: *UTD.*

Developmental history: *Last checkup was 2 weeks ago and showed normal weight, height, hearing/vision, and developmental milestones.*

Physical Examination

None.

Differential Diagnosis

1. *Viral URI*
2. *Pneumonia*
3. *Meningitis*
4. *UTI*
5. *Otitis media*
6. *Gastroenteritis*
7. *Occult bacteremia*

Diagnostic Workup

1. *Pneumatic otoscopy*
2. *Tympanometry*
3. *CBC with differential, blood culture, UA and urine culture*
4. *LP—CSF analysis*
5. *CT—head*
6. *CXR*
7. *Bronchoscopy*
8. *Serum antibody titers*
9. *U/S—renal*
10. *Voiding cystourethrogram*

CASE DISCUSSION

Differential Diagnosis

- **Viral URI:** Clues suggesting this diagnosis as the source of fever include rhinorrhea and recent exposure to a sibling with URI. It is probably viral, self-limited, and benign, but lower respiratory tract infection must first be ruled out in light of the child's apparent dyspnea and tachypnea.

- **Pneumonia:** Fever, rhinorrhea, tachypnea, and dyspnea support this diagnosis, although cough is not present. The physical exam may find retractions, nasal flaring, grunting, dullness on chest percussion, and rales.

- **Meningitis:** Findings are often subtle and nonspecific and may be limited to fever, irritability, and poor feeding, as seen in this case. The physical exam may reveal a bulging fontanelle. Meningeal signs may not be obvious in infants (nuchal rigidity and focal neurologic signs are more commonly seen in older children).

- **UTI:** Infants with UTI may not have symptoms referable to the urinary tract. Infants who do may have dribbling or colic before and during voiding. Patients with high fever and CVA tenderness are presumed to have pyelonephritis until proven otherwise.

- **Otitis media:** Otalgia and ear drainage can suggest this diagnosis in an ill, febrile child but are often not present (as in this case). The physical exam is key and may reveal a hyperemic, bulging TM; loss of TM landmarks; and decreased TM mobility.

- **Gastroenteritis:** This patient has fever but no GI symptoms. Viral infection typically causes vomiting and/or watery diarrhea, whereas bacterial infection may cause fever, tenesmus, bloody diarrhea, and severe abdominal pain.

- **Occult bacteremia:** This is an important consideration for children with high fever (> 102°F/38.9°C) and no obvious source. There is a relatively high proportion of children with no identifiable fever source who will have a positive blood culture, which can progress to sepsis if untreated. An extensive workup (see below) is not necessarily indicated in this case, as fever is < 102°F (38.9°C).

Diagnostic Workup

- **Pneumatic otoscopy:** Key to look for the decreased TM mobility seen in otitis media.

- **Tympanometry:** Useful in infants older than six months of age; confirms abnormal TM mobility in otitis media.

- **CBC with differential, blood culture, UA, and urine culture:** Constitutes the "septic" or occult bacteremia workup in children with unexplained high fever. Notably, a WBC count > 15,000/μL suggests occult bacteremia. UTI may be occult and must be investigated.

- **LP—CSF analysis:** Should be performed if there is any concern for meningitis. CSF analysis includes cell count and differential, glucose, protein, Gram stain, culture, latex agglutination for common bacterial antigens, and occasionally PCR for specific viruses.

- **CT—head:** Used mainly to rule out brain abscess or hemorrhage.

- **CXR:** To diagnose pneumonia.

- **Bronchoscopy:** A diagnostic aid in severe or refractory pneumonia cases.

- **Serum antibody titers:** To identify causative viruses in pediatric infections (not commonly used).

- **U/S—renal:** To look for anatomic anomalies that predispose to UTI.

- **Voiding cystourethrogram:** To look for vesicoureteral reflux in UTI.

CASE 8
DOORWAY INFORMATION

Opening Scenario

The mother of Maria Sterling, an 18-month-old female child, comes to the office complaining that her child has a fever.

Examinee Tasks

1. Take a focused history.

2. Explain your clinical impression and workup plan to the mother.

3. Write the patient note after leaving the room.

Checklist/SP Sheet

Patient Description

The patient's mother offers the history; the child is at home.

Notes for the SP

Show concern regarding your child's situation.

Challenging Questions to Ask

- "Do you think that I did the right thing by coming here and telling you about my child's fever?"

- "Is my child going to be okay?"

Sample Examinee Response

"You absolutely did the right thing by coming in today. Maria may have an infection that needs antibiotics; we need to examine her here in the office and then decide whether she needs any tests and/or treatment."

Examinee Checklist

Building the Doctor-Patient Relationship

Entrance

☐ Examinee knocked on the door before entering.

☐ Examinee introduced self by name.

☐ Examinee identified his/her role or position.

☐ Examinee correctly used patient's name.

☐ Examinee made eye contact with the SP.

Reflective Listening

☐ Examinee asked an open-ended question and actively listened to the response.

☐ Examinee asked the SP to list his/her concerns and listened to the response without interrupting.

☐ Examinee summarized the SP's concerns, often using the SP's own words.

Information Gathering

☐ Examinee elicited data efficiently and accurately.

✓ Question	Patient Response
☐ Chief complaint	My child has a fever.
☐ Onset	Two days ago.
☐ Temperature	I measured it, and it was 101°F rectally.
☐ Runny nose	No.
☐ Ear pulling/ear discharge	Yes, she has been pulling at her right ear for 2 days.
☐ Cough	No.
☐ Shortness of breath	No.
☐ Difficulty swallowing	She seems to have trouble swallowing but I'm not sure.
☐ Rash	Yes, she has a rash on her face and chest.
☐ Description of the rash	Tiny red dots, some slightly elevated, over the chest, back, belly, and face. There is no rash on her arms or legs.
☐ Onset of rash and progression	It started two days ago on her face and then spread to her chest, back, and belly.
☐ Nausea/vomiting	No.
☐ Change in bowel habits or in stool color or consistency	No.
☐ Change in urinary habits or in urine smell or color	No.
☐ Shaking (seizures)	No.
☐ How has the child looked (lethargic, irritated, playful, etc.)?	She looks tired. She is not playing with her toys today and is not watching TV the way she usually does.
☐ Appetite changes	She is not eating much but is able to drink milk.
☐ Ill contacts	No.
☐ Day care center	Yes.
☐ Ill contacts in day care center	I don't know.
☐ Vaccinations	Up to date.
☐ Last checkup	One month ago, and everything was normal.
☐ Birth history	It was a 40-week vaginal delivery with no complications.
☐ Child weight, height, and language development	Normal.
☐ Eating habits	Whole milk and solid food; I did not breast-feed my child.
☐ Sleeping habits	She has not slept well for two days.
☐ Hearing problems	No.
☐ Vision problems	No.
☐ Current medications	Tylenol.

☑ Question	Patient Response
☐ Past medical history	Three months ago she had an ear infection that was treated successfully with amoxicillin.
☐ Past surgical history	None.
☐ Drug allergies	No.

Connecting with the Patient

☐ Examinee recognized the SP's emotions and responded with PEARLS.

Physical Examination

None.

Closure

☐ Examinee discussed initial diagnostic impressions.

☐ Examinee discussed initial management plans:

    ☐ Follow-up tests.

☐ Examinee asked if the SP had any other questions or concerns.

Sample Closure

Mrs. Sterling, it appears that your child is suffering from an infection that may be viral or bacterial. She may be suffering from an ear infection or meningitis. A physical exam and some blood tests will be needed to identify the source of infection and the type of virus or bacteria involved. Although most viral infections clear on their own, bacterial infections require antibiotics; however, such infections generally respond well to treatment. Do you have any questions for me?

Patient Note

History

_____
_____
_____
_____
_____
_____
_____
_____
_____

Physical Examination

_____
_____
_____
_____
_____
_____
_____
_____
_____
_____

Differential Diagnosis

1. _____
2. _____
3. _____
4. _____
5. _____

Diagnostic Workup

1. _____
2. _____
3. _____
4. _____
5. _____

History

HPI: *History obtained from mother. Patient is 18-month-old female c/o fever × 2 days.*

- *Temperature recorded rectally 101°F.*
- *Tired and not playing with toys or watching TV as usual.*
- *Pulling at right ear.*
- *Difficulty swallowing and sleeping × 2 days.*
- *Loss of appetite.*
- *Maculopapular facial rash that spread over the chest, back, and abdomen sparing the arms and legs.*
- *Attends day care center, no known history of sick contacts.*
- *No cough or ear discharge.*

ROS: *Negative except as above.*

Allergies: *NKDA.*

Medications: *Tylenol.*

PMH: *Otitis media 3 months ago, treated with amoxicillin.*

Birth history: *40-Week vaginal delivery with no complications.*

Dietary history: *Formula milk and solid food. She was not breast-fed.*

Immunization history: *UTD.*

Developmental history: *Last checkup was 1 month ago and showed normal weight, height, hearing, vision, and developmental milestones.*

Physical Examination

None.

Differential Diagnosis

1. *Otitis media*
2. *Meningococcal meningitis*
3. *Scarlet fever*
4. *Fifth disease or other viral exanthem*
5. *Varicella*

Diagnostic Workup

1. *Pneumatic otoscopy*
2. *Tympanometry*
3. *LP—CSF analysis*
4. *Platelets, PT/PTT, D-dimer, fibrin split products, fibrinogen*
5. *CBC with differential, blood culture, UA and urine culture*
6. *Throat culture*
7. *Parvovirus B19 IgM antibody*
8. *Skin lesion scrapings*
9. *Varicella antibody titer*

Examinee Checklist

Building the Doctor-Patient Relationship

Entrance

☐ Examinee knocked on the door before entering.

☐ Examinee introduced self by name.

☐ Examinee identified his/her role or position.

☐ Examinee correctly used patient's name.

☐ Examinee made eye contact with the SP.

Reflective Listening

☐ Examinee asked an open-ended question and actively listened to the response.

☐ Examinee asked the SP to list his/her concerns and listened to the response without interrupting.

☐ Examinee summarized the SP's concerns, often using the SP's own words.

Information Gathering

☐ Examinee elicited data efficiently and accurately.

☐ Examinee offered the SP a glass of water or a tissue during the severe bout of coughing.

☑ Question	Patient Response
☐ Chief complaint	Cough.
☐ Onset	One week ago.
☐ Preceding symptoms/events	Runny nose, fever, sore throat two weeks ago for one week, which then resolved.
☐ Fever/chills	Mild fever, but I didn't take my temperature; no chills.
☐ Sputum production	Small amounts of white mucus.
☐ Blood in sputum	No.
☐ Chest pain	Yes, I feel a sharp pain when I cough or take a deep breath.
☐ Location	Right chest.
☐ Quality	It is like a knife. I can't take a deep breath.
☐ Alleviating/exacerbating factors	It increases when I take a deep breath and when I cough. I feel better when I sleep on my right side.
☐ Radiation of pain	No.
☐ Severity on a scale	8/10.
☐ Night sweats	No.
☐ Exposure to TB	None.
☐ Pet, animal exposure	None.
☐ Recent travel	None.

☑ Question	Patient Response
☐ Last PPD	Never had it.
☐ Associated symptoms (shortness of breath, wheezing, abdominal pain, nausea/vomiting, diarrhea/ constipation)	None.
☐ Weight/appetite changes	No.
☐ Current medications	Tylenol.
☐ Past medical history	I had gonorrhea two years ago and was treated with a course of antibiotics.
☐ Past surgical history	None.
☐ Family history	My father and mother are alive and in good health.
☐ Occupation	Pizza delivery person.
☐ Alcohol use	I drink a lot on the weekends. I never count.
☐ Have you ever felt a need to cut down on drinking?	No.
☐ Have you ever felt annoyed by criticism of your drinking?	No.
☐ Have you ever felt guilty about your drinking?	No.
☐ Have you ever had a drink early in the morning ("eye opener") to steady your nerves or get rid of a hangover?	No.
☐ Illicit drug use	Never.
☐ Tobacco	Yes, I smoke one pack a day. I started when I was 15 years old.
☐ Sexual activity	Well, I've had many girlfriends. Every Saturday night, I pick up a new girl from the nightclub.
☐ Use of condoms	Nope, I don't enjoy it with a condom.
☐ Drug allergies	No.

Connecting with the Patient

☐ Examinee recognized the SP's emotions and responded with PEARLS.

Physical Examination

☐ Examinee washed his/her hands.

☐ Examinee asked permission to start the exam.

☐ Examinee used respectful draping.

☐ Examinee did not repeat painful maneuvers.

☑ Question	Patient Response
☐ Night sweats	Yes.
☐ Chest pain	No.
☐ Shortness of breath	Yes, when I walk up the stairs.
☐ Exposure to TB	Yes, I work in a nursing home, and several of our residents are under treatment for TB.
☐ Recent travel	None.
☐ Last PPD	Last year, before I started working in the nursing home. It was negative.
☐ Associated symptoms (wheezing, abdominal pain, nausea/vomiting, diarrhea/constipation)	None.
☐ Appetite changes	Yes, I don't have an appetite.
☐ Weight changes	Yes, I've lost six pounds in the past two months.
☐ Fatigue	Yes, I don't have the energy that I had before.
☐ Since when	Two months ago.
☐ Current medications	Cough syrup "over the counter," multivitamins, albuterol inhaler.
☐ Past medical history	Chronic bronchitis.
☐ Past surgical history	Tonsillectomy and adenoidectomy, age 11.
☐ Family history	My father died of old age. My mother is alive and has Alzheimer's.
☐ Occupation	Nurse's aide.
☐ Alcohol use	None.
☐ Illicit drug use	Never.
☐ Tobacco	No, I stopped smoking two weeks ago.
☐ Duration	I've smoked for the past 35 years.
☐ Amount	One to two packs a day.
☐ Sexual activity	With my husband.
☐ Drug allergies	No.

Connecting with the Patient

☐ Examinee recognized the SP's emotions and responded with PEARLS.

Physical Examination

☐ Examinee washed his/her hands.

☐ Examinee asked permission to start the exam.

☐ Examinee used respectful draping.

☐ Examinee did not repeat painful maneuvers.

☑ Exam Component	Maneuver
☐ Head and neck exam	Inspected mouth, throat, lymph nodes
☐ CV exam	Auscultation
☐ Pulmonary exam	Auscultation, palpation, percussion
☐ Abdominal exam	Auscultation, palpation
☐ Extremities	Inspection

Closure

☐ Examinee discussed initial diagnostic impressions.

☐ Examinee discussed initial management plans:

  ☐ Follow-up tests.

☐ Examinee asked if the SP had any other questions or concerns.

Sample Closure

Mrs. McLean, your cough may be due to a lung infection that can be treated with antibiotics, or it may result from something more serious such as cancer. We will need to obtain some blood and sputum tests as well as a chest x-ray in order to identify the source of your cough. In addition, we may find it necessary to conduct more sophisticated tests in the future. The fact that you work in a nursing home puts you at risk for acquiring tuberculosis, so we are going to test you for that as well. I would also recommend that you adhere to standard respiratory precautions while working with patients who are infected with TB. Do you have any questions for me?

Patient Note

History

Physical Examination

Differential Diagnosis

1.
2.
3.
4.
5.

Diagnostic Workup

1.
2.
3.
4.
5.

History

HPI: *54 yo F with PMH chronic bronchitis c/o worsening cough × 1 month.*

- *Chronic cough for years.*
- *2 teaspoons of yellowish phlegm with streaks of blood.*
- *Dyspnea on exertion.*
- *Fever and sweats at night.*
- *Fatigue.*
- *Decreased appetite, 6-lb weight loss over 2 months.*

- *Exposure to TB as nurse's aide working in nursing home.*
- *Last PPD: 1 year ago and negative.*
- *No chest pain, chills, or wheezing.*
- *No recent travel.*

ROS: *Negative except as above.*
Allergies: *NKDA.*
Medications: *OTC cough syrup, multivitamins, albuterol inhaler.*
PMH: *Per HPI.*
PSH: *Tonsillectomy and adenoidectomy, age 11.*
SH: *1–2 PPD for 35 years; stopped smoking 2 weeks ago. No EtOH. Sexually active with husband only.*
FH: *Noncontributory.*

Physical Examination

Patient is in no acute distress.
VS: *WNL.*
HEENT: *Mouth and pharynx WNL.*
Neck: *No JVD, no lymphadenopathy.*
Chest: *Clear breath sounds bilaterally; no rhonchi, rales, or wheezing; tactile fremitus normal.*
Heart: *Apical impulse not displaced; RRR; normal S1/S2; no murmurs, rubs, or gallops.*
Abdomen: *Soft, nontender, ⊕ BS, no hepatosplenomegaly.*
Extremities: *No clubbing, cyanosis, or edema.*

Differential Diagnosis

1. *Pulmonary tuberculosis*
2. *Lung cancer*
3. *Lung abscess*
4. *Atypical pneumonia*
5. *Typical pneumonia*
6. *COPD exacerbation*
7. *Wegener granulomatosis*

Diagnostic Workup

1. *PPD*
2. *CBC*
3. *Blood cultures*
4. *Sputum Gram stain, AFB smear, routine and mycobacterial sputum cultures, and cytology*
5. *CXR—PA and lateral*
6. *CT—chest*
7. *c-ANCA*
8. *Bronchoscopy*
9. *Lung biopsy*

CASE DISCUSSION

Differential Diagnosis

- **Pulmonary TB:** Clinical suspicion is high for this given the constitutional symptoms, hemoptysis, and recent exposure to active TB. The patient should be placed in respiratory isolation immediately.

- **Lung cancer:** As noted above, constitutional symptoms and hemoptysis in a long-time smoker are worrisome for cancer.

- **Lung abscess:** A lung abscess due to anaerobic bacteria is usually associated with a gradual onset of fatigue, fever, night sweats, cough producing a foul-smelling expectoration, and weight loss. Symptoms evolve over a period of weeks or months (the time course in this case favors abscess over uncomplicated pneumonia). Other bacterial causes of lung abscess typically present more acutely.

- **Atypical pneumonia:** Refers to infection by *Mycoplasma pneumoniae*, *Chlamydia pneumoniae*, and *Legionella* species. These can all present similarly with an insidious onset of fever, malaise, headache, myalgia, sore throat, hoarseness, chest pain, and nonproductive cough. Sputum may be blood-streaked. GI symptoms may be prominent in *Legionella* infection, and severe ear pain due to bullous myringitis may complicate up to 5% of *Mycoplasma* infections. The presence of weight loss and night sweats makes atypical pneumonia less likely in this case.

- **Typical pneumonia:** Classic bacterial pneumonia begins with abrupt onset of fever, chills, pleuritic chest pain, and productive cough. Remember that signs of pulmonary consolidation on physical exam are absent in up to two-thirds of documented cases. The more subacute time course seen here makes this diagnosis less likely.

- **COPD exacerbation:** This patient's baseline productive cough is due to COPD/chronic bronchitis secondary to tobacco exposure. Exacerbations of chronic bronchitis are more acute and involve increased sputum production and/or increased wheezing and dyspnea. Night sweats and weight loss are not typical features of this diagnosis.

- **Wegener granulomatosis:** This rare small-vessel vasculitis usually develops over 4–12 months and classically involves the triad of upper respiratory tract, lower respiratory tract, and renal disease (which usually does not cause symptoms before the diagnosis is established). Constitutional symptoms are common. The absence of chronic upper respiratory complaints (eg, sinusitis or nasal crusting) makes this diagnosis less likely.

- **Other etiologies:** Other common, benign causes of chronic cough include postnasal drip, GERD, asthma, and ACE inhibitors.

Diagnostic Workup

- **PPD (tuberculin skin test):** Identifies individuals who have been infected with *Mycobacterium tuberculosis*, but does not distinguish between active and latent infection.

- **CBC:** To identify leukocytosis in infection (nonspecific).

- **Blood cultures:** May be useful in severe pneumonia to identify causative pathogenic bacteria.

- **Sputum Gram stain, AFB smear, routine and mycobacterial sputum cultures, and cytology:** To identify a causative agent of infection or to help detect malignancy.

- **CXR—PA and lateral:** To look for apical cavitary disease in TB reactivation, noncalcified nodules in lung cancer, a cavity with an air-fluid level in lung abscess, a patchy infiltrative pattern in atypical pneumonia, lobar consolidation in typical pneumonia, and infiltrates, nodules, masses, or cavities in Wegener granulomatosis.

- **CT—chest:** May demonstrate lesions unseen on CXR, and aids in characterizing the size, shape, and composition of lung and mediastinal pathology. Can also guide diagnostic procedures (eg, percutaneous transthoracic biopsies) and assist in staging.

- **c-ANCA:** Highly specific (> 90%) and sensitive for active Wegener granulomatosis.

- **Bronchoscopy:** Useful in diagnosing and staging lung cancer and in diagnosing infections.

- **Lung biopsy:** Can lead to definitive diagnosis. A range of techniques can be used depending on the location of the tumor.

Opening Scenario

Gail Abbott, a 52-year-old female, comes to the office complaining of yellow eyes and skin.

Vital Signs

BP: 130/80 mm Hg

Temp: 98.3°F (36.8°C)

RR: 15/minute

HR: 70/minute, regular

Examinee Tasks

1. Take a focused history.

2. Perform a focused physical exam (do not perform rectal, genitourinary, or female breast exam).

3. Explain your clinical impression and workup plan to the patient.

4. Write the patient note after leaving the room.

Checklist/SP Sheet

Patient Description

Patient is a 52 yo F.

Notes for the SP

- Sit up on the bed.

- Show signs of scratching.

- Exhibit RUQ tenderness on palpation.

- If ERCP, ultrasound, or MRI is mentioned, ask for an explanation.

Challenging Questions to Ask

"My father had pancreatic cancer. Could I have it, too?"

Sample Examinee Response

"It's possible; that's why we always rule it out in patients with yellow eyes or skin. Your family history does put you at slightly increased risk, and we won't know anything for certain until we run some tests."

Examinee Checklist

Building the Doctor-Patient Relationship

Entrance

☐ Examinee knocked on the door before entering.

☐ Examinee introduced self by name.

☐ Examinee identified his/her role or position.

☐ Examinee correctly used patient's name.

☐ Examinee made eye contact with the SP.

Reflective Listening

☐ Examinee asked an open-ended question and actively listened to the response.

☐ Examinee asked the SP to list his/her concerns and listened to the response without interrupting.

☐ Examinee summarized the SP's concerns, often using the SP's own words.

Information Gathering

☐ Examinee elicited data efficiently and accurately.

☑ Question	Patient Response
☐ Chief complaint	Yellow eyes and skin.
☐ Onset	Three weeks ago.
☐ Color of stool	Light.
☐ Color of urine	Dark.
☐ Pruritus	I started itching two months ago; Benadryl used to help but not anymore.
☐ Abdominal pain	Sometimes.
☐ Onset	It was around the same time that I noticed the change in the color of my eyes and skin.
☐ Constant/intermittent	Well, I don't have the pain all the time. It comes and goes.
☐ Frequency	At least once every day.
☐ Progression	It is the same.
☐ Severity on a scale	When I have the pain, it is 3/10, and then it may go down to 0.
☐ Location	It is here (points to the RUQ).
☐ Radiation	No.
☐ Quality	Dull.
☐ Alleviating factors	Tylenol. I take four pills every day just to make sure I do not feel the pain.
☐ Exacerbating factors	None.
☐ Relationship of food to pain	None.
☐ Previous episodes of similar pain	No.
☐ Nausea/vomiting	Sometimes I feel nauseated when I am in pain, but no vomiting.
☐ Diarrhea/constipation	No.
☐ Colonoscopy	Never.
☐ Blood transfusion	Yes, when I had a C-section 20 years ago.

☑ Question	Patient Response
☐ Fever, night sweats	No.
☐ Fatigue	Yes, recently.
☐ Weight changes	No.
☐ Appetite changes	I have no appetite.
☐ Joint pain	No.
☐ Travel history	I went to Mexico for a brief vacation about two months ago.
☐ Immunization before travel	No.
☐ Current medications	Tylenol, Synthroid.
☐ Similar episodes	No.
☐ Past medical history	Hypothyroidism.
☐ Past surgical history	I had two C-sections at ages 25 and 30 and a tubal ligation at age 35.
☐ Family history	My father died at 55 of pancreatic cancer. My mother is alive and healthy.
☐ Occupation	I work in a travel agency.
☐ Illicit drug use	No.
☐ Tobacco	No.
☐ Sexual activity	Yes, with my husband.
☐ Drug allergies	Penicillin, causes rash.
☐ How much alcohol do you drink?/Tell me about your use of alcohol.	One or two glasses of wine every day for 30 years.
☐ Have you ever felt a need to cut down on drinking?	No.
☐ Have you ever felt annoyed by criticism of your drinking?	No.
☐ Have you ever felt guilty about your drinking?	No, I heard that alcohol protects against heart disease.
☐ Have you ever had a drink early in the morning ("eye opener") to steady your nerves or get rid of a hangover?	No.
☐ Affecting job/relationships/legal problems	No.

Connecting with the Patient

☐ Examinee recognized the SP's emotions and responded with PEARLS.

Physical Examination

☐ Examinee washed his/her hands.

☐ Examinee asked permission to start the exam.

☐ Examinee used respectful draping.

☐ Examinee did not repeat painful maneuvers.

☑ Exam Component	Maneuver
☐ HEENT	Inspected sclerae, under tongue
☐ CV exam	Auscultation
☐ Pulmonary exam	Auscultation
☐ Abdominal exam	Inspection, auscultation, palpation (including Murphy sign), percussion, measurement of liver span
☐ Extremities	Checked for asterixis, edema
☐ Skin	Looked for spider nevi, cutaneous telangiectasias, palmar erythema

Closure

☐ Examinee discussed initial diagnostic impressions.

☐ Examinee discussed initial management plans:

    ☐ Follow-up tests.

☐ Examinee asked if the SP had any other questions or concerns.

Sample Closure

Mrs. Abbott, the symptoms you describe are usually due to a disorder either in the liver itself or bile ducts, which are physically close to your liver. We will have to run some blood tests and conduct imaging studies such as ultrasound to get a better idea of what is going on. Once we find the cause of your problem, we can come up with an appropriate treatment plan. Until then, I recommend that you stop drinking and limit your use of Tylenol, as both may harm your liver. Do you have any questions for me?

Patient Note

History

_____
_____
_____
_____
_____
_____
_____
_____
_____
_____

Physical Examination

_____
_____
_____
_____
_____
_____
_____
_____
_____
_____

Differential Diagnosis

1. _____
2. _____
3. _____
4. _____
5. _____

Diagnostic Workup

1. _____
2. _____
3. _____
4. _____
5. _____

Patient Note

History

HPI: *52 yo F c/o yellow skin and eyes × 3 weeks.*

- *Light-colored stool and dark urine.*
- *3/10 RUQ pain, dull, intermittent (daily), no radiation, unrelated to meals, relieved by Tylenol.*
- *Fatigue.*
- *Anorexia.*
- *Pruritus.*
- *Nausea.*
- *Recent travel to Mexico.*
- *History of blood transfusion 20 years ago.*
- *No diarrhea, constipation, or weight loss.*

ROS: *Negative except as above.*
Allergies: *Penicillin, causes rash.*
Medications: *Tylenol, Synthroid.*
PMH: *Hypothyroidism.*
PSH: *2 C-sections, tubal ligation.*
SH: *No smoking, 1–2 glasses of wine/day for 30 years, CAGE 0/4, no illicit drugs. Sexually active with husband only.*
FH: *Father died of pancreatic cancer at age 55.*

Physical Examination

Patient is in no acute distress.
VS: *WNL.*
HEENT: *Sclerae icteric.*
Chest: *Clear breath sounds bilaterally.*
Heart: *RRR; normal S1/S2; no murmurs, rubs, or gallops.*
Abdomen: *Soft, nondistended, C-section scar. Mild RUQ tenderness without rebound or guarding, ⊖ Murphy's, ⊕ BS, no organomegaly or masses. No evidence of ascites.*
Extremities: *No asterixis, no edema.*
Skin: *Jaundice, excoriations due to scratching, no spiders/telangiectasias/palmar erythema.*

Differential Diagnosis

1. *Extrahepatic biliary obstruction:*
   Pancreatic cancer
   Choledocholithiasis
   Cholangiocarcinoma
   Carcinoma of the ampulla
   Sphincter of Oddi dysfunction
2. *Viral hepatitis*
3. *Acetaminophen liver toxicity*
4. *Alcoholic hepatitis*
5. *Primary biliary cirrhosis*

Diagnostic Workup

1. *AST/ALT/bilirubin/alkaline phosphatase*
2. *CBC*
3. *PT/PTT*
4. *Viral hepatitis serologies*
5. *Acetaminophen level*
6. *U/S—abdomen*
7. *CT—abdomen*
8. *MRCP/ERCP*

CASE DISCUSSION

Differential Diagnosis

Jaundice results from hyperbilirubinemia, the cause of which may be hepatic or nonhepatic. The presence of a change in stool and urine color excludes unconjugated hyperbilirubinemia (eg, that associated with hemolysis or Gilbert syndrome). Thus, the predominantly conjugated hyperbilirubinemia suspected in this patient may be due to hepatocellular disease, drugs, sepsis, hereditary disorders such as Dubin-Johnson syndrome, or extrahepatic biliary obstruction. Cholangitis is ruled out by the absence of fever and chills associated with episodes of abdominal pain.

- **Extrahepatic biliary obstruction:** The patient's family history puts her at increased risk for pancreatic cancer, which classically presents with painless jaundice. However, her intermittent pain (suggesting intermittent biliary obstruction) narrows the differential to choledocholithiasis (stone in the common bile duct), cholangiocarcinoma, carcinoma of the ampulla, or sphincter of Oddi dysfunction.

- **Viral hepatitis:** The patient is at risk for hepatitis A (in light of her trip to Mexico) and chronic hepatitis C (remote blood transfusion). The intermittent nature of her RUQ pain makes acute hepatitis less likely.

- **Acetaminophen liver toxicity:** This should be suspected in acute liver injury; even moderate amounts of acetaminophen may overwhelm the metabolic capacity of a damaged liver (usually in alcoholics and in patients with chronic hepatitis or cirrhosis).

- **Alcoholic hepatitis:** The patient's symptoms are consistent with this diagnosis. Hepatomegaly is often present. Although she reports drinking only one or two glasses of wine daily, patients often underreport alcohol consumption.

- **Primary biliary cirrhosis:** This usually occurs in women aged 40–60 years, often with pruritus as a presenting symptom. However, jaundice is usually a late finding and is not associated with RUQ pain.

Diagnostic Workup

- **AST/ALT/bilirubin/alkaline phosphatase:** These levels can help differentiate a hepatocellular process (primarily associated with increased AST and ALT) from a cholestatic process (primarily associated with increased bilirubin and alkaline phosphatase).

- **CBC:** A low platelet count is often seen in chronic liver disease, due to portal hypertension and subsequent splenomegaly.

- **PT/PTT:** A coagulopathy is often seen in advanced liver disease, due to synthetic dysfunction and subsequent clotting factor deficiencies.

- **Viral hepatitis serologies:** Hepatitis A IgM antibody should be checked to document recent infection. Other screening tests include hepatitis B surface antigen and hepatitis C antibody.

- **Acetaminophen level:** Used to diagnose acetaminophen overdose.

- **U/S—abdomen:** Used to diagnose biliary obstruction, stones, or intrahepatic tumors.

- **CT—abdomen:** A CT scan provides information similar to that above but is more expensive.

- **MRCP/ERCP:** Can identify the cause, location, and extent of biliary obstruction. ERCP is invasive but has the advantage of being both a diagnostic and a therapeutic tool in many cases. MRCP is a noninvasive MRI-based diagnostic substitute.

CASE 12
DOORWAY INFORMATION

Opening Scenario

Virginia Black, a 65-year-old female, comes to the clinic complaining of forgetfulness and confusion.

Vital Signs

BP: 135/90 mm Hg

Temp: 98.0°F (36.7°C)

RR: 16/minute

HR: 76/minute, regular

Examinee Tasks

1. Take a focused history.

2. Perform a focused physical exam (do not perform rectal, genitourinary, or female breast exam).

3. Explain your clinical impression and workup plan to the patient.

4. Write the patient note after leaving the room.

Checklist/SP Sheet

Patient Description

Patient is a 65 yo F, widowed with one daughter.

Notes for the SP

- The examinee will name three objects for you and ask you to recall them after a few minutes. Pretend that you are unable to do so.

- If asked, give the examinee a list of your current medications (a piece of paper with "nitroglycerin patch, hydrochlorothiazide, and aspirin" written on it).

- Pretend that you have some weakness in your left arm.

- Show an increase in DTRs of the left arm and leg.

Challenging Questions to Ask

"Do you think I have Alzheimer disease?"

Sample Examinee Response

"At this time I don't know; we still need to run some tests. Are you concerned about having Alzheimer disease?"

Examinee Checklist

Building the Doctor-Patient Relationship

Entrance

☐ Examinee knocked on the door before entering.

☐ Examinee introduced self by name.

☐ Examinee identified his/her role or position.

☐ Examinee correctly used patient's name.

☐ Examinee made eye contact with the SP.

Reflective Listening

☐ Examinee asked an open-ended question and actively listened to the response.

☐ Examinee asked the SP to list his/her concerns and listened to the response without interrupting.

☐ Examinee summarized the SP's concerns, often using the SP's own words.

Information Gathering

☐ Examinee elicited data efficiently and accurately.

☑ Question	Patient Response
☐ Chief complaint	Difficulty remembering things.
☐ Onset	I can't remember exactly, but my daughter told me that I started forgetting last year.
☐ Progression	My daughter has told me that it is getting worse.
☐ Things that are difficult to remember	Turning off the stove, my phone number, my keys, the way home, the names of my friends.
☐ Daily activities (bathing, feeding, toileting, dressing, transferring into and out of chairs and bed)	I have some trouble with these, and I need help sometimes.
☐ Shopping	Well, I stopped shopping, since I've lost my way home so many times. My daughter shops for me.
☐ Cooking	I stopped cooking because I often leave the stove on and accidentally started a fire once.
☐ Housework	I live with my daughter and she does most of it.
☐ Paying the bills	My daughter does this for me.
☐ Gait problems	No.
☐ Urinary incontinence	No.
☐ Feeling (sad, depressed)	I feel upset because of all of this.
☐ Difficulty sleeping	No.
☐ Headaches	No.
☐ Lightheadedness or feeling faint	Only if I stand up too quickly.
☐ Passing out	No.
☐ Falls	Yes, sometimes.
☐ Head trauma	I think so; I had a large bruise on the side of my head a while back.
☐ Did you see a doctor for that fall?	No, it was just a bruise.

☑ Question	Patient Response
☐ Any shaking or seizures	No.
☐ Visual changes	No.
☐ Weakness/numbness/paresthesias	Yes, I have weakness in my left arm from a stroke I had a long time ago.
☐ Speech difficulties	No.
☐ Heart problems	I had a heart attack a long time ago.
☐ Chest pain, shortness of breath, abdominal pain, nausea/vomiting, diarrhea/constipation	No.
☐ Weight changes	I've lost weight. I don't know how much.
☐ Appetite changes	I don't have an appetite.
☐ High blood pressure	Yes, for a long time.
☐ Current medications	I don't know their names. (Give the list to the examinee if he asks for it.)
☐ Past medical history	I think that's enough, isn't it?
☐ Past surgical history	I had a bowel obstruction a long time ago, and they removed part of my intestine.
☐ Family history	My father and mother died healthy a long time ago.
☐ Occupation	I retired after the death of my husband.
☐ Alcohol use	No.
☐ Illicit drug use	No.
☐ Tobacco	No.
☐ Social history	I live with my daughter.
☐ Sexual activity	Not since the death of my husband one year ago.
☐ Support systems (family, friends)	I have many friends who care about me, besides my daughter.
☐ Drug allergies	No.

Connecting with the Patient

☐ Examinee recognized the SP's emotions and responded with PEARLS.

Physical Examination

☐ Examinee washed his/her hands.

☐ Examinee asked permission to start the exam.

☐ Examinee used respectful draping.

☐ Examinee did not repeat painful maneuvers.

☑ Exam Component	Maneuver
☐ Eye exam	Inspected pupils, fundus
☐ Neck exam	Carotid auscultation
☐ CV exam	Auscultation, orthostatic vital signs
☐ Pulmonary exam	Auscultation
☐ Abdominal exam	Palpation
☐ Neurologic exam	Mini-mental status exam, cranial nerves, motor exam, DTRs, gait, Romberg sign, sensory exam

Closure

☐ Examinee discussed initial diagnostic impressions.

☐ Examinee discussed initial management plans:

    ☐ Follow-up tests.

    ☐ Need to obtain history directly from other family members.

    ☐ Need to evaluate home safety and supervision.

    ☐ Need to obtain community resources to help the patient at home.

☐ Examinee offered support throughout the illness.

☐ Examinee asked if the SP had any other questions or concerns.

Sample Closure

Mrs. Black, your symptoms can be due to a number of disorders that can affect the brain, many of which are treatable. We need to run some tests to identify the cause of your problem. I would also like to ask your permission to speak with your family. They can help me with your diagnosis, and I can answer any questions they might have about what is happening to you and how they can help. I would also like you and your family to meet with the social worker to assess at-home supervision and safety measures. The social worker will inform you of resources that are available in the community to help you. If you would like, I can remain in close contact with you and your family to provide additional help and support. Do you have any questions for me?

Patient Note

History

_____
_____
_____
_____
_____
_____
_____
_____
_____

Physical Examination

_____
_____
_____
_____
_____
_____
_____
_____
_____
_____
_____

Differential Diagnosis

1. _____
2. _____
3. _____
4. _____
5. _____

Diagnostic Workup

1. _____
2. _____
3. _____
4. _____
5. _____

Patient Note

History

HPI: *65 yo F c/o difficulty remembering × 1 year, after death of husband.*

- *Progressively worsening memory.*
- *Affects daily activities (bathing, feeding, toileting, dressing, transferring into and out of chairs and bed, shopping, cooking, managing money, using the telephone, cleaning the house).*
- *Transient orthostatic lightheadedness with frequent falls, 1 head injury without medical attention.*
- *Upset due to memory difficulty.*
- *Weight loss, no appetite.*
- *No headache, visual changes, gait problems, difficulty sleeping, or urinary incontinence.*

ROS: *Residual weakness in left arm after a stroke.*

Allergies: *NKDA.*

Medications: *HCTZ, aspirin, transdermal nitroglycerin.*

PMH: *Hypertension, stroke, MI. The patient cannot remember exactly when she had them.*

PSH: *Partial bowel resection due to obstruction many years ago.*

SH: *No smoking, no EtOH, no illicit drugs. She is a widow, is retired, lives with her daughter, and has a good support system (family, friends).*

FH: *Noncontributory.*

Physical Examination

Patient is in no acute distress.

VS: *WNL, no orthostatic changes.*

HEENT: *Normocephalic, atraumatic, PERRLA, no funduscopic abnormalities.*

Neck: *Supple, no carotid bruits.*

Chest: *Clear breath sounds bilaterally.*

Heart: *RRR; normal S1/S2; no murmurs, rubs, or gallops.*

Abdomen: *Soft, nondistended, nontender, no hepatosplenomegaly.*

Neuro: *Mental status: Alert and oriented × 3, spells backward but can't recall 3 objects. Cranial nerves: 2–12 intact. Motor: Strength 5/5 in all muscle groups except 3/5 in left arm. DTRs: Asymmetric 3+ in left upper and lower extremities, 1+ in the right, ⊖ Babinski bilaterally. Cerebellar: ⊖ Romberg. Gait: Normal. Sensation: Intact to pinprick and soft touch.*

Differential Diagnosis

1. *Alzheimer disease*
2. *Vascular ("multi-infarct") dementia*
3. *Depression with pseudodementia*
4. *Hypothyroidism*
5. *Vitamin B_{12} deficiency*
6. *Subdural hematoma*

Diagnostic Workup

1. *CBC*
2. *Electrolytes, calcium, glucose, BUN/Cr*
3. *Serum B_{12}, TSH, RPR*
4. *CT—head or MRI—brain*
5. *EEG or SPECT*

CASE DISCUSSION

Differential Diagnosis

Dementia is an acquired, progressive impairment in cognitive function that includes amnesia plus some degree of aphasia, apraxia, agnosia, and/or impaired executive function. It is critical to obtain additional history from nondemented family members to establish an accurate time course of cognitive decline. The dementia syndromes are primarily clinical diagnoses reached after any partially reversible causes have been excluded.

- **Alzheimer disease:** This is the most common cause of dementia. It usually has an insidious onset, with steady, progressive decline in cognitive function over years. The earliest findings are impairment in memory and visuospatial abilities. Alzheimer disease is a clinical diagnosis.

- **Vascular ("multi-infarct") dementia:** This often coexists with Alzheimer disease, and given the patient's history of atherosclerotic vascular disease (eg, stroke, MI), it could certainly be contributing in this case. There is classically more of a stepwise deterioration in vascular dementia compared to the steady cognitive decline seen in Alzheimer. Also, there may be an earlier loss of executive function and personality changes in vascular dementia.

- **Depression with pseudodementia:** The time course of cognitive decline following the death of the patient's husband may indicate depression, which can present atypically in the elderly and may mimic or, more commonly, coexist with dementia. However, it is more likely that her cognitive decline has been progressive for several years but became more noticeable to her children after her husband died.

- **Hypothyroidism:** This can cause neuropsychiatric symptoms (often a late finding) and must be ruled out in patients with dementia. However, there are no classic signs or symptoms to suggest hypothyroidism in this case.

- **Vitamin B$_{12}$ deficiency:** A prior bowel resection (eg, of the terminal ileum) may put the patient at risk for this deficiency. It can cause depression, irritability, paranoia, confusion, and dementia but is usually associated with other neurologic symptoms, such as paresthesias and leg weakness. On occasion, dementia may precede the characteristic megaloblastic anemia.

- **Subdural hematoma:** This should be ruled out given the patient's history of falls and head trauma. Even though her cognitive decline spans at least a year, it is possible that a comorbid chronic subdural hematoma could have exacerbated her mental status changes in recent weeks or months.

Diagnostic Workup

- **CBC:** Used to look for macrocytic anemia in vitamin B$_{12}$ deficiency.

- **Electrolytes, calcium, glucose, BUN/Cr:** To screen for medical conditions that can present with cognitive dysfunction (eg, hypernatremia, hypercalcemia, hyperglycemia, uremia).

- **Serum B$_{12}$, TSH, RPR:** To screen for partially reversible causes of dementia (RPR can be restricted to patients who manifest signs of neurosyphilis).

- **CT—head:** Used to look for a crescent-shaped, hyperdense extra-axial mass in subdural hematoma, intracerebral masses, strokes, or dilated ventricles (as in normal pressure hydrocephalus).

- **MRI—brain:** The most sensitive exam to look for focal CNS lesions or atrophy.

- **EEG or SPECT:** Used in rare cases to help differentiate delirium from depression or dementia.

Opening Scenario

Raymond Stern, a 56-year-old male, comes to the clinic for diabetes follow-up.

Vital Signs

BP: 139/85 mm Hg

Temp: 98.0°F (36.7°C)

RR: 15/minute

HR: 75/minute, regular

Examinee Tasks

1. Take a focused history.

2. Perform a focused physical exam (do not perform rectal, genitourinary, or female breast exam).

3. Explain your clinical impression and workup plan to the patient.

4. Write the patient note after leaving the room.

Checklist/SP Sheet

Patient Description

Patient is a 56 yo M.

Notes for the SP

- Pretend that you have a loss of sharp and dull sensations, vibration sense, and position sense in both feet ("stocking" distribution).
- Pretend to have a normal knee jerk and absent ankle reflex.

Challenging Questions to Ask

"Will I lose my feet, doctor?"

Sample Examinee Response

"Amputation is a last resort in patients with diabetes who develop an infection in their feet, and, fortunately, we are not at that point. The nerve damage to your feet is uncomfortable, but it alone will not lead to amputation as long as you take the proper measures to protect your feet from injury. If we continue to keep your blood sugars and cholesterol well controlled, we should be able to avoid amputation. We'll discuss more on how to do that later in the visit."

Examinee Checklist

Building the Doctor-Patient Relationship

Entrance

☐ Examinee knocked on the door before entering.

☐ Examinee introduced self by name.

☐ Examinee identified his/her role or position.

☐ Examinee correctly used patient's name.

☐ Examinee made eye contact with the SP.

Reflective Listening

☐ Examinee asked an open-ended question and actively listened to the response.

☐ Examinee asked the SP to list his/her concerns and listened to the response without interrupting.

☐ Examinee summarized the SP's concerns, often using the SP's own words.

Information Gathering

☐ Examinee elicited data efficiently and accurately.

☑ Question	Patient Response
☐ Chief complaint	I am here for a diabetes checkup. The last time I saw my doctor was six months ago.
☐ Onset	I have had diabetes mellitus for the past 25 years.
☐ Treatment	NPH insulin, 20 units in the morning and 15 units in the evening.
☐ Compliance with medications	I never miss any doses.
☐ Last blood sugar reading	Three days ago, and it was 135.
☐ Blood sugar monitoring	I have a blood sugar monitor at home, and I check my blood sugar twice a week. It usually ranges between 120 and 145.
☐ Last HbA$_{1c}$	The last was six months ago, and it was 7.
☐ Last time eyes were checked	One year ago, and there were no signs of diabetic eye disease.
☐ How he is feeling today	Good.
☐ Medication side effects	No.
☐ Heart symptoms (chest pain, palpitations)	Sometimes I feel my heart racing, and I start sweating.
☐ Description of these symptoms	It happens rarely if I miss a meal. I feel better after drinking orange juice.
☐ Pulmonary complaints (shortness of breath, cough)	No.
☐ Neurologic complaints (headaches, dizziness, weakness, numbness)	I have tingling and numbness in my feet all the time, especially at night; it's gotten worse over the past two months.
☐ Polyuria, dysuria, hematuria	No.
☐ Abdominal complaints (pain, dyspepsia, nausea)	No.
☐ Change in bowel habits	No.
☐ Visual problems (blurred vision)	No.
☐ Foot infection	No.

Reflective Listening

☐ Examinee asked an open-ended question and actively listened to the response.

☐ Examinee asked the SP to list his/her concerns and listened to the response without interrupting.

☐ Examinee summarized the SP's concerns, often using the SP's own words.

Information Gathering

☐ Examinee elicited data efficiently and accurately.

☑ Question	Patient Response
☐ Chief complaint	I feel dizzy.
☐ Describe the meaning of dizziness	Well, I feel as if the room were spinning around me.
☐ Onset	Two days ago.
☐ Progression	It is getting worse.
☐ Constant/intermittent	It comes and goes.
☐ Duration	It lasts for 20–30 minutes.
☐ Timing	It can happen anytime.
☐ Positions that can elicit the dizziness (lying down, sitting, standing up)	When I get up from bed or lie down to sleep, but as I said, it can happen anytime.
☐ Positions that can relieve the dizziness	None.
☐ Tinnitus	No.
☐ Hearing loss (which ear, when)	Yes, I have difficulty hearing you in my left ear. This started yesterday.
☐ Fullness or pressure in the ears	No.
☐ Discharge from the ears	No.
☐ Falls	No, sometimes I feel unsteady as if I were going to fall down, but I don't fall.
☐ Nausea/vomiting	Yes, I feel nauseated, and I vomited several times.
☐ Recent infections	I have had really bad diarrhea. I've had it for the past three days, but it is much better today.
☐ Fever	No.
☐ Description of stool	It was a watery diarrhea with no blood.
☐ Abdominal pain	No.
☐ URI (runny nose, sore throat, cough)	No.
☐ Headaches	No.
☐ Head trauma	No.
☐ Current medications	Furosemide, captopril.

☑ Question	Patient Response
☐ Past medical history	High blood pressure, diagnosed seven years ago.
☐ Past surgical history	Appendectomy.
☐ Family history	No similar problem in the family.
☐ Occupation	Executive director of an insurance company.
☐ Alcohol use	Yes, I drink 2–3 beers a week.
☐ Illicit drug use	No.
☐ Tobacco	No.
☐ Sexual activity	Yes, with my wife.
☐ Drug allergies	No.

Connecting with the Patient

☐ Examinee recognized the SP's emotions and responded with PEARLS.

Physical Examination

☐ Examinee washed his/her hands.

☐ Examinee asked permission to start the exam.

☐ Examinee used respectful draping.

☐ Examinee did not repeat painful maneuvers.

☑ Exam Component	Maneuver
☐ HEENT	Inspected for nystagmus, funduscopic exam, otoscopy, assessed hearing, Rinne and Weber tests, inspected mouth and throat
☐ CV exam	Auscultation, orthostatic vital signs
☐ Neurologic exam	Cranial nerves, motor exam, DTRs, gait, Romberg sign, tilt test (eg, Dix-Hallpike maneuver)

Closure

☐ Examinee discussed initial diagnostic impressions.

☐ Examinee discussed initial management plans:

    ☐ Follow-up tests.

☐ Examinee asked if the SP had any other questions or concerns.

Sample Closure

Mr. Albright, the dizziness you are experiencing may be due to a problem in your ears or brain, or it may result from low blood pressure. We will have to run some tests to pinpoint the source of your symptoms. These may include blood tests, a hearing evaluation, and an MRI that will provide detailed images of your brain. Until we find the cause of your problem, it is important that you are careful when you stand up quickly or walk unaccompanied, and you should be sure to make use of hand railings whenever possible. Do you have any questions for me?

Patient Note

History

_____
_____
_____
_____
_____
_____
_____
_____
_____

Physical Examination

_____
_____
_____
_____
_____
_____
_____
_____
_____
_____
_____
_____

Differential Diagnosis

1. _____

2. _____

3. _____

4. _____

5. _____

Diagnostic Workup

1. _____

2. _____

3. _____

4. _____

5. _____

History

HPI: *53 yo M c/o intermittent dizziness × 2 days.*

- *Sensation of room spinning around him.*
- *Occurs during day when getting up or lying down.*
- *Episodes last 20–30 minutes and are progressively getting worse.*
- *Left-sided hearing loss since yesterday.*
- *Nausea and vomiting.*
- *Watery, nonbloody diarrhea × 3 days that has since resolved.*
- *No tinnitus, fullness in ear, ear discharge, headache, or head trauma.*
- *No recent URI.*

ROS: *Negative except as above.*

Allergies: *NKDA.*

Medications: *Furosemide, captopril.*

PMH: *Hypertension, diagnosed 7 years ago.*

PSH: *Appendectomy.*

SH: *No smoking, 2–3 beers/week, no illicit drugs.*

FH: *Noncontributory.*

Physical Examination

Patient is in no acute distress.

VS: *WNL, no orthostatic changes.*

HEENT: *NC/AT, PERRLA, EOMI without nystagmus, no papilledema, no cerumen, TMs normal, mouth and oropharynx normal.*

Heart: *RRR; normal S1/S2; no murmurs, rubs, or gallops.*

Neuro: *Cranial nerves: 2–12 grossly intact except for decreased hearing acuity in the left ear. ⊕ Rinne (air conduction > bone conduction on the left), Weber no lateralization, ⊖ tilt test. Motor: Strength 5/5 throughout. DTRs: 2+ intact, symmetric, ⊖ Babinski bilaterally. Cerebellar: ⊖ Romberg, finger to nose normal. Gait: Normal.*

Differential Diagnosis

1. *Ménière disease*
2. *Orthostatic hypotension due to dehydration*
3. *Benign paroxysmal positional vertigo*
4. *Labyrinthitis*
5. *Perilymphatic fistula*
6. *Acoustic neuroma*

Diagnostic Workup

1. *Dix-Hallpike maneuver*
2. *VDRL/RPR*
3. *Audiometry*
4. *MRI—brain*
5. *Brain stem auditory evoked potentials*
6. *Electronystagmography*

CASE DISCUSSION

Differential Diagnosis

Vertigo signals vestibular disease, whereas lightheadedness and dysequilibrium are usually nonvestibular in origin. A central vestibular system lesion (eg, vertebrobasilar insufficiency, brain stem and cerebellar tumors, MS) is unlikely in this patient given the presence of hearing loss and an otherwise normal neurologic exam. Vertigo syndromes due to peripheral lesions are discussed below. These cases are often accompanied by nausea and vomiting, and vertigo may be so severe that the patient is unable to walk or stand.

- **Ménière disease:** This classically presents with episodic vertigo (usually lasting 1–8 hours) and low-frequency hearing loss as well as with features not seen in this case, such as tinnitus and a sensation of aural fullness. Symptoms result from distention of the endolymphatic compartment of the inner ear. Syphilis and head trauma are two known causes.

- **Orthostatic hypotension due to dehydration:** Risk factors for dehydration in this case include diarrhea and loop diuretic use. However, the patient does not complain of lightheadedness and is not objectively orthostatic.

- **Benign paroxysmal positional vertigo (BPPV):** This describes transient vertigo following changes in head position but is not associated with hearing loss.

- **Labyrinthitis:** This frequently follows a viral infection (usually URI) and is accompanied by hearing loss and tinnitus, but vertigo is usually continuous and lasts several days to a week.

- **Perilymphatic fistula:** This is a rare cause of vertigo and sensorineural hearing loss, usually resulting from head trauma or extensive barotrauma. Episodes of vertigo are fleeting, generally lasting seconds.

- **Acoustic neuroma:** Acoustic neuroma more commonly causes continuous dysequilibrium rather than episodic vertigo. As noted above, central lesions are unlikely in patients with vertigo, hearing loss, and an otherwise normal neurologic exam. However, an intracranial mass lesion must be ruled out in any patient with unilateral hearing loss.

Diagnostic Workup

- **Dix-Hallpike maneuver:** Used to diagnose BPPV (look for nystagmus, reproduction of vertigo).
- **VDRL/RPR:** To rule out syphilis, which can cause Ménière disease.
- **Audiometry:** Used to assess hearing function.
- **MRI—brain:** Required for the evaluation of central vestibular lesions.
- **Brain stem auditory evoked potentials:** Used to help diagnose central vestibular disease.
- **Electronystagmography:** Used to document characteristics of nystagmus that may differentiate central from peripheral vestibular system lesions.

CASE 15
DOORWAY INFORMATION

Opening Scenario

Gary Mitchell, a 46-year-old male, comes to the office complaining of fatigue.

Vital Signs

BP: 120/85 mm Hg

Temp: 98.2°F (36.8°C)

RR: 12/minute

HR: 65/minute, regular

Examinee Tasks

1. Take a focused history.

2. Perform a focused physical exam (do not perform rectal, genitourinary, or female breast exam).

3. Explain your clinical impression and workup plan to the patient.

4. Write the patient note after leaving the room.

Checklist/SP Sheet

Patient Description

Patient is a 46 yo M.

Notes for the SP

- Look sad, and don't smile.
- Speak and move slowly.
- Start yawning as the examinee enters the room.

Challenging Questions to Ask

- "I think that life is full of misery. Why do we have to live?"
- "I am afraid that I might have AIDS."

Sample Examinee Response

This patient clearly has more to say. Silence is appropriate here, or some small encouragement for the patient to continue talking. Alternatively, say, "It sounds as if you're losing hope. Have you thought about hurting yourself or tried to do so?" Or, "Tell me more about your concern about AIDS."

Examinee Checklist

Building the Doctor-Patient Relationship

Entrance

☐ Examinee knocked on the door before entering.

☐ Examinee introduced self by name.

☐ Examinee identified his/her role or position.

☐ Examinee correctly used patient's name.

☐ Examinee made eye contact with the SP.

Reflective Listening

☐ Examinee asked an open-ended question and actively listened to the response.

☐ Examinee asked the SP to list his/her concerns and listened to the response without interrupting.

☐ Examinee summarized the SP's concerns, often using the SP's own words.

Information Gathering

☐ Examinee elicited data efficiently and accurately.

☐ Examinee explored the SP's concern about AIDS (eg, "Tell me more about that.").

☑ Question	Patient Response
☐ Chief complaint	Feeling tired, no energy.
☐ Onset	Three months ago.
☐ Associated events	I was in a car accident, and I failed to save my friend from the car before it blew up.
☐ Injuries related to the accident	No.
☐ Progression of the fatigue during the day	Same throughout the day.
☐ Affecting job/performance	Yes, I can't concentrate on my work anymore. I don't have the energy to work.
☐ Appetite changes	Loss of appetite.
☐ Weight changes	I have gained 6 pounds over the past three months.
☐ Feeling of depression	Yes, I feel sad and depressed all the time.
☐ Suicidal thoughts/plans/attempts	I think of death sometimes but have had no plans or attempts.
☐ Feelings of blame or guilt	No, it was an accident. I tried to help my friend but couldn't.
☐ Sleeping problems (falling asleep, staying asleep, early waking)	Well, I don't have problems falling asleep, but I wake up sometimes because of nightmares. I always see the accident, my friend calling for help, and the car blowing up. I feel so scared and helpless. I wake up very early in the morning and feel sleepy all day.
☐ Snoring	Yes.
☐ Loss of concentration	Yes, I can't concentrate on my work.
☐ Associated symptoms (fever, chills, chest pain, shortness of breath, abdominal pain, diarrhea/constipation)	No.
☐ Cold intolerance	Yes.
☐ Skin/hair changes	My hair is falling out more than usual.
☐ Current medications	None.

☑ Question	Patient Response
☐ Past medical history	Well, I had some burning during urination. I don't really remember the diagnosis that the doctor reached, but it started with the letter C. I took antibiotics for one week. This was five months ago.
☐ Past surgical history	None.
☐ Family history	My parents are alive and in good health.
☐ Occupation	Accountant.
☐ Alcohol use	Two to three beers a month.
☐ Illicit drug use	Never.
☐ Tobacco	One pack a day for 25 years.
☐ Exercise	No.
☐ Diet	The usual. I haven't changed anything in my diet in more than 10 years.
☐ Sexual activity	Not interested anymore. I have a girlfriend, and we have been together for the past six months. I don't use condoms because they make me feel uncomfortable. I have had several sexual partners in the past.
☐ Drug allergies	No.

Connecting with the Patient

☐ Examinee recognized the SP's emotions and responded with PEARLS.

Physical Examination

☐ Examinee washed his/her hands.

☐ Examinee asked permission to start the exam.

☐ Examinee used respectful draping.

☐ Examinee did not repeat painful maneuvers.

☑ Exam Component	Maneuver
☐ Head and neck exam	Inspected conjunctivae, mouth and throat, lymph nodes; examined thyroid gland
☐ CV exam	Auscultation
☐ Pulmonary exam	Auscultation
☐ Abdominal exam	Auscultation, palpation, percussion
☐ Extremities	Inspection, checked DTRs

Closure

☐ Examinee discussed initial diagnostic impressions.

☐ Examinee discussed initial management plans:

    ☐ Follow-up tests.

    ☐ Lifestyle modification (diet, exercise, relaxation techniques, smoking cessation).

    ☐ Safe sex practices.

    ☐ HIV testing and consent.

    ☐ Depression counseling:

        ☐ Sources of support (eg, trusted friends and loved ones) and information about community groups.

        ☐ Possible need for referral to a psychiatrist.

        ☐ Suicide contract (ie, contact your physician or go to the ED for any suicidal thoughts or plans).

☐ Examinee asked if the SP had any other questions or concerns.

Sample Closure

Mr. Mitchell, it appears that your life has been very stressful lately, and my suspicion is that you may be clinically depressed. Before I make a definitive diagnosis, however, I would like to order some blood tests, including one for HIV, as you have risk factors for sexually transmitted diseases. Depending on the results of these tests, I may also ask you to participate in a sleep study, in which doctors can observe how you breathe while you are sleeping. Once we have completed these tests, we should have a better idea of what is causing your fatigue. In the meantime, I strongly recommend that you quit smoking, exercise regularly, and participate in activities that you find relaxing. I would also like you to promise me that if you feel like hurting yourself, you will call someone who can help you or go immediately to an emergency department. Do you have any questions for me?

Patient Note

History

_____
_____
_____
_____
_____
_____
_____
_____
_____

Physical Examination

_____
_____
_____
_____
_____
_____
_____
_____
_____
_____
_____

Differential Diagnosis

1. _____

2. _____

3. _____

4. _____

5. _____

Diagnostic Workup

1. _____

2. _____

3. _____

4. _____

5. _____

Patient Note

History

HPI: *46 yo M c/o fatigue × 3 months.*

- *Fatigue began after unsuccessful attempt to save his friend after a car accident.*
- *Constant fatigue throughout the day.*
- *Low energy.*
- *Decreased concentration, which is negatively affecting job as accountant.*
- *Decreased appetite but gained 6 lbs.*
- *Early awakening and difficulty staying asleep due to recurrent nightmares about accident.*
- *Feels sleepy throughout the day.*
- *Feelings of being depressed and helpless.*
- *Suicidal ideation but no suicide plans/attempts.*
- *Snores.*
- *Cold intolerance.*
- *Hair loss.*
- *Loss of interest in sex.*
- *No constipation.*
- *No feelings of blame or guilt.*

ROS: *Negative except as above.*
Allergies: *NKDA.*
Medications: *None.*
PMH: *Urethritis (possibly chlamydia), treated 5 months ago.*
SH: *1 PPD for 25 years, 2 beers/month. History of unprotected sex with multiple female partners.*
FH: *Noncontributory.*

Physical Examination

Patient is in no acute distress, looks tired with a flat affect, speaks and moves slowly.
VS: *WNL.*
HEENT: *No conjunctival pallor, mouth and pharynx WNL.*
Neck: *No lymphadenopathy, thyroid normal.*
Chest: *Clear breath sounds bilaterally.*
Heart: *RRR; normal S1/S2; no murmurs, rubs, or gallops.*
Abdomen: *Soft, nondistended, nontender, ⊕ BS, no hepatosplenomegaly.*
Extremities: *No edema, normal DTRs in lower extremities.*

Differential Diagnosis

1. *Depression*
2. *Adjustment disorder with depressed mood*
3. *Hypothyroidism*
4. *Obstructive sleep apnea*
5. *Post-traumatic stress disorder*
6. *HIV infection*

Diagnostic Workup

1. *CBC*
2. *TSH*
3. *Ambulatory nocturnal pulse oximetry*
4. *Polysomnography*
5. *HIV antibody*
6. *MRI—brain*

CASE DISCUSSION

Differential Diagnosis

Fatigue is a common, nonspecific complaint with many etiologies ranging from simple overexertion to serious diseases such as cancer.

- **Depression:** Many classic symptoms are present in this patient. The mnemonic **SIG E CAPS** helps recall them: **S**leep disturbance, decreased **I**nterest, feelings of **G**uilt, decreased **E**nergy/depressed mood, decreased **C**oncentration, change in **A**ppetite, **P**sychomotor agitation or slowing, and **S**uicidal ideation.

- **Adjustment disorder with depressed mood:** The stress of witnessing a friend's death may lead to maladaptive behavior, with depression as the predominant symptom.

- **Hypothyroidism:** This should be ruled out in a patient with fatigue for months. The cold intolerance, hair loss, and weight gain are additional nonspecific symptoms that suggest this diagnosis.

- **Obstructive sleep apnea:** Although the patient snores, this diagnosis is less likely given that his excessive daytime somnolence is occurring in the context of many other depressive symptoms. Nonetheless, obstructive sleep apnea is common and underdiagnosed, and it does occur in nonobese patients.

- **Post-traumatic stress disorder (PTSD):** This is characterized by (1) reexperiencing a traumatic event (eg, flashbacks); (2) avoidance of stimuli associated with the trauma; and (3) increased arousal (eg, anxiety, sleep disturbance, hypervigilance). Despite having nightmares about the accident, this patient does not sufficiently manifest the last two features of the disorder.

- **HIV infection:** Given his history of STDs, the patient should also be tested for this. However, it is highly unlikely that HIV infection accounts for his current depression (unless there are frontal lobe lesions due to infection or malignancy).

Diagnostic Workup

- **CBC:** To rule out anemia.
- **TSH:** A screening test for hypothyroidism.
- **Ambulatory nocturnal pulse oximetry:** An initial test to evaluate possible obstructive sleep apnea.
- **Polysomnography:** To diagnose obstructive sleep apnea.
- **HIV antibody:** To rule out HIV infection.
- **MRI—brain:** To rule out the exceedingly rare possibility that the patient's symptoms are due to an intracranial mass lesion.

Opening Scenario

Jessica Lee, a 32-year-old female, comes to the office complaining of fatigue.

Vital Signs

BP: 120/85 mm Hg

Temp: 98.2°F (36.8°C)

RR: 13/minute

HR: 80/minute, regular

Examinee Tasks

1. Take a focused history.

2. Perform a focused physical exam (do not perform rectal, genitourinary, or female breast exam).

3. Explain your clinical impression and workup plan to the patient.

4. Write the patient note after leaving the room.

Checklist/SP Sheet

Patient Description

Patient is a 32 yo F, married with two children.

Notes for the SP

- Look anxious and pale.
- Exhibit bruises on the face and arms that elicit pain when touched.

Challenging Questions to Ask

"I am drinking a lot of water, doctor. What do you think the reason is?"

Sample Examinee Response

"At this point I don't know for sure, but I want to run some tests. Drinking a lot of water could be the first signs of diabetes and we will need to check for that."

Examinee Checklist

Building the Doctor-Patient Relationship

Entrance

☐ Examinee knocked on the door before entering.

☐ Examinee introduced self by name.

☐ Examinee identified his/her role or position.

☐ Examinee correctly used patient's name.

☐ Examinee made eye contact with the SP.

Reflective Listening

☐ Examinee asked an open-ended question and actively listened to the response.

☐ Examinee asked the SP to list his/her concerns and listened to the response without interrupting.

☐ Examinee summarized the SP's concerns, often using the SP's own words.

Information Gathering

☐ Examinee elicited data efficiently and accurately.

☑ Question	Patient Response
☐ Chief complaint	Feeling tired, weak, no energy.
☐ Onset	Five months ago.
☐ Associated events	None.
☐ Progression of the fatigue during the day	I feel okay in the morning; then gradually I start feeling more and more tired and weak.
☐ Change in vision (double vision) during the day	No.
☐ Affecting job/performance	Yes, I don't have energy to work.
☐ Appetite changes	I have a very good appetite.
☐ Weight changes	No.
☐ Feeling of depression	Sometimes I feel sad.
☐ Cause of bruises	I fell down the stairs and hurt myself (looks anxious). It is my fault. I don't always pay attention.
☐ Being physically or emotionally hurt or abused by anybody	Well, sometimes when my husband gets angry with me, but he loves me very much, and he promises not to do it again.
☐ Feeling safe/afraid at home	Sometimes I feel afraid, especially when my husband gets drunk.
☐ Are the children being abused or threatened?	Well, he slapped my younger son the other day for breaking a glass. He should be more attentive.
☐ Suicidal thoughts/plans/attempts	No.
☐ Feelings of blame or guilt	Yes, I think I am being awkward. It is my fault.
☐ Presence of guns at home	No.
☐ Any family members who know about the abuse	No.
☐ Emergency plan	No.
☐ Sleeping problems (falling asleep, staying asleep, early waking, snoring)	No.
☐ Loss of concentration	Yes, I can't concentrate on my work.
☐ Menstrual period	Regular and heavy; lasts seven days.
☐ Last menstrual period	Two weeks ago.

☑ Question	Patient Response
☐ Urinary symptoms	I recently started to wake up at night to urinate.
☐ Polyuria	Yes, I have to go to the bathroom more often during the day.
☐ Pain during urination or change in the color of urine	No.
☐ Polydipsia	Yes, I feel thirsty all the time, and I drink a lot of water.
☐ Associated symptoms (fever, chills, chest pain, shortness of breath, abdominal pain, diarrhea/constipation, cold intolerance, skin/hair changes)	None.
☐ Current medications	None.
☐ Past medical history	None.
☐ Past surgical history	I fell and broke my arm a year ago.
☐ Family history	My father had diabetes and died of a heart attack. My mother is in a nursing home with Alzheimer's.
☐ Occupation	Nurse.
☐ Alcohol use	No.
☐ Illicit drug use	Never.
☐ Tobacco	No.
☐ Exercise	No.
☐ Diet	I am a vegetarian.
☐ Sexual activity	I don't feel any desire for sex, but we do it when my husband wants.
☐ Drug allergies	No.

Connecting with the Patient

☐ Examinee recognized the SP's emotions and responded with PEARLS.

Physical Examination

☐ Examinee washed his/her hands.

☐ Examinee asked permission to start the exam.

☐ Examinee used respectful draping.

☐ Examinee did not repeat painful maneuvers.

☑ *Exam Component*	*Maneuver*
☐ Head and neck exam	Inspected conjunctivae, mouth and throat, lymph nodes; examined thyroid gland
☐ CV exam	Auscultation
☐ Pulmonary exam	Auscultation
☐ Abdominal exam	Auscultation, palpation, percussion
☐ Extremities	Inspection, motor exam, DTRs

Closure

☐ Examinee discussed initial diagnostic impressions.

☐ Examinee discussed initial management plans:

   ☐ Follow-up tests.

   ☐ Domestic violence counseling:

      ☐ "I care about your safety and I am always available for help and support."

      ☐ "Everything we discuss is confidential, but I must involve child protective services if your children are being abused."

      ☐ Support group information, including contact numbers or Web sites.

      ☐ Safety planning.

☐ Examinee asked if the SP had any other questions or concerns.

Sample Closure

Ms. Lee, I am concerned about your safety and your relationship with your husband. I would like you to know that I am available for help and support whenever you need it. Although everything we discuss is confidential, I must involve child protective services if I have reason to believe that your children are being abused. I will bring back some telephone numbers and contact information for you regarding where to go for help if you or your children are in a crisis or if you just want someone to talk to. I am also concerned about your frequent urination and thirst. I will run a simple blood test to see if you have any problems with your blood sugar or your hormones. Do you have any questions?

Patient Note

History

Physical Examination

Differential Diagnosis

1.
2.
3.
4.
5.

Diagnostic Workup

1.
2.
3.
4.
5.

History

HPI: *32 yo F c/o fatigue and weakness × 5 months.*

- *Fatigue increases throughout the day.*
- *Loss of energy and concentration, which is affecting job as nurse.*
- *Patient admits that husband, who is an alcoholic, has beaten her.*
- *At least 1 episode of physical abuse directed at youngest son.*
- *Patient attempts to defend husband's actions.*
- *Feels guilty.*
- *Self-blame.*
- *Has not reported abuse.*
- *No emergency plan.*
- *Feels sad but denies suicidal ideation.*
- *Polyuria, polydipsia, nocturia × 5 months.*
- *LMP 2 weeks ago, menstrual period is regular, q28 days, lasting 7 days of heavy flow.*
- *No dysuria or change in color of urine.*
- *No constipation, cold intolerance, or change in appetite or weight.*
- *No sleep problems.*

ROS: *Negative except as above.*
Allergies: *NKDA.*
Medications: *None.*
SH: *No smoking, no EtOH. Sexually active with her husband; decreased sexual desire.*
FH: *Diabetic father died from a heart attack; mother is in a nursing home with Alzheimer disease.*

Physical Examination

Patient is in no acute distress, looks anxious.
VS: *WNL.*
HEENT: *Pale conjunctivae.*
Neck: *No lymphadenopathy, thyroid normal.*
Chest: *Clear breath sounds bilaterally.*
Heart: *RRR; normal S1/S2; no murmurs, rubs, or gallops.*
Abdomen: *Soft, nondistended, nontender, ⊕ BS, no hepatosplenomegaly.*
Extremities: *Muscle strength 5/5 throughout; DTRs 2+; symmetric, painful bruises on both arms.*

Differential Diagnosis

1. *Domestic violence*
2. *Depression*
3. *Diabetes mellitus*
4. *Diabetes insipidus*
5. *Anemia*
6. *Myasthenia gravis*
7. *Hypothyroidism*

Diagnostic Workup

1. *CBC, iron level, TIBC, ferritin, serum B_{12}*
2. *Electrolytes*
3. *UA*
4. *Serum glucose, HbA_{1c}*
5. *TSH*
6. *MRI—brain (pituitary protocol)*
7. *DDAVP nasal spray test (vasopressin)*

CASE DISCUSSION

Differential Diagnosis

- **Domestic violence:** The patient is clearly a victim of domestic violence and of her husband's alcoholism. This can explain many of her symptoms but not the polyuria or polydipsia.

- **Depression:** As above, depression likely coexists but does not account for the patient's recent polyuria or polydipsia (if objectively verified).

- **Diabetes mellitus (DM):** Aside from domestic violence issues, many of the patient's symptoms can be explained by new-onset diabetes. Her positive family history puts her at risk. She should also be asked about any recent vaginal yeast infections, which are a frequent complication of hyperglycemia (and may be its initial presenting symptom).

- **Diabetes insipidus (DI):** This is an uncommon disease characterized by polyuria (of low specific gravity) and polydipsia. It has many etiologies and is caused by a deficiency of or resistance to vasopressin.

- **Anemia:** This may also help explain her fatigue and weakness. Menstruating females often have an iron deficiency anemia, and strict vegans may also have anemia related to vitamin B_{12} deficiency. Conjunctival pallor on exam has a high likelihood ratio for predicting a hematocrit < 30% (hemoglobin < 10 g/dL).

- **Myasthenia gravis:** Increasing fatigue as the day progresses is highly nonspecific. By contrast, this disease involves fluctuating muscle weakness and presents with ptosis, diplopia, difficulty chewing or swallowing, respiratory difficulties, and/or limb weakness.

- **Hypothyroidism:** Nonspecific symptoms such as fatigue and weakness may suggest this common diagnosis. However, hypothyroidism does not explain polyuria, polydipsia, or the admitted physical abuse.

Diagnostic Workup

- **CBC, iron level, TIBC, ferritin, serum B_{12}:** Blood tests to investigate anemia.
- **Electrolytes:** Hypernatremia may be seen in DI.
- **UA:** Dilute urine is seen in DI, glycosuria in DM.
- **Serum glucose, HbA_{1c}:** To screen for DM.
- **TSH:** Thyroid disease must be ruled out in a patient with symptoms of depression.
- **MRI—brain (pituitary protocol):** To look for mass lesions in central DI.
- **DDAVP nasal spray test ("vasopressin challenge test"):** To confirm a clinical suspicion of central DI.

Opening Scenario

William Jordan, a 61-year-old male, comes to the office complaining of fatigue.

Vital Signs

BP: 135/85 mm Hg

Temp: 98.6°F (37°C)

RR: 13/minute

HR: 70/minute, regular

Examinee Tasks

1. Take a focused history.

2. Perform a focused physical exam (do not perform rectal, genitourinary, or female breast exam).

3. Explain your clinical impression and workup plan to the patient.

4. Write the patient note after leaving the room.

Checklist/SP Sheet

Patient Description

Patient is a 61 yo M, married with three children.

Notes for the SP

- Look weak and sad, and sit leaning forward.
- Exhibit abdominal discomfort that increases when you lie on your back.
- Show pain on palpation of the epigastric area.

Challenging Questions to Ask

"I want to go on a trip with my wife. Can we do the tests after I come back?"

Sample Examinee Response

"It doesn't sound as if you're feeling well enough to be able to enjoy a trip. Let's do some initial blood tests, and then we can see how you're feeling and decide whether we're comfortable letting you go away."

Examinee Checklist

Building the Doctor-Patient Relationship

Entrance

☐ Examinee knocked on the door before entering.

☐ Examinee introduced self by name.

☐ Examinee identified his/her role or position.

☐ Examinee correctly used patient's name.

☐ Examinee made eye contact with the SP.

Reflective Listening

☐ Examinee asked an open-ended question and actively listened to the response.

☐ Examinee asked the SP to list his/her concerns and listened to the response without interrupting.

☐ Examinee summarized the SP's concerns, often using the SP's own words.

Information Gathering

☐ Examinee elicited data efficiently and accurately.

☑ Question	Patient Response
☐ Chief complaint	Feeling tired, weak, low energy.
☐ Onset	Six months ago.
☐ Associated events	None.
☐ Progression of the fatigue during the day	The same throughout the day.
☐ Affecting job/performance	Yes, I don't have energy for my daily 30-minute walk with my dog, and even at work I am not as energetic as before.
☐ Appetite changes	I have a poor appetite.
☐ Weight changes	I lost 8 pounds during the past six months.
☐ Change in bowel habits	No, I have a bowel movement 2-3 times a week. It has been like this for the past 10 years.
☐ Blood in stool	No.
☐ Abdominal pain or discomfort	Yes, I do feel some discomfort here (points to the epigastric area).
☐ Onset of discomfort	Four months ago; it increased gradually.
☐ Quality	Vague, deep.
☐ Severity on a scale	4/10.
☐ Alleviating/exacerbating factors	Nothing makes it worse, but I feel better when I lean forward.
☐ Relationship to food	No.
☐ Radiation	I feel the discomfort reaching my back.
☐ Nausea/vomiting	Sometimes I feel nauseated.
☐ Feeling of depression	Yes, I feel sad.
☐ Reason for feeling sad	I don't know, really.
☐ Suicidal thoughts/plans/attempts	No.
☐ Feelings of blame, guilt, worthlessness	No.
☐ Sleeping problems (falling asleep, staying asleep, early waking, snoring)	I wake up unusually early in the morning. It has been like this for the past two months.

☑ Question	Patient Response
☐ Loss of concentration	Yes, I can't concentrate anymore while watching the news or playing cards with my friends.
☐ Loss of interest	I don't enjoy playing cards with my friends anymore. I feel that life is boring.
☐ Associated symptoms (fever/chills, chest pain, cough, shortness of breath, cold intolerance, skin/hair changes)	None.
☐ Current medications	Tylenol, but it is not helping.
☐ Past psychiatric history	No.
☐ Past medical history	No.
☐ Past surgical history	Appendectomy at age 16.
☐ Family history	My father died in a car accident and had diabetes, and my mother died of breast cancer.
☐ Occupation	Police officer, retired one year ago.
☐ Alcohol use	One or two beers 2–3 times a week.
☐ Illicit drug use	Never.
☐ Tobacco	I stopped it six months ago after 30 years of smoking 1 pack a day (because I felt disgusted, and smoking made me feel sick).
☐ Exercise	I walk 30 minutes every day.
☐ Diet	Regular; I like junk food.
☐ Sexual activity	Sexually active with my wife.
☐ Drug allergies	No.

Connecting with the Patient

☐ Examinee recognized the SP's emotions and responded with PEARLS.

Physical Examination

☐ Examinee washed his/her hands.

☐ Examinee asked permission to start the exam.

☐ Examinee used respectful draping.

☐ Examinee did not repeat painful maneuvers.

☑ *Exam Component*	*Maneuver*
☐ Head and neck exam	Inspected conjunctivae, mouth and throat, lymph nodes; examined thyroid gland
☐ CV exam	Auscultation
☐ Pulmonary exam	Auscultation
☐ Abdominal exam	Auscultation, percussion, palpation (including rebound tenderness and Murphy sign)
☐ Extremities	Inspection, palpation

Closure

☐ Examinee discussed initial diagnostic impressions.

☐ Examinee discussed initial management plans:

   ☐ Follow-up tests.

   ☐ Depression counseling:

      ☐ Support system at home (friends, family).

      ☐ Support systems in the hospital and community.

      ☐ Coping skills: Exercise, relaxation techniques, spending more time with family and friends.

☐ Examinee asked if the SP had any other questions or concerns.

Sample Closure

Mr. Jordan, your symptoms are consistent with a few different diagnoses. They may be caused by an ulcer that would resolve with a course of antibiotics and acid suppressors, or they may have a more serious cause, such as pancreatic cancer. I am going to schedule you for an abdominal ultrasound that may reveal the source of your pain, and I will also run some blood tests. I know you are concerned about your upcoming vacation, but the results of your tests should be back within a few days, and they should give us a good idea what is wrong with you. In the meantime, our social worker can meet with you to help you find ways to cope with the stress you have been experiencing in your life. Do you have any questions for me?

Patient Note

History

Physical Examination

Differential Diagnosis

1.
2.
3.
4.
5.

Diagnostic Workup

1.
2.
3.
4.
5.

History

HPI: *61 yo M c/o fatigue and weakness. The patient notes that the fatigue and weakness started 6 months ago. He feels tired all day. He has poor appetite and lost 8 lbs in the past 6 months. He also complains of occasional nausea and of a vague, deep epigastric discomfort that radiates to the back. This discomfort started 4 months ago and has gradually increased to a severity of 4/10. The discomfort decreases when he leans forward and increases when he lies on his back. There is no relationship of the pain to food. No change in bowel movements or blood in the stool. He feels sad sometimes, has lost interest in things that he used to enjoy, wakes up unusually early in the morning, and complains of low energy and concentration that have affected his daily activities and work. The patient denies suicidal ideation or plans. No feelings of guilt or worthlessness.*

ROS: *Negative except as above.*
Allergies: *NKDA.*
Medications: *Tylenol.*
PMH: *None.*
PSH: *Appendectomy at age 16.*
SH: *1 PPD for 30 years; stopped 6 months ago. Drinks 1–2 beers 2–3 times/week. Sexually active with his wife.*
FH: *Father with diabetes, died accidentally. Mother died from breast cancer.*

Physical Examination

Patient is in no acute distress, looks sad.
VS: *WNL.*
HEENT: *No conjunctival pallor, mouth and pharynx normal.*
Neck: *Supple, no JVD, no lymphadenopathy, thyroid normal.*
Chest: *Clear breath sounds bilaterally.*
Heart: *RRR; normal S1/S2; no murmurs, rubs, or gallops.*
Abdomen: *Soft, nondistended, mild epigastric tenderness, no rebound tenderness, ⊖ Murphy, ⊕ BS, no hepatosplenomegaly.*
Extremities: *No edema.*

Differential Diagnosis

1. *Depression*
2. *Pancreatic cancer*
3. *Chronic pancreatitis*
4. *Peptic ulcer disease*
5. *Hypothyroidism*

Diagnostic Workup

1. *CBC, stool for occult blood*
2. *Glucose*
3. *Amylase, lipase*
4. *AST/ALT/bilirubin/alkaline phosphatase*
5. *TSH*
6. *AXR*
7. *CT or U/S—abdomen*
8. *Upper endoscopy*

CASE DISCUSSION

Differential Diagnosis

- **Depression:** The patient has many classic symptoms of depression (**SIG E CAPS;** see Case 15). Although it may be a somatic symptom of depression, his abdominal pain is of significant concern and warrants a thorough medical evaluation.

- **Pancreatic cancer:** The pattern and location of pain are worrisome for pancreatic disease, and weight loss raises a concern for malignancy. Depression may be its initial manifestation. Diarrhea, presumably due to malabsorption, is also an occasional early finding (not seen in this case).

- **Chronic pancreatitis:** The pattern and location of pain are consistent with this diagnosis, but usually there is a history of recurrent episodes of similar pain. The patient's alcohol use should be explored further, as alcoholism accounts for 70%–80% of chronic pancreatitis.

- **Peptic ulcer disease:** Suspect this diagnosis in any patient with epigastric pain, although the complaint is neither sensitive nor specific enough to make a reliable diagnosis. It is important to note that many patients deny any relationship of the pain to meals. Weight loss, however, is unusual in uncomplicated ulcer disease and may suggest gastric malignancy.

- **Hypothyroidism:** Nonspecific symptoms such as fatigue and weakness may suggest this common diagnosis. Abdominal pain is unusual.

Diagnostic Workup

- **CBC, stool for occult blood:** To screen for blood loss in peptic ulcer.

- **Glucose:** To screen for pancreatic endocrine dysfunction (ie, diabetes mellitus).

- **Amylase, lipase:** Nonspecific, but can be elevated in chronic pancreatitis or malignancy.

- **AST/ALT/bilirubin/alkaline phosphatase:** To look for evidence of obstructive jaundice (often seen in pancreatic cancer).

- **TSH:** Thyroid disease must be ruled out in a patient with symptoms of depression.

- **AXR:** To look for pancreatic calcification in chronic pancreatitis.

- **CT or U/S—abdomen:** To diagnose pancreatic cancer or other pathology.

- **Upper endoscopy:** To diagnose ulcer disease.

Opening Scenario

Kelly Clark, a 35-year-old female, comes to the ED complaining of headache.

Vital Signs

BP: 135/90 mm Hg

Temp: 98.6°F (37°C)

RR: 16/minute

HR: 76/minute, regular

Examinee Tasks

1. Take a focused history.

2. Perform a focused physical exam (do not perform rectal, genitourinary, or female breast exam).

3. Explain your clinical impression and workup plan to the patient.

4. Write the patient note after leaving the room.

Checklist/SP Sheet

Patient Description

Patient is a 35 yo F, married with three children.

Notes for the SP

Hold the right side of your head during the encounter and look as if you are in severe pain.

Challenging Questions to Ask

"Do you have anything that will make me feel better? Please, doctor, I am in pain."

Sample Examinee Response

"Yes, we have many options for medicines to relieve your pain, but first I need to learn as much as I can about your pain so that I can recommend the best medicine."

Examinee Checklist

Building the Doctor-Patient Relationship

Entrance

☐ Examinee knocked on the door before entering.

☐ Examinee introduced self by name.

☐ Examinee identified his/her role or position.

☐ Examinee correctly used patient's name.

☐ Examinee made eye contact with the SP.

Reflective Listening

☐ Examinee asked an open-ended question and actively listened to the response.

☐ Examinee asked the SP to list his/her concerns and listened to the response without interrupting.

☐ Examinee summarized the SP's concerns, often using the SP's own words.

Information Gathering

☐ Examinee elicited data efficiently and accurately.

☑ Question	Patient Response
☐ Chief complaint	Headache.
☐ Onset	Two weeks ago.
☐ Constant/intermittent	Well, I don't have the pain all the time. It comes and goes.
☐ Frequency	At least once a day.
☐ Progression	It is getting worse (2–3 times a day).
☐ Severity on a scale	When I have the pain, it is 9/10 and prevents me from working.
☐ Location	It is here (points to the whole right side of the head).
☐ Duration	One or two hours.
☐ Radiation (changes its location)	No.
☐ Quality	Sharp and pounding.
☐ Aura (warning that the headache is about to come)	No.
☐ Timing (the same time every day/ morning/evening)	The headache may come at any time. I'm having one now.
☐ Relationship with menses	No.
☐ Alleviating factors	Resting in a quiet, dark room; sleep, aspirin.
☐ Exacerbating factors	Stress, light, and noise.
☐ Nausea/vomiting	Sometimes I feel nauseated when I am in pain. Yesterday I vomited for the first time.
☐ Headache wakes you up from sleep	No.
☐ Visual changes/tears/red eye	No.
☐ Weakness/numbness	No.
☐ Speech difficulties	No.
☐ Runny nose during the attack	No.
☐ Similar episodes before	Yes, in college I had a similar headache that was accompanied by nausea.
☐ Weight/appetite changes	No.
☐ Joint pain/fatigue	Occasional aches and pains treated with ibuprofen.

☑ Question	Patient Response
☐ Stress	Yes, I am working on a new project that I have to finish this month. Last month was a disaster. I worked hard on my designs, but they were rejected, and I have to start all over again.
☐ Head trauma	No.
☐ Last menstrual period	Two weeks ago.
☐ Current medications	Ibuprofen.
☐ Past medical history	An episode of sinusitis four months ago, treated with amoxicillin (but the pain was different from the one I have now).
☐ Past surgical history	Tubal ligation eight years ago.
☐ Family history	My father died at age 65 of a brain tumor. My mother is alive and has migraines.
☐ Occupation	Engineer.
☐ Alcohol use	No.
☐ Illicit drug use	No.
☐ Tobacco use	No.
☐ Social history	I live with my husband and three children.
☐ Sexual activity	With my husband.
☐ Use of OCPs	No, I had a tubal ligation after my third child eight years ago.
☐ Drug allergies	No.

Connecting with the Patient

☐ Examinee recognized the SP's emotions and responded with PEARLS.

Physical Examination

☐ Examinee washed his/her hands.

☐ Examinee asked permission to start the exam.

☐ Examinee used respectful draping.

☐ Examinee did not repeat painful maneuvers.

☑ Exam Component	Maneuver
☐ HEENT	Palpation (head, facial sinuses, temporomandibular joints), funduscopic exam; inspected nose, mouth, teeth, and throat
☐ Neck exam	Inspection, palpation
☐ CV exam	Auscultation
☐ Pulmonary exam	Auscultation
☐ Neurologic exam	Cranial nerves, muscle strength, DTRs

Closure

☐ Examinee discussed initial diagnostic impressions.

☐ Examinee discussed initial management plans:

   ☐ Follow-up tests.

☐ Examinee asked if the SP had any other questions or concerns.

Sample Closure

Mrs. Clark, it sounds as if your symptoms are due to a migraine headache, so the first thing I will do is prescribe some medications that will alleviate your pain. To ensure that there isn't something else going on, however, I would like to get a CT scan of your head to rule out a mass or vascular problem as the cause of your headache. A blood test may also show if you have problems other than migraine. Do you have any questions for me?

Patient Note

History

Physical Examination

Differential Diagnosis

1.
2.
3.
4.
5.

Diagnostic Workup

1.
2.
3.
4.
5.

History

HPI: *35 yo F c/o daily headaches for 2 weeks. These headaches occur 2–3 times a day and last for 1–2 hours. The pain is sharp and pounding. It is located on the right hemisphere of the head, with no radiation or preceding aura. The pain reaches 9/10 in severity and prevents the patient from continuing her activities. Headaches are exacerbated by stress, light, and noise and are alleviated by resting in a dark room, sleep, and aspirin. The pain is sometimes accompanied by nausea and vomiting. No changes in weight or appetite.*

ROS: *Occasional aches and pains.*

Allergies: *NKDA.*

Medications: *Ibuprofen.*

PMH: *Headaches at age 20, accompanied by nausea. One episode of sinusitis 4 months ago, treated with amoxicillin.*

PSH: *Tubal ligation 8 years ago.*

SH: *No smoking, no EtOH, no illicit drugs. Patient is an engineer, lives with husband and 3 children, and is sexually active with husband only.*

FH: *Father died of a brain tumor at age 65. Mother has migraines.*

Physical Examination

Patient is in severe pain.

VS: *WNL.*

HEENT: *NC/AT, nontender to palpation, PERRLA, EOMI, no papilledema, no nasal congestion, no pharyngeal erythema or exudates, dentition good.*

Neck: *Supple, no lymphadenopathy.*

Chest: *Clear breath sounds bilaterally.*

Heart: *RRR; normal S1/S2; no murmurs, rubs, or gallops.*

Neuro: *Mental status: Alert and oriented × 3, good concentration. Cranial nerves: 2–12 grossly intact. Motor: Strength 5/5 throughout. DTRs: 2+ intact, symmetric.*

Differential Diagnosis

1. *Migraine*
2. *Tension headache*
3. *Depression*
4. *Pseudotumor cerebri*
5. *Intracranial mass lesion*
6. *Cluster headache*
7. *Sinusitis*

Diagnostic Workup

1. *CBC*
2. *CT—head or MRI—brain*
3. *LP*
4. *CT—sinus*

CASE DISCUSSION

Differential Diagnosis

- **Migraine:** Despite lacking an aura, the patient's presentation is classic for this diagnosis.

- **Tension headache:** This is often associated with stress but is usually bilateral and squeezing. It lasts from hours to days and gets worse as the day progresses.

- **Depression:** Headaches may be worse on arising in the morning and are associated with other symptoms of depression.

- **Pseudotumor cerebri:** Headaches can be focal but are usually accompanied by diplopia and other visual symptoms. Exam should reveal papilledema but can be normal during the first few days after onset of illness.

- **Intracranial mass lesion:** One-third of patients with brain tumors present with a primary complaint of headache. Headache is nonspecific and may mimic features of migraine. Certain brain tumors may have a familial basis.

- **Cluster headache:** This involves unilateral periorbital pain, often accompanied by ipsilateral nasal congestion, rhinorrhea, lacrimation, redness of the eye, and/or Horner syndrome. Episodes of daily pain occur in clusters and often awaken patients at night. However, this rarely occurs in women (a similar entity seen in women is termed *chronic paroxysmal hemicrania*).

- **Sinusitis:** This is a rare cause of headache. There are no signs or symptoms of sinus or respiratory infection in this case.

Diagnostic Workup

- **CBC:** To look for leukocytosis, a nonspecific sign of infection or inflammation. Mild normocytic anemia and thrombocytosis may also be seen in temporal arteritis.

- **CT—head or MRI—brain:** Headache syndromes are largely clinical diagnoses. Neuroimaging is generally reserved for patients with acute severe headache, chronic unexplained headache, or abnormalities on neurologic exam. MRI provides greater anatomic detail, but CT is preferred to rule out acute bleeds.

- **LP:** To look for elevated opening pressure in pseudotumor. CSF is otherwise normal. RBCs and xanthochromia can be seen in subarachnoid hemorrhage (perform if suspicion is high despite a negative CT scan).

- **CT—sinus:** To look for sinusitis.

Opening Scenario

Carl Fisher, a 57-year-old male, comes to the ED complaining of bloody urine.

Vital Signs

BP: 130/80 mm Hg

Temp: 98.5°F (36.9°C)

RR: 13/minute

HR: 72/minute, regular

Examinee Tasks

1. Take a focused history.

2. Perform a focused physical exam (do not perform rectal, genitourinary, or female breast exam).

3. Explain your clinical impression and workup plan to the patient.

4. Write the patient note after leaving the room.

Checklist/SP Sheet

Patient Description

Patient is a 57 yo M.

Notes for the SP

- Show pain when the examinee checks for CVA tenderness on the right.

- If the examinee mentions prostate disease, ask, "What's prostate disease?"

Challenging Questions to Ask

"They told me this is because of my old age. Is that true?"

Sample Examinee Response

"No. Bloody urine is rarely normal."

Examinee Checklist

Building the Doctor-Patient Relationship

Entrance

☐ Examinee knocked on the door before entering.

☐ Examinee introduced self by name.

☐ Examinee identified his/her role or position.

☐ Examinee correctly used patient's name.

☐ Examinee made eye contact with the SP.

Reflective Listening

☐ Examinee asked an open-ended question and actively listened to the response.

☐ Examinee asked the SP to list his/her concerns and listened to the response without interrupting.

☐ Examinee summarized the SP's concerns, often using the SP's own words.

Information Gathering

☐ Examinee elicited data efficiently and accurately.

☑ Question	Patient Response
☐ Chief complaint	I have blood in my urine, doctor.
☐ How did he know it was blood?	It was bright red and later had some clots.
☐ Onset	Yesterday morning.
☐ Progression	That was the only time it has ever happened; my urine is back to normal.
☐ Pain/burning on urination	None.
☐ Fever	None.
☐ Abdominal/flank pain	None.
☐ Polyuria, frequency	Yes.
☐ Straining during urination	Yes.
☐ Nocturia	Yes.
☐ Weak stream	Yes.
☐ Dribbling	Yes.
☐ Onset of the previous symptoms	Two years ago. They told me I am getting old; am I?
☐ History of renal stones	No.
☐ Associated symptoms (nausea/vomiting, diarrhea/constipation)	None.
☐ Constitutional symptoms (weight loss, appetite changes, night sweats)	None.
☐ Previous similar episodes	No.
☐ Current medications	Allopurinol.
☐ Past medical history	Gout.
☐ Past surgical history	Appendectomy at age 23.
☐ Family history	My father died at age 80 because of a kidney problem. My mother is alive and healthy.
☐ Occupation	Painter.
☐ Alcohol use	A couple of beers after work, 2–3 times a week.

☑ Question	Patient Response
☐ Illicit drug use	No.
☐ Tobacco	Yes, I have smoked 1 pack a day for 30 years.
☐ Sexual activity	I have a new girlfriend; I met her last month in the bar.
☐ Sexual orientation	Women only.
☐ Use of condoms	Sometimes, if they're available.
☐ History of STDs	I have herpes. The last attack was several months ago. The lesions stay for several days and resolve without treatment.
☐ HIV test	Never.
☐ Drug allergies	No.

Connecting with the Patient

☐ Examinee recognized the SP's emotions and responded with PEARLS.

Physical Examination

☐ Examinee washed his/her hands.

☐ Examinee asked permission to start the exam.

☐ Examinee used respectful draping.

☐ Examinee did not repeat painful maneuvers.

☑ Exam Component	Maneuver
☐ CV exam	Auscultation
☐ Pulmonary exam	Auscultation
☐ Abdominal exam	Auscultation, palpation, percussion, checked for CVA tenderness
☐ Extremities	Inspection

Closure

☐ Examinee discussed initial diagnostic impressions.

☐ Examinee discussed initial management plans:

   ☐ Follow-up tests: Examinee mentioned the need for a genital exam and a rectal exam for the prostate.

☐ Examinee asked if the SP had any other questions or concerns.

Sample Closure

Mr. Fisher, the blood in your urine could be caused by a variety of factors, so I would like to do a few tests to elicit an answer. First I will draw some blood, and then I will perform a genital exam as well as a rectal exam to assess your prostate. I will then order a urine test to look for signs of infection. Depending on the results we obtain, I may also order some imaging studies to determine if there is a stone in your urinary tract, an anatomic abnormality, or a tumor. Do you have any questions for me?

Patient Note

History

_____
_____
_____
_____
_____
_____
_____
_____
_____

Physical Examination

_____
_____
_____
_____
_____
_____
_____
_____
_____
_____

Differential Diagnosis

1. _____
2. _____
3. _____
4. _____
5. _____

Diagnostic Workup

1. _____
2. _____
3. _____
4. _____
5. _____

Patient Note

History

HPI: *57 yo male c/o 1 episode of painless hematuria yesterday morning. He has no fever, no abdominal or flank pain, and no dysuria. No history of renal stones. He has a 2-year history of straining on urination, polyuria, nocturia, weak urinary stream, and dribbling. No nausea, vomiting, diarrhea, or constipation. No change in appetite or weight loss. No previous similar episodes.*

ROS: *Negative except as above.*

Allergies: *NKDA.*

Medications: *Allopurinol.*

PMH: *Gout; genital herpes that recurred several months ago.*

PSH: *Appendectomy, age 23.*

SH: *1 PPD for 30 years, 2 beers 2–3 times/week, no illicit drugs. Works as a painter. Heterosexual, has a new partner, and uses condoms occasionally.*

FH: *Father died from kidney disease at age 80.*

Physical Examination

Patient is in no acute distress.

VS: *WNL.*

Chest: *Clear breath sounds bilaterally.*

Heart: *RRR; normal S1/S2; no murmurs, rubs, or gallops.*

Abdomen: *Soft, nondistended, nontender, ⊕ BS, no hepatosplenomegaly. Mild right CVA tenderness.*

Extremities: *No edema.*

Differential Diagnosis

1. *Bladder cancer*
2. *Urolithiasis*
3. *BPH*
4. *Prostate cancer*
5. *Renal cell carcinoma*
6. *Glomerulonephritis*
7. *UTI*

Diagnostic Workup

1. *Genital exam*
2. *Rectal exam*
3. *UA*
4. *Urine culture*
5. *Urine cytology*
6. *BUN/Cr*
7. *PSA*
8. *U/S—renal*
9. *Cystoscopy*
10. *CT—abdomen/pelvis*
11. *IVP*

CASE DISCUSSION

Differential Diagnosis

A useful mnemonic for the differential diagnosis of hematuria is **HITTERS**—etiologies include **H**ematologic or coagulation disorders, **I**nfection, **T**rauma, **T**umor, **E**xercise, **R**enal disorder, and **S**tones. Gynecologic sources may need to be excluded in women. The passage of clots often localizes the source of bleeding to the lower urinary tract. Gross hematuria in adults represents malignancy until proven otherwise.

- **Bladder cancer:** Hematuria and irritative voiding symptoms are consistent with this diagnosis, and the patient's cigarette smoking and possible occupational exposure to industrial solvents are risk factors. However, the finding of right CVA tenderness is unusual and could be a sign of upper urinary tract disease.

- **Urolithiasis:** Despite the presence of hematuria and CVA tenderness, this very common diagnosis is unlikely in the absence of sudden, severe colicky flank pain. Pain may migrate to the groin and is not alleviated by changes in position.

- **BPH:** The patient's urinary symptoms are classic for this diagnosis except that hematuria (if present) is usually microscopic. Again, CVA tenderness may signal upper urinary tract pathology.

- **Prostate cancer:** As above, this diagnosis is plausible but is hard to reconcile with the presence of CVA tenderness (could postulate metastasis to a right posterior rib).

- **Renal cell carcinoma:** The classic triad is hematuria, flank pain, and a palpable mass. Constitutional symptoms may be prominent. The patient's other urinary symptoms may be due to coexisting BPH.

- **Glomerulonephritis:** The absence of hypertension or signs of volume overload (eg, edema) argues against intrinsic renal disease. However, remember that IgA nephropathy is the most common acute glomerulonephritis and most commonly presents with an episode of gross hematuria. Presentation is usually concurrent with URI, GI symptoms, or a flulike illness.

- **UTI:** This can cause hematuria but is uncommon in males. The patient has no other symptoms to suggest acute infection.

Diagnostic Workup

- **Genital exam:** To exclude a urologic source of bleeding in men.

- **Rectal exam:** To detect masses as well as prostatic enlargement or nodules.

- **UA:** To assess hematuria, pyuria, bacteriuria, etc. Dysmorphic RBCs or casts are signs of glomerular disease. The absence of hematuria does not rule out urolithiasis.

- **Urine culture:** To exclude UTI.

- **Urine cytology:** Has variable sensitivity in detecting bladder cancers, depending on the tumor's grade and stage. Examine three voided samples to maximize sensitivity.

- **BUN/Cr:** To evaluate kidney function.

- **PSA:** The serum level correlates with the volume of both benign and malignant prostatic tissue. Can be normal in about 20% of patients who have nonmetastatic prostate cancer.

- **U/S—renal:** Can detect bladder and renal masses and stones, but is operator dependent and is less sensitive in detecting ureteral disease.

- **Cystoscopy:** The gold standard for the diagnosis of bladder cancer.

- **CT—abdomen/pelvis:** To evaluate the urinary tract. Can identify neoplasms and a variety of benign conditions such as stones.

- **IVP:** Provides an assessment of the kidneys, ureters, and bladder but is generally being replaced by CT—urogram to avoid contrast administration.

CASE 20
DOORWAY INFORMATION

Opening Scenario

James Miller, a 54-year-old male, comes to the clinic for hypertension follow-up.

Vital Signs

BP: 135/90 mm Hg

Temp: 98.0°F (36.7°C)

RR: 16/minute

HR: 70/minute, regular

Examinee Tasks

1. Take a focused history.

2. Perform a focused physical exam (do not perform rectal, genitourinary, or female breast exam).

3. Explain your clinical impression and workup plan to the patient.

4. Write the patient note after leaving the room.

Checklist/SP Sheet

Patient Description

Patient is a 54 yo M.

Notes for the SP

Don't mention impotence unless the examinee asks whether you are having any side effects from your medications or whether you have any other concerns.

Challenging Questions to Ask

"I think it is my age. Isn't that right, doctor?"

Sample Examinee Response

"No, I don't think it's because of your age. I worry more about your medications. However, testosterone levels can decrease with age, and we will check for that."

Examinee Checklist

Building the Doctor-Patient Relationship

Entrance

☐ Examinee knocked on the door before entering.

☐ Examinee introduced self by name.

☐ Examinee identified his/her role or position.

☐ Examinee correctly used patient's name.

☐ Examinee made eye contact with the SP.

Reflective Listening

☐ Examinee asked an open-ended question and actively listened to the response.

☐ Examinee asked the SP to list his/her concerns and listened to the response without interrupting.

☐ Examinee summarized the SP's concerns, often using the SP's own words.

Information Gathering

☐ Examinee elicited data efficiently and accurately.

☑ Question	Patient Response
☐ Chief complaint	I am here to check on my blood pressure.
☐ Onset	Last year I found out that I have hypertension.
☐ Treatment	The doctor started me on hydrochlorothiazide, but my blood pressure stayed high. He added propranolol six months ago.
☐ Compliance with medications	Well, sometimes I forget to take the pills, but in general I take them regularly.
☐ Last blood pressure checkup	Six months ago.
☐ How he is feeling today	Good.
☐ Home monitoring of blood pressure	No.
☐ Any other symptoms (fatigue, headaches, dizziness, blurred vision, nausea, palpitations, chest pain, shortness of breath, urinary changes, weakness, bowel movement changes, sleep problems)	No.
☐ Medication side effects	Over the past four months I started having problems in my sexual performance. A friend told me it is the propranolol, but I think it is my age. Isn't that right, doctor?
☐ Description of the problem	I have a weak erection.
☐ Severity on 1–10 scale, where 1 is flaccid and 6 is adequate for penetration	About a 4.
☐ Early-morning or nocturnal erections	No.
☐ Libido	That's weak, too, doc. I'm just not as interested in sex as I used to be.
☐ Marital or work problems	No, my wife is great and I am very happy in my job.
☐ Feelings of depression	No.
☐ Feelings of anxiety or stress	No.
☐ Any leg or buttock pain while walking or resting	No.
☐ Weight changes	No.
☐ Appetite changes	No.

☑ Question	Patient Response
☐ Diabetes	No.
☐ History of hypercholesterolemia	Yes, it was diagnosed last year.
☐ Previous heart problems	No.
☐ History of TIA or stroke	No.
☐ Current medications	Propranolol, hydrochlorothiazide, lovastatin.
☐ Past medical history	None.
☐ Past surgical history	None.
☐ Family history	My father died at age 50 of a heart attack. My mother is healthy, but she has Alzheimer disease. She is in a nursing home now.
☐ Occupation	Schoolteacher.
☐ Diet	I eat a lot of junk food.
☐ Exercise	No.
☐ Alcohol use	Yes, 3–4 beers a week.
☐ Illicit drug use	No.
☐ Tobacco	No.
☐ Social history	I am married and live with my wife.
☐ Sexual activity	I had a wonderful sex life with my wife until four months ago, when I started having this problem that I told you about. I think I am getting old.
☐ Drug allergies	No.

Connecting with the Patient

☐ Examinee recognized the SP's emotions and responded with PEARLS.

Physical Examination

☐ Examinee washed his/her hands.

☐ Examinee asked permission to start the exam.

☐ Examinee used respectful draping.

☐ Examinee did not repeat painful maneuvers.

☑ Exam Component	Maneuver
☐ Head and neck exam	Funduscopic exam, carotid auscultation
☐ CV exam	Palpation, auscultation
☐ Pulmonary exam	Auscultation
☐ Abdominal exam	Auscultation, palpation
☐ Extremities	Inspection, palpatation of peripheral pulses
☐ Neurologic exam	DTRs, Babinski sign, sensation and strength in bilateral lower extremities

Closure

☐ Examinee discussed initial diagnostic impressions.

☐ Examinee discussed initial management plans:

  ☐ Follow-up tests: Examinee mentioned the need for genital and rectal exams.

  ☐ Lifestyle modification (diet, exercise, alcohol cessation).

  ☐ Changing propranolol to another antihypertensive medication that does not cause erectile dysfunction.

☐ Examinee asked if the SP had any other questions or concerns.

Sample Closure

Mr. Miller, your blood pressure level was 135/90 when we measured it earlier today, which is close to our target of 130/80. However, it would be even better if we could get it down to around 120/80. Fortunately, that should be feasible with lifestyle changes such as decreasing your salt and fat intake and increasing the amount of exercise you are doing. As for your problems with your erection, this is a very common side effect of one of the blood pressure medications you are taking. For this reason, I would like to give you a medication other than propranolol to control your blood pressure. I am also going to order some blood tests to make sure that your problem is not due to any other medical condition. In addition, I would like to perform a genital exam as well as a rectal exam to assess your prostate. Do you have any questions for me?

Patient Note

History

Physical Examination

Differential Diagnosis

1.

2.

3.

4.

5.

Diagnostic Workup

1.

2.

3.

4.

5.

Patient Note

History

HPI: 54 yo M presents for follow-up of his hypertension that was diagnosed last year. He was initially started on HCTZ; propranolol was added 6 months ago. He is fairly compliant with his medications. He does not monitor his blood pressure at home. His last blood pressure checkup was 6 months ago. He is feeling well except for erectile dysfunction and decreased libido noted 4 months ago. No leg claudication or any previous history of heart problems, stroke, TIA, or diabetes. No marital or work problems. No depression, anxiety, appetite or weight changes, or history of trauma.

ROS: Negative except as above.

Allergies: NKDA.

Medications: HCTZ, propranolol, lovastatin.

PMH: Hypertension, hypercholesterolemia diagnosed 1 year ago.

PSH: None.

SH: No smoking, 3–4 beers/week, no illicit drugs. Works as a schoolteacher; married and lives with his wife.

FH: Father died of a heart attack at age 50. Mother is in a nursing home due to Alzheimer disease.

Physical Examination

Patient is in no acute distress.

VS: WNL.

HEENT: No funduscopic abnormalities.

Neck: No carotid bruits, no JVD.

Chest: Clear breath sounds bilaterally.

Heart: Apical impulse not displaced; RRR; normal S1/S2; no murmurs, rubs, or gallops.

Abdomen: Soft, nondistended, nontender, ⊕ BS, no bruits, no organomegaly.

Extremities: No edema, no hair loss or skin changes. Radial, brachial, femoral, dorsalis pedis, and posterior tibialis 2+ and symmetric.

Neuro: Motor: Strength 5/5 in bilateral lower extremities. Sensation: Intact to pinprick and soft touch in lower extremities. DTRs: Symmetric 2+ in lower extremities, ⊖ Babinski bilaterally.

Differential Diagnosis

1. Drug-induced erectile dysfunction (ED)
2. Hypogonadism
3. ED caused by vascular disease
4. Depression
5. Alcohol-related ED
6. Peyronie disease

Diagnostic Workup

1. Genital exam
2. Rectal exam
3. Serum glucose
4. Testosterone
5. LH/FSH
6. Prolactin, TSH
7. Ferritin
8. MRI—brain
9. Doppler U/S—penis
10. Dynamic cavernosography
11. BUN/Cr, electrolytes, cholesterol, UA, ECG

CASE DISCUSSION

Differential Diagnosis

- **Drug-induced erectile dysfunction (ED):** Antihypertensives (but rarely diuretics) and alcohol are commonly associated with ED. β-Blockers may also result in loss of libido.

- **Hypogonadism:** Testosterone deficiency has many underlying etiologies but, as with other endocrine problems, is attributable to either central (due to insufficient gonadotropin secretion by the pituitary) or end-organ disease (pathology in the testes themselves). In addition to diminished libido and possible ED, there are often associated symptoms such as hot flushes, fatigue, and depression.

- **ED caused by vascular disease:** Hypertension and hyperlipidemia are risk factors for atherosclerotic vascular disease, but there are no historical or physical findings (eg, angina, leg claudication, diminished pulses, hair loss, or thin, shiny skin) to suggest its presence in this case. For example, arterial insufficiency involving the terminal aorta is a common cause of ED but is usually accompanied by vascular claudication of the legs (Leriche syndrome).

- **Depression:** Psychogenic causes can lead to loss of libido and loss of erections and are suggested when nocturnal or early-morning erections are preserved (not seen in this case). This patient denies other depressive symptoms, but further exploration of his feelings about his demented, nursing-home-bound mother may be more revealing.

- **Alcohol-related ED:** The use of alcohol (as well as tobacco and illicit drugs) is associated with an increased risk of ED.

- **Peyronie disease:** Fibrous plaque of the tunica albuginea can lead to penile scarring and ED.

Diagnostic Workup

- **Genital exam:** To rule out Peyronie disease (eg, see penile scarring or plaque formation).

- **Rectal exam:** To detect masses or prostatic abnormalities.

- **Serum glucose:** To screen for diabetes, a possible contributor to ED.

- **Testosterone level:** To screen for hypogonadism.

- **LH/FSH:** Gonadotropin levels should be checked in patients with low or borderline testosterone levels. Levels are elevated ("hypergonadotropic") in the setting of testicular pathology and are low ("hypogonadotropic") in the setting of pituitary or hypothalamic disease.

- **Prolactin, TSH:** To screen for other abnormalities of pituitary function in patients with hypogonadotropic hypogonadism.

- **Ferritin:** To screen for hemochromatosis, a common condition; ED can be an early manifestation due to iron deposition in the pituitary gland causing hypogonadotropic hypogonadism.

- **MRI—brain:** To rule out a pituitary or hypothalamic lesion in patients presenting with hypogonadotropic hypogonadism.

- **Doppler U/S—penis:** To assess blood flow in the cavernous arteries.

- **Dynamic cavernosography:** To determine the site and extent of venous leak (suspected in patients with normal arterial inflow).

- **BUN/Cr, electrolytes, cholesterol, UA, ECG:** Useful in the longitudinal care of hypertension and hyperlipidemia. To screen for kidney disease, for LVH or prior silent MIs, for response to cholesterol-lowering medication, and for complications of medical therapy (eg, diuretic-induced hypokalemia).

Opening Scenario

Kathleen Moore, a 33-year-old female, comes to the clinic complaining of knee pain.

Vital Signs

BP: 130/80 mm Hg

Temp: 99.5°F (37.5°C)

RR: 16/minute

HR: 76/minute, regular

Examinee Tasks

1. Take a focused history.

2. Perform a focused physical exam (do not perform rectal, genitourinary, or female breast exam).

3. Explain your clinical impression and workup plan to the patient.

4. Write the patient note after leaving the room.

Checklist/SP Sheet

Patient Description

Patient is a 33 yo F, divorced with two daughters.

Notes for the SP

- Pretend to have pain when the examinee moves your left knee in all directions.
- Do not allow the examinee to fully flex or extend your left knee.
- Paint your left knee red to make it look inflamed.

Challenging Questions to Ask

"Do you think I will be able to walk on my knee like before?"

Sample Examinee Response

"Most likely, but that depends on the underlying problem and your response to treatment."

Examinee Checklist

Building the Doctor-Patient Relationship

Entrance

☐ Examinee knocked on the door before entering.

☐ Examinee introduced self by name.

☐ Examinee identified his/her role or position.

☐ Examinee correctly used patient's name.

☐ Examinee made eye contact with the SP.

Reflective Listening

☐ Examinee asked an open-ended question and actively listened to the response.

☐ Examinee asked the SP to list his/her concerns and listened to the response without interrupting.

☐ Examinee summarized the SP's concerns, often using the SP's own words.

Information Gathering

☐ Examinee elicited data efficiently and accurately.

☑ Question	Patient Response
☐ Chief complaint	Left knee pain.
☐ Onset	Two days ago.
☐ Function	I can't move it. I use a cane to walk.
☐ Redness	Yes.
☐ Swelling of the joint	Yes.
☐ Alleviating factors	Rest and Tylenol help a little bit.
☐ Exacerbating factors	Moving my knee and walking.
☐ History of trauma to the knee	No.
☐ Other joint pain	Yes, my wrists and fingers are always painful and stiff. Five years ago I had a painful, swollen big toe on my left foot.
☐ Duration of the pain in the fingers	Six months.
☐ Stiffness in the morning/duration	Yes, for an hour.
☐ Photosensitivity	No.
☐ Rashes	No.
☐ Oral ulcers	I had many in my mouth last month, but they've resolved now.
☐ Fatigue	Yes, I've had no energy to work and have felt tired all the time for the past six months.
☐ Fever/chills	I feel hot now, but I have no chills.
☐ Hair loss	No.
☐ Cold temperature causing problems with the fingers	Sometimes my fingers become pale and then blue when they are exposed to cold weather or cold water.
☐ Heart symptoms (chest pain, palpitations)	No.
☐ Pulmonary complaints (shortness of breath, cough)	No.

☑ Question	Patient Response
☐ Neurologic complaints (seizures, weakness, numbness)	No.
☐ Urinary problems (hematuria)	No.
☐ Abdominal pain	No.
☐ History of recent tick bite	No.
☐ Pregnancies	I have two daughters. Both were delivered by C-section.
☐ Miscarriages/abortions	I had two spontaneous abortions a long time ago.
☐ Last menstrual period	Two weeks ago.
☐ Weight changes	I've lost about 10 pounds over the past six months.
☐ Appetite changes	I don't have a good appetite.
☐ Current medications	I used Tylenol to relieve my pain, but it is not working as well anymore.
☐ Past medical history	None.
☐ Past surgical history	Two C-sections at ages 23 and 25.
☐ Family history	My mother has rheumatoid arthritis and is living in a nursing home. I don't know my father.
☐ Occupation	Waitress.
☐ Alcohol use	I don't drink a lot, usually 2–4 beers a week except for weekends, when I don't count.
☐ CAGE questions	No (to all four).
☐ Last alcohol ingestion	Four days ago.
☐ Illicit drug use	No.
☐ Tobacco	Yes, one pack a day for the past 20 years.
☐ Sexual activity	I am sexually active with a new boyfriend whom I met two months ago.
☐ Use of condoms	Occasionally.
☐ Number of sexual partners during the past year	Four.
☐ Active with men, women, or both	Men only.
☐ Vaginal discharge	No.
☐ History of STDs	Yes, I had gonorrhea one year ago. I took antibiotics and was fine.
☐ Drug allergies	No.

Connecting with the Patient

☐ Examinee recognized the SP's emotions and responded with PEARLS.

Physical Examination

☐ Examinee washed his/her hands.

☐ Examinee asked permission to start the exam.

☐ Examinee used respectful draping.

☐ Examinee did not repeat painful maneuvers.

☑ Exam Component	Maneuver
☐ Mouth exam	Inspection
☐ Musculoskeletal exam	Inspection and palpation (compared both knees, including range of motion); examined other joints (shoulders, elbows, wrists, hands, fingers, hips, ankles)
☐ Hair and skin exam	Inspection
☐ CV exam	Auscultation
☐ Pulmonary exam	Auscultation
☐ Abdominal exam	Auscultation, palpation, percussion

Closure

☐ Examinee discussed initial diagnostic impressions.

☐ Examinee discussed initial management plans:

   ☐ Follow-up tests: Examinee mentioned the need for a pelvic exam.

☐ Examinee discussed safe sex practices.

☐ Examinee asked if the SP had any other questions or concerns.

Sample Closure

Ms. Moore, there are a few things that could be causing your knee pain, such as gout, an infection, or rheumatoid arthritis. To find out, I would like to draw fluid from your knee and then draw some blood. Sometimes infections from the pelvis can spread to other parts of your body, such as your knee, and for that reason I would also like to do a pelvic exam. These tests will likely reveal the source of your pain. You mentioned earlier that you don't always use condoms. I know condoms may be difficult to use regularly, but they are important in helping to control the spread of STDs. Do you have any questions for me?

Patient Note

History

_____

_____

_____

_____

_____

_____

_____

_____

Physical Examination

_____

_____

_____

_____

_____

_____

_____

_____

_____

_____

_____

Differential Diagnosis

1. _____

2. _____

3. _____

4. _____

5. _____

Diagnostic Workup

1. _____

2. _____

3. _____

4. _____

5. _____

History

HPI: *33 yo F c/o left knee pain that started 2 days ago and is causing difficulty walking. She has swelling and redness in her left knee and mild fever but no chills. She denies trauma. She has a history of fatigue and painful wrists and fingers and has experienced 1-hour morning stiffness over the past 6 months. She also recalls multiple oral ulcers that resolved last month. She describes Raynaud phenomenon but denies rash, photosensitivity, hair loss, or recent tick bites. She recalls a 10-lb weight loss over the past 6 months and has no appetite.*

ROS: *Negative except as above.*

Allergies: *NKDA.*

Medications: *Tylenol.*

PMH: *Episode of acute left big toe arthritis 5 years ago; gonorrhea 1 year ago.*

PSH: *Two C-sections.*

SH: *1 PPD for 20 years. Usually drinks 2–4 beers/week; on weekends drinks more; last ingestion 4 days ago; CAGE 0/4. No illicit drugs. Sexually active with multiple partners; inconsistent condom use.*

FH: *Mother has rheumatoid arthritis and lives in a nursing home.*

Physical Examination

Patient is in no acute distress but favors the left knee.

VS: *WNL.*

HEENT: *No oral lesions.*

Chest: *Clear breath sounds bilaterally.*

Heart: *RRR; normal S1/S2; no murmurs, rubs, or gallops.*

Abdomen: *Soft, nondistended, ⊕ BS, no hepatosplenomegaly.*

Extremities: *Erythema, tenderness, pain, and restricted range of motion on flexion and extension of left knee compared to right knee. Shoulder, elbow, wrist, hand, finger, hip, and ankle joints WNL bilaterally.*

Differential Diagnosis

1. Gout
2. Pseudogout
3. SLE
4. Rheumatoid arthritis
5. Gonococcal septic arthritis
6. Nongonococcal septic arthritis
7. Osteoarthritis

Diagnostic Workup

1. Pelvic exam and cervical cultures
2. Knee aspiration and synovial fluid analysis
3. XR—left knee and both hands
4. CBC
5. ANA, anti-dsDNA, RF
6. Blood culture

CASE DISCUSSION

Differential Diagnosis

- **Gout:** This acute, usually monoarticular, crystal-induced arthritis rarely occurs in premenopausal women, but the patient's history of first MTP arthritis ("podagra") is classic for gout. Alcohol ingestion causes hyperuricemia and may precipitate an acute attack. Foot, ankle, and knee joints are also commonly affected. Gout does not explain her hand arthralgias, but osteoarthritis is common and may coexist.

- **Pseudogout:** Another crystal-induced arthritis, pseudogout frequently involves the knees and wrists but is usually seen in patients older than 60 years of age.

- **SLE:** Joint symptoms (usually symmetric peripheral arthralgias), constitutional symptoms, and Raynaud phenomenon may be early manifestations of this disease. Unilateral knee involvement is not typical. The diagnosis requires at least 4 of the following 11 criteria: malar ("butterfly") rash, discoid rash, symmetric arthritis, photosensitivity, oral ulcers, serositis, renal disease, CNS involvement, hematologic disorders (her fatigue may be due to anemia), immunologic abnormalities (her history of spontaneous abortions may signal the presence of antiphospholipid antibodies), or ANA positivity. More testing needs to be done before SLE can be diagnosed in this case.

- **Rheumatoid arthritis:** This is suggested in a patient with a positive family history, symmetric small joint arthritis (eg, fingers, wrists), prolonged morning stiffness, and systemic symptoms (low-grade fever, anorexia, weight loss, fatigue, and weakness). However, this patient's hand joints were not red, warm, swollen, or tender on exam. Monoarthritis is also uncommon but is occasionally seen early in the course of the disease.

- **Gonococcal septic arthritis:** This occurs in healthy hosts, most commonly young women (women are much more likely than men to have asymptomatic genitourinary gonococcal infection, which allows the bug to mutate and disseminate). The knee is the most frequently involved joint, but the monoarthritis (or tenosynovitis) is usually preceded by a few days of migratory polyarthralgias. Also, this patient does not have the characteristic rash, which consists of small necrotic pustules on the extremities (including the palms and soles).

- **Nongonococcal septic arthritis:** This occurs suddenly, usually affects the knee or wrist, and is most commonly caused by S. aureus. However, it is a disease of an abnormal host; previous joint damage and IV drug use are key risk factors not present in this case.

- **Osteoarthritis:** Onset is insidious, joint stiffness brief, and joint inflammation minimal, all of which are incongruent with this patient's presentation. Also, osteoarthritis spares the wrist and MCP joints and is not associated with constitutional symptoms.

Diagnostic Workup

- **Pelvic exam and cervical cultures:** Necessary to investigate gonococcal infection and are often positive in the absence of symptoms (urine, anorectal, and throat cultures may also be necessary).

- **Knee aspiration, Gram stain, culture, and inspection for crystals:** In most cases of acute monoarthritis, joint aspiration must be performed to rule out septic arthritis. Inflammatory joint synovial fluid contains >3,000 WBCs/μL, and septic joint fluid often contains >50,000 cells/μL. The demonstration of needle-shaped, negatively birefringent crystals or rhomboid-shaped, weakly positively birefringent crystals confirms gout or pseudogout, respectively.

- **XR—left knee and both hands:** Specific changes in rheumatoid arthritis include symmetric joint space narrowing, marginal bony erosions, and periarticular demineralization. However, x-rays are usually normal during the first 6 months of illness. In gout, look for punched-out cortical erosions and a sclerotic joint margin. In pseudogout, look for calcified articular cartilage ("chondrocalcinosis"). In osteoarthritis, look for joint space narrowing, marginal osteophytes, subchondral osteosclerosis, and occasionally subchondral cysts.

- **CBC:** Look for anemia, leukopenia, and/or thrombocytopenia in SLE, or leukocytosis in acute gout and septic arthritis.

- **Immunologic tests:** ANA is a highly sensitive (but nonspecific) screening test for SLE. A negative test essentially excludes the disease. If ANA is positive, investigate antibody against double-stranded DNA (anti-dsDNA), antibody against the Smith antigen, anticardiolipin antibodies, and lupus anticoagulant to help confirm SLE. RF is present in > 75% of patients with rheumatoid arthritis.

- **Blood culture:** An important test in septic arthritis.

Opening Scenario

Charles Andrews, a 66-year-old male, comes to the clinic complaining of a tremor.

Vital Signs

BP: 135/90 mm Hg

Temp: 98.6°F (37°C)

RR: 16/minute

HR: 70/minute, regular

Examinee Tasks

1. Take a focused history.

2. Perform a focused physical exam (do not perform rectal, genitourinary, or female breast exam).

3. Explain your clinical impression and workup plan to the patient.

4. Write the patient note after leaving the room.

Checklist/SP Sheet

Patient Description

Patient is a 66 yo M.

Notes for the SP

■ Exhibit mild muscle rigidity in your wrists and arms—that is, when the examinee tries to move your wrists and arms, stiffen them and move them slowly.

■ Lean your back forward slightly and walk in small, shuffling steps.

■ Exhibit a resting hand tremor (pill rolling) that disappears with movement.

Challenging Questions to Ask

"Do you think I will get better?"

Sample Examinee Response

"I think your tremor will improve with medication, but I don't know how long the improvement will last. The tremor may be a sign of a larger movement disorder called Parkinson disease, and we need to do more evaluation to explore that possibility."

Examinee Checklist

Building the Doctor-Patient Relationship

Entrance

☐ Examinee knocked on the door before entering.

☐ Examinee introduced self by name.

☐ Examinee identified his/her role or position.

☐ Examinee correctly used patient's name.

☐ Examinee made eye contact with the SP.

Reflective Listening

☐ Examinee asked an open-ended question and actively listened to the response.

☐ Examinee asked the SP to list his/her concerns and listened to the response without interrupting.

☐ Examinee summarized the SP's concerns, often using the SP's own words.

Information Gathering

☐ Examinee elicited data efficiently and accurately.

☑ Question	Patient Response
☐ Chief complaint	I have a tremor in this hand (points to right hand).
☐ Location	Only in the right hand.
☐ Duration	I noticed it about six months ago, but it seems to be getting worse recently.
☐ Context	It shakes when I'm just sitting around doing nothing. It usually stops when I hold out the remote control to change the channel.
☐ Alleviating factors	None.
☐ Exacerbating factors	It seems more severe when I am really tired.
☐ Associated symptoms (falls, headaches, TIA symptoms, drooling, changes in voice or handwriting, difficulty with ADLs/IADLs, depression, constipation, rash, etc)	No, I don't think so. My wife says I've slowed down, but I think that's just because I retired last year. (If asked what your wife means, say that she is frustrated because it is your job to push the grocery cart, but you can't keep up with her in the store anymore.)
☐ Prior history of similar symptoms	Well, back in college I occasionally had a hand tremor after pulling an all-nighter and drinking lots of coffee. The tremor was in both hands, but it was worse in the right. It seemed faster than the one I have now.
☐ Caffeine intake	One cup of coffee every morning. I used to drink three cups a day, but I've cut back over the past few months.
☐ Alcohol use	None. Both of my parents were alcoholics, so I never touch it.
☐ Past medical history	High cholesterol, treated with diet. Asthma, treated with an albuterol inhaler as needed.
☐ History of head trauma	No.
☐ Family history	My parents died in a car accident in their 40s, and my sister is healthy.
☐ Social history	I am married and live with my wife.
☐ Occupation	Retired chemistry professor.
☐ Exercise	No, I'm really not very active anymore.

CASE DISCUSSION

Differential Diagnosis

- **Parkinson disease (PD):** This is the most common cause of resting tremor (ie, it is evident with the affected body part supported and completely at rest but improves or subsides with voluntary activity), although some patients with PD also have a postural-action tremor that is indistinguishable from essential tremor (ET, see below). Tremor is usually low frequency (4–6 Hz), begins in one upper extremity, and may later involve the other extremities as well. Leg tremor is more commonly due to PD than to ET. The face, lips, and jaw may be involved, but in contrast to ET, PD does not produce head tremor. Along with the tremor, the patient's bradykinesia and rigidity suggest PD.

- **Essential tremor (ET):** This is the most common neurologic cause of postural tremor (ie, tremor that is apparent when the arms are held outstretched) or action tremor (ie, tremor that increases at the end of goal-directed activity such as finger-to-nose testing). Approximately 50% of cases are familial. Tremor is usually high frequency and often asymmetrically involves the distal upper extremity. The head, voice, chin, trunk, and legs can also be involved. ET is not associated with other neurologic signs and is improved following the ingestion of small amounts of alcohol. Differentiation from the classic resting tremor of PD is usually straightforward, as in this case.

- **Physiologic tremor:** This refers to a very low-amplitude, high-frequency (10–12 Hz) tremor present in normal individuals. The tremor is often not visible, but when enhanced by medications or other medical conditions, it is the most common cause of postural and action tremors. Conditions that can enhance physiologic tremor include anxiety, excitement, sleep deprivation/fatigue, hypoglycemia, caffeine intake, alcohol withdrawal, thyrotoxicosis, fever, and pheochromocytoma.

- **Midbrain lesion:** Midbrain injury due to stroke, trauma, or demyelinating disease is a rare cause of a solitary asymmetric resting tremor.

- **Drug-induced tremor:** Many medications can enhance physiologic tremor, notably β-agonists (such as albuterol), nicotine, theophylline, TCAs, lithium, valproic acid, and corticosteroids. Mercury and arsenic exposure may also contribute to tremor. Neuroleptics and metoclopramide can cause drug-induced parkinsonism, but tremor is often absent in these cases.

- **Psychogenic tremor:** This often manifests with varying frequency and either becomes more irregular or subsides entirely when the patient is asked to perform a complex, repetitive motor task with the contralateral limb.

- **Wilson's disease:** This can cause resting tremor (among other manifestations) but is not considered in patients older than 40 years of age.

- **Hyperthyroidism:** This is associated with fine tremor along with a variety of other classic signs and symptoms.

Diagnostic Workup

- **TSH:** To screen for hyperthyroidism.

- **Heavy metal screen:** To screen for mercury and arsenic toxicity via urine or blood tests.

- **MRI—brain:** To rule out a structural lesion, particularly in the midbrain or basal ganglia.

- **Ceruloplasmin, slit lamp examination for Kayser-Fleischer rings, AST/ALT, CBC, 24-hour urinary copper, liver biopsy:** These tests constitute the screening tests (and diagnostic tests, in the case of liver biopsy) used to evaluate for suspected Wilson's disease. As noted previously, the patient's advanced age precludes consideration of Wilson's disease in this case.

Opening Scenario

Jay Keller, a 49-year-old male, comes to the ED complaining of passing out a few hours earlier.

Vital Signs

BP: 135/90 mm Hg

Temp: 98.0°F (36.7°C)

RR: 16/minute

HR: 76/minute, regular

Examinee Tasks

1. Take a focused history.

2. Perform a focused physical exam (do not perform rectal, genitourinary, or female breast exam).

3. Explain your clinical impression and workup plan to the patient.

4. Write the patient note after leaving the room.

Checklist/SP Sheet

Patient Description

Patient is a 49 yo M, married with three children.

Notes for the SP

None.

Challenging Questions to Ask

"Do you think I have a brain tumor?"

Sample Examinee Response

"I think it's unlikely. To make absolutely sure, however, we will do a CT scan, which is a special x-ray test of the brain. That will help us see the structure of the brain and rule out any bleeding or tumor."

Examinee Checklist

Building the Doctor-Patient Relationship

Entrance

☐ Examinee knocked on the door before entering.

☐ Examinee introduced self by name.

☐ Examinee identified his/her role or position.

☐ Examinee correctly used patient's name.

☐ Examinee made eye contact with the SP.

Reflective Listening

☐ Examinee asked an open-ended question and actively listened to the response.

☐ Examinee asked the SP to list his/her concerns and listened to the response without interrupting.

☐ Examinee summarized the SP's concerns, often using the SP's own words.

Information Gathering

☐ Examinee elicited data efficiently and accurately.

☑ Question	Patient Response
☐ Chief complaint	I passed out.
☐ Describe what happened	This morning I was taking the groceries to the car with my wife when I suddenly fell down and blacked out.
☐ Loss of consciousness before, during, or after the fall	I think I lost consciousness and then fell down on the ground.
☐ Duration of loss of consciousness	My wife told me that I did not respond to her for several minutes.
☐ Palpitations before the fall	Yes, just before I fell down, my heart started racing.
☐ Sensing something unusual before losing consciousness (sounds, lights, smells, etc)	No.
☐ Spinning/lightheadedness	I felt lightheaded right before the fall.
☐ Shaking (seizure)	Yes, my wife told me that my arms and legs started shaking after I fell down.
☐ Duration of shaking	She said around 30 seconds.
☐ Bit tongue	No.
☐ Lost control of the bladder	No.
☐ Weakness/numbness	No.
☐ Speech difficulties	No.
☐ Confusion after regaining consciousness	No.
☐ Headaches	No.
☐ Chest pain, shortness of breath	No.
☐ Abdominal pain, nausea/vomiting, diarrhea/constipation	No.
☐ Head trauma	No.
☐ Similar falls, lightheadedness, or passing out before	No.
☐ Gait abnormality	No.
☐ Weight changes	No.

☑ Question	Patient Response
☐ Appetite changes	No.
☐ Current medications	Hydrochlorothiazide, captopril, aspirin, atenolol.
☐ Past medical history	High blood pressure for the past 15 years; heart attack one year ago.
☐ Past surgical history	Appendectomy.
☐ Family history	My father died from a heart attack at age 55, and my mother died in good health.
☐ Occupation	Clerk in a video store.
☐ Alcohol use	Yes, I drink 3–4 beers a week.
☐ CAGE questions	No (to all four).
☐ Illicit drug use	No.
☐ Tobacco	No, I stopped a year ago. I had smoked one pack a day for the previous 25 years.
☐ Sexual activity	Yes, with my wife.
☐ Drug allergies	No.

Connecting with the Patient

☐ Examinee recognized the SP's emotions and responded with PEARLS.

Physical Examination

☐ Examinee washed his/her hands.

☐ Examinee asked permission to start the exam.

☐ Examinee used respectful draping.

☐ Examinee did not repeat painful maneuvers.

☑ Exam Component	Maneuver
☐ Head and neck exam	Inspection (head, mouth), carotid auscultation and palpation, thyroid exam
☐ CV exam	Palpation, auscultation, orthostatic vital signs
☐ Pulmonary exam	Auscultation
☐ Extremities	Palpated peripheral pulses
☐ Neurologic exam	Mental status, cranial nerves (including funduscopic exam), motor exam, DTRs, cerebellar, Romberg test, gait, sensory exam

Closure

☐ Examinee discussed initial diagnostic impressions.

☐ Examinee discussed initial management plans:

    ☐ Follow-up tests.

☐ Examinee asked if the SP had any other questions or concerns.

Sample Closure

Mr. Keller, I need to run some tests to determine the reason you passed out this morning, so I am going to get a CT scan of your head to look for bleeding or masses, and I will then order some blood tests to look for infections or electrolyte abnormalities. You mentioned that your heart was racing just before you passed out, so I will also ask you to wear a heart monitor for 24 hours. Doing so is just like having a constant ECG, and it will allow us to detect any abnormal heartbeats you might have. We will start with these tests and then go from there. Do you have any questions for me?

Patient Note

History

_____
_____
_____
_____
_____
_____
_____
_____

Physical Examination

_____
_____
_____
_____
_____
_____
_____
_____
_____
_____

Differential Diagnosis

1. _____
2. _____
3. _____
4. _____
5. _____

Diagnostic Workup

1. _____
2. _____
3. _____
4. _____
5. _____

History

HPI: *49 yo M c/o 1 episode of syncope that occurred a few hours ago. He was taking the groceries to the car with his wife when he suddenly felt lightheaded, had palpitations, lost consciousness, and fell down. He was unconscious for several minutes. His wife recalls that his arms and legs started shaking for 30 seconds after he fell down. He denies subsequent confusion, weakness or numbness, speech difficulties, tongue biting, or incontinence.*

ROS: *Negative except as above.*

Allergies: *NKDA.*

Medications: *HCTZ, captopril, aspirin, atenolol.*

PMH: *Hypertension for the past 15 years; MI 1 year ago.*

PSH: *Appendectomy.*

SH: *1 PPD for 25 years; quit smoking 1 year ago. Drinks 3–4 beers/week, CAGE 0/4, no illicit drugs.*

FH: *Father died from an MI at age 55.*

Physical Examination

Patient is in no acute distress.

VS: *WNL, no orthostatic changes.*

HEENT: *NC/AT, PERRLA, no funduscopic abnormalities, no tongue trauma.*

Neck: *Supple, no carotid bruits, 2+ carotid pulses with good upstroke bilaterally, thyroid normal.*

Chest: *Clear breath sounds bilaterally.*

Heart: *Apical impulse not displaced; RRR; normal S1/S2; no murmurs, rubs, or gallops.*

Extremities: *Symmetric 2+ brachial, radial, and dorsalis pedis pulses bilaterally.*

Neuro: *Cranial nerves: 2–12 grossly intact. Motor: Strength 5/5 throughout. Sensation: Intact to pin-prick and soft touch bilaterally. DTRs: Symmetric 2+ in upper and lower extremities, ⊖ Babinski bilaterally. Cerebellar: Romberg, finger to nose normal. Gait: Normal.*

Differential Diagnosis

1. *Convulsive syncope*
2. *Vasovagal syncope*
3. *Cardiac arrhythmia*
4. *Drug-induced orthostatic hypotension*
5. *Seizure*
6. *Aortic stenosis*

Diagnostic Workup

1. *CBC, electrolytes*
2. *CXR*
3. *CT—head or MRI—brain*
4. *ECG and Holter monitor*
5. *Echocardiography*
6. *Prolactin*
7. *EEG*

CASE DISCUSSION

Differential Diagnosis

- **Convulsive syncope:** Seizure-like activity often occurs after syncope and is due to global cerebral hypoperfusion. There is no EEG correlate, and a seizure workup is not required.

- **Vasovagal syncope:** This often occurs in the setting of emotional stress or pain and may be due to excessive vagal tone with resulting hypotension. Syncope is often heralded by nausea, sweating, tachycardia, pallor, and feeling "faint." This is also the mechanism of syncope in postmicturition syncope.

- **Cardiac arrhythmia:** Cardiac syncope typically occurs without warning, although a history of palpitations may indicate the presence of an underlying arrhythmia. This patient's history of MI increases his risk of developing ventricular tachycardia, and β-blocker therapy may contribute to bradyarrhythmia.

- **Drug-induced orthostatic hypotension:** The patient's antihypertensive medications increase his risk for orthostatic hypotension and syncope. However, lightheadedness and syncope in this condition is usually postural (ie, occurs when getting up from a lying or seated position), and this patient's orthostatic vital signs were normal.

- **Seizure:** Seizures usually occur unpredictably in a manner unrelated to posture or exertion. They may stem from a variety of causes, including metabolic factors, trauma, vascular factors, and brain tumors. Tonic-clonic seizures are often accompanied by tongue biting, incontinence, and prolonged confusion or drowsiness postictally.

- **Aortic stenosis:** This and other mechanical causes (eg, hypertrophic obstructive cardiomyopathy, atrial myxoma) are commonly exertional or postexertional and occur without warning. The lack of a murmur and other physical findings makes this unlikely in this case.

Diagnostic Workup

- **CBC, electrolytes:** To rule out anemia, evidence of hyperviscosity, or electrolyte imbalance that could lead to arrhythmia or other causes of syncope.

- **CXR:** To rule out lung mass, cardiomyopathy, or other pathology.

- **CT—head:** The test of choice to exclude intracranial hemorrhage. Also rules out tumor, trauma, prior stroke, or abscess.

- **MRI—brain:** Provides better anatomic detail than CT. Indicated when focal neurologic signs and symptoms are present. MRA is helpful when vertebrobasilar insufficiency is suspected (ie, when syncope is accompanied by other brain stem signs).

- **ECG and Holter or event monitor:** To evaluate possible arrhythmia.

- **Echocardiography:** To rule out mechanical causes of syncope (eg, severe aortic stenosis, atrial myxoma, severe LVH with small residual cavity size, and hypertrophic obstructive cardiomyopathy).

- **Prolactin:** Often elevated within 30–60 minutes of a generalized seizure (it is useless after that time interval). Must be compared to baseline prolactin levels.

- **EEG:** To evaluate suspected seizure activity.

Opening Scenario

Kristin Grant, a 30-year-old female, comes to the office complaining of weight gain.

Vital Signs

BP: 120/85 mm Hg

Temp: 98.0°F (36.7°C)

RR: 13/minute

HR: 65/minute, regular

BMI: 30

Examinee Tasks

1. Take a focused history.

2. Perform a focused physical exam (do not perform rectal, genitourinary, or female breast exam).

3. Explain your clinical impression and workup plan to the patient.

4. Write the patient note after leaving the room.

Checklist/SP Sheet

Patient Description

Patient is a 30 yo F.

Notes for the SP

None.

Challenging Questions to Ask

"I want to go back to smoking because I believe that I have started gaining weight since I quit."

Sample Examinee Response

"I understand that controlling your weight is important to you, but the health risks of smoking far outweigh those associated with weight gain. We also need to determine if something else is contributing to your weight gain and, if so, discuss strategies to deal with it."

Examinee Checklist

Building the Doctor-Patient Relationship

Entrance

☐ Examinee knocked on the door before entering.

☐ Examinee introduced self by name.

☐ Examinee identified his/her role or position.

☐ Examinee correctly used patient's name.

☐ Examinee made eye contact with the SP.

Reflective Listening

☐ Examinee asked an open-ended question and actively listened to the response.

☐ Examinee asked the SP to list his/her concerns and listened to the response without interrupting.

☐ Examinee summarized the SP's concerns, often using the SP's own words.

Information Gathering

☐ Examinee elicited data efficiently and accurately.

☑ Question	Patient Response
☐ Chief complaint	I am gaining weight.
☐ Onset	Three months ago.
☐ Weight gained	20 Pounds.
☐ Cold intolerance	Yes.
☐ Skin/hair changes	My hair is falling out more than usual, and I feel that my skin has become dry.
☐ Voice change	No.
☐ Constipation	No.
☐ Appetite changes	I have a good appetite.
☐ Fatigue	No.
☐ Depression	No.
☐ Sleeping problems (falling asleep, staying asleep, early waking, snoring)	No.
☐ Associated symptoms (fever/chills, chest pain, shortness of breath, abdominal pain, diarrhea)	No.
☐ Last menstrual period	One week ago.
☐ Frequency of menstrual periods	I used to get my period every four weeks, but recently I've been getting it every six weeks or more. The period lasts seven days.
☐ Start of change in cycle	Six months ago.
☐ Pads/tampons changed a day	It was 2–3 a day, but the blood flow is becoming less, and I use only one a day now.
☐ Age at menarche	Age 13.
☐ Pregnancies	I have one child; he is 10 years old.
☐ Problems during pregnancy/delivery	No, it was a normal delivery, and my child is healthy.
☐ Miscarriages/abortions	None.
☐ Hirsutism	No.

☑ Question	Patient Response
☐ Current medications	Lithium.
☐ Past medical history	I have bipolar disorder. I was started on lithium 6 months ago; I haven't had any problems since then.
☐ Past surgical history	None.
☐ Family history of obesity	My mother and sister are obese.
☐ Occupation	Housekeeper.
☐ Alcohol use	None.
☐ Illicit drug use	Never.
☐ Tobacco	I quit smoking three months ago. I had smoked two packs a day for 10 years.
☐ Exercise	No.
☐ Diet	The usual. I haven't changed anything in my diet in more than 10 years. Donuts, lots of coffee during the day, chicken, steak, Chinese food, and salad.
☐ Sexual activity	With my husband.
☐ Contraceptives	My husband had a vasectomy two years ago.
☐ Drug allergies	No.

Connecting with the Patient

☐ Examinee recognized the SP's emotions and responded with PEARLS.

Physical Examination

☐ Examinee washed his/her hands.

☐ Examinee asked permission to start the exam.

☐ Examinee used respectful draping.

☐ Examinee did not repeat painful maneuvers.

☑ Exam Component	Maneuver
☐ Head exam	Inspected conjunctivae, mouth, and throat
☐ Neck exam	Palpated lymph nodes, thyroid gland
☐ CV exam	Auscultation
☐ Pulmonary exam	Auscultation
☐ Abdominal exam	Auscultation, palpation, percussion
☐ Extremities	Inspected for edema, checked DTRs

Closure

☐ Examinee discussed initial diagnostic impressions.

☐ Examinee discussed initial management plans:

　☐ Follow-up tests.

　☐ Lifestyle modification (diet, exercise, relaxation techniques, smoking cessation support).

☐ Examinee asked if the SP had any other questions or concerns.

Sample Closure

Mrs. Grant, most smokers gain an average of 5 pounds when they quit. You have gained 20 pounds. This may have resulted from your smoking cessation, but bear in mind that the health risk posed by smoking is far worse than the risk you might incur from excessive weight gain. In addition, there may be other reasons for your weight gain; for example, it may be related to your thyroid gland or it may be a side effect of the lithium you're taking. I would like to draw some blood to measure your thyroid function and lithium levels. In the meantime, in addition to stopping smoking, you should continue to promote a healthier lifestyle. Try to decrease the fatty foods you eat and increase the healthy ones, such as fruits and vegetables. Exercising only 30 minutes three times a week can also improve your health. Do you have any questions for me?

Patient Note

History

Physical Examination

Differential Diagnosis

1.
2.
3.
4.
5.

Diagnostic Workup

1.
2.
3.
4.
5.

History

HPI: *30 yo F c/o weight gain of 20 lbs over the past 3 months after she stopped smoking. She has a good appetite and reports no change in her diet. For 6 months she has experienced oligomenorrhea and hypomenorrhea, dry skin, and cold intolerance. The patient denies voice change, constipation, hirsutism, depression, fatigue, or sleep problems.*

OB/GYN: *Last menstrual period last week. See HPI for other.*

ROS: *Negative except as above.*

Allergies: *NKDA.*

Medications: *Lithium, started 6 months ago.*

PMH: *Bipolar disorder, diagnosed 6 months ago.*

SH: *2 PPD for 10 years; stopped 3 months ago. No alcohol, no illicit drugs. Sexually active with husband only. Doesn't exercise.*

Diet: *Consists mainly of donuts, lots of coffee during the day, chicken, steak, Chinese food, and salad.*

FH: *Mother and sister are obese.*

Physical Examination

Patient is in no acute distress.

VS: *WNL.*

HEENT: *No conjunctival pallor, mouth and pharynx WNL.*

Neck: *No lymphadenopathy, thyroid normal.*

Chest: *Clear breath sounds bilaterally.*

Heart: *RRR; normal S1/S2; no murmurs, rubs, or gallops.*

Abdomen: *Soft, nontender, nondistended, ⊕ BS, no hepatosplenomegaly.*

Extremities: *No edema, normal DTRs in lower extremities bilaterally.*

Differential Diagnosis

1. *Smoking cessation*
2. *Hypothyroidism*
3. *Lithium-related obesity*
4. *Familial obesity*
5. *Pregnancy*
6. *Cushing syndrome*

Diagnostic Workup

1. *TSH*
2. *Urine hCG*
3. *Glucose, cholesterol, triglycerides*
4. *Dexamethasone suppression test*
5. *24-Hour urine free cortisol*
6. *Lithium level*

CASE DISCUSSION

Differential Diagnosis

- **Smoking cessation:** Weight gain occurs in most patients following smoking cessation but usually averages only 2 kg (4.4 lb). However, major weight gain such as that seen in this case may occur. Patients generally report increased appetite and calorie consumption.

- **Hypothyroidism:** The patient has classic symptoms of hypothyroidism, and it needs to be ruled out as a cause of her weight gain.

- **Lithium-related obesity:** Weight gain is a common side effect of lithium therapy and may contribute in this case.

- **Familial obesity:** There are probably strong genetic influences on the development of obesity, but a positive family history does not account for acute weight gain.

- **Pregnancy:** Regardless of the menstrual history given by the patient, pregnancy should be suspected in a woman of childbearing age who has unexplained weight gain.

- **Cushing syndrome:** This is a rare cause of unexplained weight gain and can usually be diagnosed by physical exam (eg, one can see hypertension, moon facies, plethora, supraclavicular fat pads, truncal obesity with thin limbs, and abdominal striae).

Diagnostic Workup

- **TSH:** To diagnose suspected hypothyroidism.

- **Urine hCG:** To rule out pregnancy.

- **Glucose, cholesterol, triglycerides:** To screen for medical complications of obesity.

- **Dexamethasone suppression test:** To screen for hypercortisolism. A suppressed morning cortisol following bedtime dexamethasone administration excludes Cushing syndrome with 98% certainty.

- **24-Hour urine free cortisol:** Performed if the dexamethasone suppression test is abnormal. Helps confirm hypercortisolism.

Opening Scenario

Patricia Garrison, a 36-year-old female, comes to the office complaining of not having menstrual periods recently.

Vital Signs

BP: 120/85 mm Hg

Temp: 98.0°F (36.7°C)

RR: 13/minute

HR: 65/minute, regular

Examinee Tasks

1. Take a focused history.

2. Perform a focused physical exam (do not perform rectal, genitourinary, or female breast exam).

3. Explain your clinical impression and workup plan to the patient.

4. Write the patient note after leaving the room.

Checklist/SP Sheet

Patient Description

Patient is a 36 yo F.

Notes for the SP

None.

Challenging Questions to Ask

"Am I going through menopause?"

Sample Examinee Response

"I doubt it. It would be extremely unusual at your age. I need to learn more by asking you about other symptoms and examining you, and then we can discuss possible reasons you are not having periods."

Examinee Checklist

Building the Doctor-Patient Relationship

Entrance

☐ Examinee knocked on the door before entering.

☐ Examinee introduced self by name.

☐ Examinee identified his/her role or position.

☐ Examine correctly used patient's name.

☐ Examinee made eye contact with the SP.

Reflective Listening

☐ Examinee asked an open-ended question and actively listened to the response.

☐ Examinee asked the SP to list his/her concerns and listened to the response without interrupting.

☐ Examinee summarized the SP's concerns, often using the SP's own words.

Information Gathering

☐ Examinee elicited data efficiently and accurately.

☑ Question	Patient Response
☐ Chief complaint	I haven't had a period in three months.
☐ Menstrual history	I used to have regular periods every month lasting for 4–5 days, but over the past year I started having them less frequently—every 5–6 weeks lasting for seven days.
☐ Pads/tampons changed a day	It was 2–3 a day, but the blood flow is becoming less, and I use only 1 a day now.
☐ Age at menarche	Age 14.
☐ Weight changes	I have gained 15 pounds over the past year.
☐ Cold intolerance	No.
☐ Skin/hair changes	Actually, I noticed some facial hair recently that I am plucking.
☐ Voice change	No.
☐ Change in bowel habits	No.
☐ Appetite changes	I have a good appetite.
☐ Fad diet or diet pills	No, I've been a vegetarian for 10 years.
☐ Fatigue	No.
☐ Depression/anxiety/stress	No.
☐ Hot flashes	No.
☐ Vaginal dryness/itching	No.
☐ Sleeping problems (falling asleep, staying asleep, early waking, snoring)	No.
☐ Urinary frequency	No.
☐ Nipple discharge	Yes, just last week I noticed some milky discharge from my left breast.
☐ Visual changes	No.
☐ Headache	No.
☐ Abdominal pain	No.
☐ Sexual activity	Once a week on average with my husband.
☐ Contraceptives	The same pills for eight years.

☑ Question	Patient Response
☐ Pregnancies	I have one child; he is 10 years old.
☐ Problems during pregnancy/delivery	No, it was a normal delivery, and my child is healthy.
☐ Miscarriages/abortions	No.
☐ Last Pap smear	Ten months ago. It was normal.
☐ History of abnormal Pap smears	No.
☐ Current medications	None.
☐ Past medical history	None.
☐ Past surgical history	None.
☐ Family history	My father and mother are healthy; my mother began menopause at age 55.
☐ Occupation	Nurse.
☐ Alcohol use	None.
☐ Illicit drug use	Never.
☐ Tobacco	No.
☐ Exercise	I run two miles three times a week.
☐ Drug allergies	No.

Connecting with the Patient

☐ Examinee recognized the SP's emotions and responded with PEARLS.

Physical Examination

☐ Examinee washed his/her hands.

☐ Examinee asked permission to start the exam.

☐ Examinee used respectful draping.

☐ Examinee did not repeat painful maneuvers.

☑ Exam Component	Maneuver
☐ Neck exam	Examined thyroid gland
☐ CV exam	Auscultation
☐ Pulmonary exam	Auscultation
☐ Abdominal exam	Auscultation, palpation, percussion
☐ Extremities	Inspection
☐ Neurologic exam	Visual fields, extraocular movements, checked DTRs

Closure

☐ Examinee discussed initial diagnostic impressions.

☐ Examinee discussed initial management plans:

    ☐ Follow-up tests: Examinee mentioned the need for pelvic and breast exams.

☐ Examinee asked if the SP had any other questions or concerns.

Sample Closure

Ms. Garrison, there are a few reasons you may not be having regular periods. The first thing we need to do is determine whether you are pregnant. We can do that with a simple urine test. The other thing we need to do is conduct breast and pelvic exams, especially since you have had some nipple discharge, and look for any signs of menopause. Menopause is highly unlikely at your age, but on rare occasions it may occur. A blood test to measure your hormone levels will also help us determine if you are menopausal or have a hormonal imbalance. This will give us a good start in figuring out why you haven't had your period, and we will go from there. Do you have any questions for me?

CASE DISCUSSION

Differential Diagnosis

- **Pregnancy:** This is the most common cause of secondary amenorrhea in women of childbearing age and should be ruled out during the initial evaluation.

- **Hyperprolactinemia:** This causes menstrual cycle disturbances, galactorrhea, and infertility. It may result from a variety of conditions, including pregnancy, hypothyroidism, renal failure, and cirrhosis, or it can be a side effect of medications. Roughly 70% of women with secondary amenorrhea and galactorrhea will have hyperprolactinemia.

- **Polycystic ovary syndrome (PCOS):** This manifests variably as hirsutism, obesity, virilization, infertility, and glucose intolerance. About one-half of patients have amenorrhea (due to chronic anovulation). The patient's oligomenorrhea and hirsutism in the context of recent weight gain suggest this diagnosis.

- **Thyroid disease:** Both hyper- and hypothyroidism can cause menstrual irregularities, although amenorrhea is more commonly due to hypothyroidism. Except for galactorrhea and weight gain, the patient does not have other signs or symptoms of thyroid disease.

- **Premature ovarian failure:** This refers to primary hypogonadism that occurs before age 40. Causes include autoimmunity against the ovary, pelvic radiation therapy, chemotherapy, surgical bilateral oophorectomy, and familial factors. The patient's lack of menopausal symptoms (eg, fatigue, insomnia, headache, diminished libido, depression, and hot flashes) makes this diagnosis unlikely.

- **Asherman syndrome:** This describes amenorrhea due to endometrial scarring, which can occur following uterine infections. The vaginal estrogen effect is normal.

Diagnostic Workup

- **Pelvic and breast exams:** Required to check for genital virilization (ie, clitoromegaly), uterine or adnexal enlargement, and estrogen effect (via inspection of vaginal mucosa and Pap smear) and to elicit breast discharge.

- **Urine hCG:** To rule out pregnancy.

- **LH/FSH:** PCOS is a clinical diagnosis; an increased LH/FSH ratio is often seen but is neither necessary nor sufficient to make the diagnosis. Physiologically, increased levels of estrone (derived from obesity) are believed to suppress pituitary FSH, leading to a relative increase in LH. Constant LH stimulation of the ovary then results in anovulation (and often amenorrhea). An elevated FSH (> 40) is diagnostic for premature ovarian failure.

- **Prolactin, TSH:** To screen for hyperprolactinemia and thyroid disease. Free T_4 is also useful if hyperthyroidism (or central hypothyroidism) is suspected.

- **Electrolytes, glucose, BUN/Cr, AST/ALT/bilirubin/alkaline phosphatase:** To check renal and hepatic function and to screen for evidence of hypercortisolism (eg, high sodium and low potassium).

- **Testosterone, DHEAS:** To screen for hyperandrogenism when amenorrhea is accompanied by hirsutism and virilization. Mild elevations are often due to PCOS, but high levels may be due to ovarian or adrenal tumors.

- **MRI—brain:** Required to evaluate the pituitary region in patients suspected of having amenorrhea due to a hypothalamic or pituitary etiology (eg, hyperprolactinemia).

- **Hysteroscopy:** To look for endometrial adhesions that are diagnostic for Asherman syndrome.

CASE 26
DOORWAY INFORMATION

Opening Scenario

Stephanie McCall, a 28-year-old female, comes to the office complaining of pain during sex.

Vital Signs

BP: 120/85 mm Hg

Temp: 98.0°F (36.7°C)

RR: 13/minute

HR: 65/minute, regular

Examinee Tasks

1. Take a focused history.

2. Perform a focused physical exam (do not perform rectal, genitourinary, or female breast exam).

3. Explain your clinical impression and workup plan to the patient.

4. Write the patient note after leaving the room.

Checklist/SP Sheet

Patient Description

Patient is a 28 yo F.

Notes for the SP

None.

Challenging Questions to Ask

When asked about vaginal discharge, ask, "Do you think I have a sexually transmitted disease?"

Sample Examinee Response

"There are many causes of vaginal discharge, only some of which are due to sexually transmitted infections. I will try to look for clues by asking you more questions and examining you, and we will definitely send a sample of the discharge to the lab to check for infection."

Examinee Checklist

Building the Doctor-Patient Relationship

Entrance

☐ Examinee knocked on the door before entering.

☐ Examinee introduced self by name.

☐ Examinee identified his/her role or position.

☐ Examinee correctly used patient's name.

☐ Examinee made eye contact with the SP.

Reflective Listening

☐ Examinee asked an open-ended question and actively listened to the response.

☐ Examinee asked the SP to list his/her concerns and listened to the response without interrupting.

☐ Examinee summarized the SP's concerns, often using the SP's own words.

Information Gathering

☐ Examinee elicited data efficiently and accurately.

☑ Question	Patient Response
☐ Chief complaint	I have been experiencing pain during sex.
☐ Onset	Three months ago.
☐ Describe pain	Aching and burning.
☐ Timing	It happens every time I try to have sex.
☐ Location	In the vaginal area. It starts on the outside, and I feel it on the inside with deep thrusting.
☐ Vaginal discharge	Yes, recently.
☐ Color/amount/smell	White, small amount every day (I don't have to wear a pad); it smells like fish.
☐ Itching	Yes, a little bit.
☐ Douching	No.
☐ Last menstrual period	Two weeks ago.
☐ Frequency of menstrual periods	Regular, every month; lasts for three days.
☐ Pads/tampons changed a day	Three.
☐ Painful periods	Yes, they have started to be painful over the past year.
☐ Postcoital or intermenstrual bleeding	No.
☐ Sexual partner	I have had the same boyfriend for the past year; before that, I had a relationship with my ex-boyfriend for five years.
☐ Contraception	I am using the patch.
☐ Sexual desire	Good.
☐ Conflicts with partner	No, we are pretty close.
☐ Feeling safe at home	Yes, I have my own apartment.
☐ History of physical, sexual, or emotional abuse	I don't usually talk about it, but I was raped in college, and that was when I contracted gonorrhea.
☐ History of vaginal infections or STDs	I had gonorrhea 10 years ago in college.
☐ Last Pap smear	Six months ago; it was normal.
☐ History of abnormal Pap smears	No.

✓ Question	Patient Response
☐ Depression/anxiety	No.
☐ Hot flashes	No.
☐ Vaginal dryness during intercourse	No.
☐ Sleeping problems	No.
☐ Urinary frequency/pain with urination	No.
☐ Pregnancies	I have never been pregnant.
☐ Current medications	None.
☐ Past medical history	None.
☐ Past surgical history	None.
☐ Family history	Both parents are healthy.
☐ Occupation	Editor for a fashion magazine.
☐ Alcohol use	A couple of beers on the weekends; sometimes a glass of wine on a romantic dinner.
☐ CAGE questions	No (to all four).
☐ Illicit drug use	Marijuana in college.
☐ Tobacco	No.
☐ Exercise	I swim and run regularly.
☐ Drug allergies	No.

Connecting with the Patient

☐ Examinee recognized the SP's emotions and responded with PEARLS.

Physical Examination

☐ Examinee washed his/her hands.

☐ Examinee asked permission to start the exam.

☐ Examinee used respectful draping.

☐ Examinee did not repeat painful maneuvers.

✓ Exam Component	Maneuver
☐ CV exam	Auscultation
☐ Pulmonary exam	Auscultation
☐ Abdominal exam	Auscultation, palpation, percussion

Closure

☐ Examinee discussed initial diagnostic impressions.

☐ Examinee discussed initial management plans:

    ☐ Follow-up tests: Examinee mentioned the need for a pelvic exam.

☐ Examinee asked if the SP had any other questions or concerns.

Sample Closure

Ms. McCall, your most likely diagnosis is an infection in the vagina or cervix. However, there are other, less common causes for your problem. I can't make a diagnosis until I do a pelvic exam and take a look at what I find under a microscope. I will also take a cervical swab and send it for gonorrhea and chlamydia testing. Do you have any questions for me?

Patient Note

History

_____
_____
_____
_____
_____
_____
_____
_____

Physical Examination

_____
_____
_____
_____
_____
_____
_____
_____
_____
_____
_____

Differential Diagnosis

1. _____
2. _____
3. _____
4. _____
5. _____

Diagnostic Workup

1. _____
2. _____
3. _____
4. _____
5. _____

History

HPI: 28 yo F c/o pain during intercourse for 3 months, located both superficially and with deep thrusting. She also noticed a small white vaginal discharge with a fishy odor, accompanied by mild vaginal pruritus. Denies postcoital or intermenstrual vaginal bleeding. She is sexually active with her boyfriend (only) for the past year, and her sexual desire is good. She feels safe at home and denies any conflicts with her partner. She also denies vaginal dryness, hot flashes, hirsutism, depression, fatigue, sleep problems, dysuria, and urinary frequency.

OB/GYN: G0P0. Last menstrual period 2 weeks ago; has regular menses but started to be painful over the past year. No history of abnormal Pap smears; most recent was 6 months ago. Uses patch for contraception.

ROS: Negative except as above.

Allergies: NKDA.

Medications: None.

PMH: History of rape 10 years ago; subsequently contracted gonorrhea.

SH: No tobacco. Drinks a couple of beers on the weekends, occasional wine, CAGE 0/4; used marijuana in college. Exercises regularly.

FH: Noncontributory.

Physical Examination

Patient is in no acute distress.

VS: WNL.

Chest: Clear breath sounds bilaterally.

Heart: RRR; normal S1/S2; no murmurs, rubs, or gallops.

Differential Diagnosis

1. Vulvovaginitis
2. Cervicitis
3. Endometriosis
4. Vulvodynia
5. Domestic violence
6. Pelvic tumor
7. Vaginismus

Diagnostic Workup

1. Pelvic exam
2. Wet mount, KOH prep, "whiff" test
3. Cervical cultures (chlamydia and gonorrhea DNA probes)
4. U/S—pelvis
5. MRI—pelvis
6. Laparoscopy

CASE DISCUSSION

Differential Diagnosis

- **Vulvovaginitis:** This describes infection or inflammation of the vagina. Etiologies include pathogens, allergic or contact reactions, or friction from intercourse. The presence of vaginal discharge (accompanied by a fishy odor and pruritus) makes this a likely diagnosis.

- **Cervicitis:** The presence of vaginal discharge and pain with deep thrusting suggests infection or inflammation of the cervix.

- **Endometriosis:** This describes abnormal ectopic endometrial tissue, which can cause inflammation and scarring in the lower pelvis. Endometriosis may account for the patient's dysmenorrhea over the past year and, if so, could also cause dyspareunia with deep thrusting. Her history of gonorrhea infection (if it caused pelvic inflammatory disease) also puts her at risk for pelvic scarring and subsequent dyspareunia (due to impaired mobility of pelvic organs).

- **Vulvodynia:** This is the leading cause of dyspareunia in premenopausal women but is not well understood. Pain may be constant or intermittent, focal or diffuse, and superficial or deep. Physical findings are often absent, making it a diagnosis of exclusion. However, vulvar erythema can be seen in a subset of vulvodynia termed *vulvar vestibulitis*.

- **Domestic violence:** Physicians must screen for this in any woman presenting with dyspareunia. Serial screening is required, as victims may not disclose this history initially.

- **Pelvic tumor:** This could account for the patient's pain with deep thrusting and possibly for her history of dysmenorrhea. However, pelvic tumors are not associated with vaginal discharge and pruritus.

- **Vaginismus:** This describes severe involuntary spasm of muscles around the introitus and often results from fear, pain, or sexual or psychological trauma. The muscle contractions generally preclude penetration. Although this patient was raped in the past, she does not describe the muscle contractions characteristic of vaginismus.

Diagnostic Workup

- **Pelvic exam:** To localize and reproduce the pain or discomfort and to determine if any pathology is present. A complete exam includes external genital inspection and palpation, a speculum exam, and bimanual and rectal exams.

- **Wet mount, KOH prep, "whiff" test:** The vaginal discharge is examined microscopically. The presence of epithelial cells covered with bacteria (clue cells) suggests bacterial vaginosis, and the presence of hyphae and spores indicates candidal infection. Motile organisms are seen in trichomonal infection. A "fishy" odor after exposure of the discharge to a drop of potassium hydroxide is characteristic of bacterial vaginosis.

- **Cervical cultures:** To diagnose chlamydia, gonorrhea, and occasionally HSV infection (the latter is characterized by the presence of vesicles or ulcers on the cervix).

- **Imaging studies:** U/S and MRI are useful to assess the size and positioning of pelvic organs and to help rule out masses or other pathology.

- **Laparoscopy:** This is the gold standard test used to confirm a clinical diagnosis of endometriosis.

Opening Scenario

Rick Meyer, a 51-year-old male construction worker, comes to the office complaining of back pain.

Vital Signs

BP: 120/85 mm Hg

Temp: 98.2°F (36.8°C)

RR: 20/minute

HR: 80/minute, regular

Examinee Tasks

1. Take a focused history.

2. Perform a focused physical exam (do not perform rectal, genitourinary, or female breast exam).

3. Explain your clinical impression and workup plan to the patient.

4. Write the patient note after leaving the room.

Checklist/SP Sheet

Patient Description

Patient is a 51 yo M who lives with his girlfriend.

Notes for the SP

- Pretend that you have paraspinal lower back tenderness when examined.
- Show normal reflexes, sensation, and strength in both lower extremities.
- Lean forward slightly when walking.

Challenging Questions to Ask

"I don't think I can go to work, doctor. Can you write a letter to my boss so that I can have some days off?"

Sample Examinee Response

"You're right; heavy construction work can worsen your back pain or cause it to heal more slowly. I will ask your boss to reassign you to light duty for a while."

Examinee Checklist

Building the Doctor-Patient Relationship

Entrance

☐ Examinee knocked on the door before entering.

☐ Examinee introduced self by name.

☐ Examinee identified his/her role or position.

☐ Examinee correctly used patient's name.

☐ Examinee made eye contact with the SP.

Reflective Listening

☐ Examinee asked an open-ended question and actively listened to the response.

☐ Examinee asked the SP to list his/her concerns and listened to the response without interrupting.

☐ Examinee summarized the SP's concerns, often using the SP's own words.

Information Gathering

☐ Examinee elicited data efficiently and accurately.

☑ Question	Patient Response
☐ Chief complaint	Pain in my back.
☐ Onset	One week ago.
☐ Associated/precipitating events	I was lifting some heavy boxes; then my back started hurting right away.
☐ Progression	It has been the same.
☐ Severity on a scale	8/10.
☐ Location	The middle of my lower back.
☐ Radiation	It radiates to my left thigh and sometimes reaches my left foot.
☐ Quality	Sharp.
☐ Alleviating factors	Lying still in bed.
☐ Exacerbating factors	Walking, sitting for a long time, coughing.
☐ Weakness/numbness	None.
☐ Difficulty urinating	I noticed that over the past six months I have had to strain in order to urinate. Sometimes I feel as if I haven't emptied my bladder fully.
☐ Urinary or fecal incontinence	No.
☐ Fever, night sweats, weight loss	No.
☐ History of back pain in the past	Well, for the past year I have been having back pain on and off, mainly when I walk. It is usually accompanied by pain in my legs. That pain goes away when I stop walking and sit down.
☐ Current medications	I take ibuprofen. It helps, but the pain is still there.
☐ Past medical history	None.
☐ Past surgical history	None.
☐ Family history	My father died of a heart attack at age 65, and my mother is healthy.
☐ Occupation	Construction worker.
☐ Alcohol use	Yes, a couple of beers on the weekends.

☑ Question	Patient Response
☐ CAGE questions	No (to all four).
☐ Illicit drug use	Never.
☐ Tobacco	Yes, one pack a day for the past 18 years.
☐ Drug allergies	Penicillin gives me a rash.

Connecting with the Patient

☐ Examinee recognized the SP's emotions and responded with PEARLS.

Physical Examination

☐ Examinee washed his/her hands.

☐ Examinee asked permission to start the exam.

☐ Examinee used respectful draping.

☐ Examinee did not repeat painful maneuvers.

☑ Exam Component	Maneuver
☐ Back exam	Inspection, palpation, range of motion
☐ Extremities	Inspection, palpation of peripheral pulses, hip exam
☐ Neurologic exam	Motor, DTRs, Babinski sign, gait (including toe and heel walking), passive straight leg raising, sensory exam

Closure

☐ Examinee discussed initial diagnostic impressions.

☐ Examinee discussed initial management plans:

    ☐ Follow-up tests: Examinee mentioned the need for a rectal exam.

☐ Examinee asked if the SP had any other questions or concerns.

Sample Closure

Mr. Meyer, I am concerned about your difficulty urinating, so I would like to do a rectal exam and assess your prostate for benign growths or cancer. I would also like to run some blood tests and order an x-ray and possibly an MRI of your back so that I can better determine the cause of your pain. In the meantime, as we discussed, I will write a note to your employer requesting that you be given only light duties while you are at work. Do you have any questions for me?

Patient Note

History

_____
_____
_____
_____
_____
_____
_____

Physical Examination

_____
_____
_____
_____
_____
_____
_____
_____
_____
_____
_____

Differential Diagnosis

1. _____
2. _____
3. _____
4. _____
5. _____

Diagnostic Workup

1. _____
2. _____
3. _____
4. _____
5. _____

Patient Note

History

HPI: *51 yo M construction worker c/o lower back pain that started after he lifted heavy boxes 1 week ago. The pain is 8/10, sharp, and radiates to the left thigh and sometimes to the left foot. Pain worsens with movement, cough, and sitting for a long time. Pain is relieved by lying still and partially by ibuprofen. He denies urinary/stool incontinence or weakness/loss of sensation in lower extremities. No fever, night sweats, or weight loss. He does report difficulty urinating and incomplete emptying of the bladder for 6 months as well as a 1-year history of intermittent lower back pain and leg pain with ambulation that resolves with sitting.*

ROS: *Negative except as above.*

Allergies: *Penicillin, causes rash.*

Medications: *Ibuprofen.*

PMH: *None.*

PSH: *None.*

SH: *1 PPD for 18 years, 1–2 beers on weekends, CAGE 0/4.*

FH: *Noncontributory.*

Physical Examination

Patient is in mild distress due to back pain.

Back: *Mild paraspinal muscle tenderness bilaterally, normal range of motion, no warmth or erythema.*

Extremities: *2+ popliteal, dorsalis pedis, and posterior tibial pulses bilaterally. Hips normal, non-tender range of motion bilaterally.*

Neuro: *Motor: Strength 5/5 throughout, including left great toe dorsiflexion. DTRs: 2+ symmetric, ⊖ Babinski bilaterally. Gait: Normal (including toe and heel walking), although he walks with back slightly bent forward. Straight leg raising ⊖ bilaterally. Sensation: Intact.*

Differential Diagnosis

1. *Disk herniation*
2. *Lumbar muscle strain*
3. *Degenerative arthritis*
4. *Lumbar spinal stenosis*
5. *Metastatic prostate cancer*
6. *Multiple myeloma*
7. *Malingering*

Diagnostic Workup

1. *Rectal exam*
2. *XR—L-spine*
3. *MRI—L-spine*
4. *PSA*
5. *CBC, calcium, BUN/Cr*
6. *Serum and urine protein electrophoresis*

CASE DISCUSSION

Differential Diagnosis

- **Disk herniation:** Low back pain radiating down the buttock and below the knee suggests nerve root irritation due to disk herniation. However, this pattern is nonspecific and can also be caused by sacroiliitis, facet joint degenerative arthritis, spinal stenosis, or other causes of sciatica. Most disk herniations occur at the L4–L5 or L5–S1 vertebral levels. These nerve roots are quickly assessed by checking the knee-jerk reflex (L4), great toe dorsiflexion (L5), and ankle-jerk reflex (S1). Ipsilateral straight leg raising that produces radicular symptoms (with the leg raised < 60 degrees) is highly sensitive but nonspecific in herniations at these levels. This patient may have disk herniation but has no objective evidence of neurologic compromise at this point.

- **Lumbar muscle strain:** This often follows strenuous or unusual exertion, but pain usually does not radiate to the extremities. Paraspinal muscle tenderness is often present.

- **Degenerative arthritis:** Degenerative back diseases are common, and classically pain is exacerbated by activity and alleviated by rest. Radicular symptoms may be present.

- **Lumbar spinal stenosis:** This is most often seen in patients older than 60 years of age. They present with gradual onset of back pain that radiates to the buttocks and legs with or without leg numbness and weakness. Pain usually occurs with walking or prolonged standing and subsides by sitting or leaning forward (as in this case).

- **Metastatic prostate cancer:** The most common cancers leading to vertebral body metastasis are prostate, breast, lung, multiple myeloma, and lymphoma. In metastatic disease, patients complain of gradual-onset back pain (or occasionally acute pain in the case of pathologic fracture) with or without neurologic symptoms. Pain may be worse at night and unrelieved by rest. This patient's urinary symptoms may be a sign of prostatic disease.

- **Multiple myeloma:** Typically, patients are older than 50 years of age. Back and bone pain may be the only presenting complaint. Anemia, neuropathy, hypercalcemia, and renal failure are also common.

- **Malingering:** This is defined as intentional faking of symptoms for secondary gain (eg, getting out of work).

Diagnostic Workup

The history and physical exam are often all that is required, as the majority of patients with low back pain will improve within four weeks. Patients who require more extensive or urgent evaluation are those suspected of having pain caused by infection, cancer, abdominal aortic aneurysm, or neurologic emergency (eg, cauda equina syndrome).

- **Rectal exam (including "saddle area" sensory exam):** To evaluate the prostate, rectal sphincter tone, and integrity of sacral nerve roots.

- **XR—L-spine:** Can show evidence of vertebral osteomyelitis, cancer, or fractures. Degenerative changes are expected in older patients and correlate poorly with clinical symptoms.

- **MRI—L-spine:** Provides the best anatomic detail and is the test of choice for suspected herniation, infection, or malignancy. Remember that asymptomatic disk herniation is common, so its presence does not necessarily correlate with clinical disease.

- **PSA:** Screening test for prostate cancer.

- **CBC, calcium, BUN/Cr:** To detect anemia, hypercalcemia, and renal failure, all of which may be clues to underlying multiple myeloma.

- **Serum and urine protein electrophoresis:** To detect a monoclonal paraprotein in myeloma.

Opening Scenario

The mother of Theresa Wheaton, a 6-month-old female child, calls the office complaining that her child has diarrhea.

Examinee Tasks

1. Take a focused history.

2. Explain your clinical impression and workup plan to the mother.

3. Write the patient note after leaving the room.

Checklist/SP Sheet

Patient Description

The patient's mother offers the history.

Notes for the SP

Show concern about your child's health, but add that you don't want to come to the office unless you have to because you do not have transportation.

Challenging Questions to Ask

"How sick is my baby?"

Sample Examinee Response

"It is hard for me to give you an accurate answer over the phone. I would like you to bring your baby here so that I can examine her and perhaps run some tests. After that, I should be able to give you a more accurate assessment."

Examinee Checklist

Building the Doctor-Patient Relationship

Entrance

☐ Examinee introduced self by name.

☐ Examinee identified his/her role or position.

☐ Examinee correctly used patient's name and identified caller and relationship of caller to patient.

Reflective Listening

☐ Examinee asked an open-ended question and actively listened to the response.

☐ Examinee asked the SP to list his/her concerns and listened to the response without interrupting.

☐ Examinee summarized the SP's concerns, often using the SP's own words.

Information Gathering

☐ Examinee elicited data efficiently and accurately.

☐ Examinee showed compassion for the SP and her child.

☑ Question	Patient Response
☐ Chief complaint	My baby has diarrhea.
☐ Onset	It started yesterday at 2 P.M.
☐ Progression	It is getting worse.
☐ Frequency of bowel movements	She has about six bowel movements per day.
☐ Description of bowel movements	Light brown, watery, large amounts.
☐ Blood in stool	No.
☐ Relationship to oral intake	None.
☐ Previous regular bowel movements	Yes.
☐ Abdominal distention	No.
☐ Appetite changes	She is not as hungry as she used to be.
☐ Activities	Not as playful as she was earlier.
☐ Awake and responsive	She is less responsive and looks drowsy.
☐ Number of wet diapers	None since yesterday.
☐ Dry mouth or sunken soft spot over the head	Yes, her mouth is dry.
☐ Treatment tried	I tried some Tylenol, but it did not help.
☐ Vigorous cry	No, her cry is weak.
☐ Recent URI	No.
☐ Fever	Yes; I took her temperature, and it was 100.5.
☐ Breathing fast	No.
☐ Nausea/vomiting	No.
☐ Rash	No.
☐ Shaking (seizures)	No.
☐ Cough, pulling ear, or crying when urine is passed	No.
☐ Day care center	Yes.
☐ Ill contacts in day care center	Not to my knowledge.
☐ Vaccinations	Up to date.
☐ Last checkup	Two weeks ago, and everything was normal.
☐ Birth history	It was an uncomplicated spontaneous vaginal delivery.
☐ Eating habits	Formula with iron; rice cereal at night; occasionally juice.
☐ Current medications	None.
☐ Past medical history	Nothing of note.

☑ Question	Patient Response
☐ Past surgical history	None.
☐ Family history	None.
☐ Drug allergies	None.

Connecting with the Patient

☐ Examinee recognized the SP's emotions and responded with PEARLS.

Physical Examination

None.

Closure

☐ Examinee discussed initial diagnostic impressions.

☐ Examinee discussed initial management plans:

   ☐ Follow-up tests.

☐ Examinee asked if the SP had any other questions or concerns.

Sample Closure

Ms. Wheaton, from the information you have given me, I am concerned that your child may be dehydrated. She hasn't urinated since yesterday, and she is weak and drowsy. It is very hard for me to assess her over the telephone, and I do not want to jeopardize her health in any way. For this reason, I am going to ask you to bring her in for a physical exam and a full assessment, and we will then proceed according to what we find on the exam. I understand that you may have problems with transportation, but we are fortunate to have a social worker here who can help you handle these issues. After we are done on the phone, I will transfer your call to him, and he can help you. Do you have any questions for me?

Patient Note

History

Physical Examination

Differential Diagnosis

1.
2.
3.
4.
5.

Diagnostic Workup

1.
2.
3.
4.
5.

Patient Note

History

HPI: *The source of information is the patient's mother. The mother of a 6-month-old F c/o her child having 1 day of diarrhea, weakness, and drowsiness. The child has had 6 watery brown bowel movements per day. There was no blood in her stool, but she has not urinated since yesterday. She received Tylenol without improvement. The mother reports the child's temperature as 100.5°F and adds that her mouth is dry. The child has no known sick contacts but is in day care. The mother denies any nausea/vomiting, lethargy, excessive sleeping, abnormal behavior, or recent URIs. The child had a normal checkup 2 weeks ago and is up to date on her immunizations. She has a diet of formula with iron and rice cereal at night with occasional juice.*

ROS: *Negative.*

Allergies: *NKDA.*

Medications: *None.*

PMH: *Uncomplicated spontaneous vaginal delivery.*

PSH: *None.*

FH: *Noncontributory.*

Physical Examination

None.

Differential Diagnosis

1. *Rotavirus*
2. *Bacterial diarrhea*
3. *Malabsorption*
4. *UTI*
5. *Intussusception*
6. *Bacteremia*

Diagnostic Workup

1. *Rotavirus enzyme immunoassay*
2. *Electrolytes*
3. *Stool leukocytes, culture, ova and parasitology, and pH*
4. *UA*
5. *AXR*
6. *Blood cultures*

CASE DISCUSSION

Differential Diagnosis

- **Rotavirus:** This is the cause of 60% of cases of acute pediatric infectious diarrhea.

- **Bacterial diarrhea:** The most common types of bacterial diarrhea, in order of frequency, are *Shigella*, *Salmonella*, *Campylobacter jejuni*, and *Yersinia enterocolitica*.

- **Malabsorption:** This condition may result from a baby's consumption of juice and may be the culprit in the current patient's case. It is important to counsel parents that juice should not be introduced into the diet of babies in this age group. Some children may have milk intolerance as well. However, milk intolerance would probably not present as acutely as is seen here.

- **UTI:** Diarrhea in infants may be a nonspecific response to an infection such as UTI or pyelonephritis.

- **Intussusception:** Given the severe nature of this disease, intussusception must be considered in the differential. The classic presentation includes abdominal pain, vomiting, and bloody stools. Some 75% of patients with intussusception have only two of these findings. Intussusception is also associated with recent viral illness and low-grade fever.

- **Bacteremia:** Bacteremia/sepsis should be ruled out in any child with high fever, drowsiness, and no urine output.

Diagnostic Workup

- **Rotavirus enzyme immunoassay:** This test is 97% sensitive and 97% specific for rotavirus infection.

- **Electrolytes:** Children with diarrhea frequently have metabolic acidosis or other electrolyte abnormalities, such as hyponatremia.

- **Stool leukocytes, culture, ova and parasitology, and pH:** WBCs in the stool would suggest an infectious etiology, and cultures may reveal a bacterial pathogen. Microscopy may reveal ova or parasites such as *Giardia*, an infection that is common among the day care population. Stool pH can distinguish a secretory from an osmotic cause of diarrhea by revealing a pH of > 6 or < 5, respectively.

- **UA:** To assess for pyelonephritis or UTI.

- **AXR:** A plain film abdominal radiograph should pick up characteristics of nonspecific bowel obstruction in intussusception.

- **Blood cultures:** To rule out bacteremia.

Opening Scenario

Paul Stout, a 75-year-old male, comes to the office complaining of hearing loss.

Vital Signs

BP: 132/68 mm Hg

Temp: 98.4°F (36.9°C)

RR: 18/minute

HR: 84/minute, regular

Examinee Tasks

1. Take a focused history.

2. Perform a focused physical exam (do not perform rectal, genitourinary, or female breast exam).

3. Explain your clinical impression and workup plan to the patient.

4. Write the patient note after leaving the room.

Checklist/SP Sheet

Patient Description

Patient is a 75 yo M.

Notes for the SP

- Ask the examinee to speak up if he or she did not speak in a loud and clear manner.
- Pretend that you have difficulty hearing in both ears.
- On physical exam, demonstrate that you have no lateralization on the Weber test (ie, show that your hearing is equal in both ears).
- Pretend that you cannot hear when spoken to from behind.

Challenging Questions to Ask

"Do you think I am going deaf?"

Sample Examinee Response

"Based on your symptoms and the results of my exam, you have some kind of hearing deficit. We need to perform more tests to figure out the cause of the problem, whether it is going to get worse, and whether we can halt its progression or improve your hearing. Now, I would like you to stop taking aspirin."

Examinee Checklist

Building the Doctor-Patient Relationship

Entrance

☐ Examinee knocked on the door before entering.

☐ Examinee introduced self by name.

☐ Examinee identified his/her role or position.

☐ Examinee correctly used patient's name.

☐ Examinee made eye contact with the SP.

Reflective Listening

☐ Examinee asked an open-ended question and actively listened to the response.

☐ Examinee asked the SP to list his/her concerns and listened to the response without interrupting.

☐ Examinee summarized the SP's concerns, often using the SP's own words.

Information Gathering

☐ Examinee elicited data efficiently and accurately.

☑ Question	Patient Response
☐ Chief complaint	I can't hear as well as I used to.
☐ Description	My wife has told me that I can't hear well, and lately I have noticed that I have been reading lips.
☐ Onset	This has been going on for one year.
☐ Progression	It has been getting worse.
☐ Location	It seems like I'm having trouble with both ears, but I'm not sure.
☐ Is hearing lost for all sounds or for anything specific?	Nothing specific.
☐ Do words sound jumbled or distorted?	Yes, especially in crowded places or when I watch television.
☐ Can you locate the source of sound?	Yes.
☐ Do you have any problems understanding speech?	No.
☐ Treatments tried	I saw my doctor one month ago, and he cleaned out some wax from my ears.
☐ Did that help you?	No.
☐ Ear pain	No.
☐ Ear discharge	No.
☐ Sensation of room spinning around you	No.
☐ Feeling of imbalance	No.

☑ Question	Patient Response
☐ Recent infections	I had a urinary infection about a year ago. My doctor gave me an antibiotic, but I don't remember its name.
☐ Ringing in the ears	Sometimes, in both ears.
☐ Trauma to the ears	No.
☐ Exposure to loud noises	Yes.
☐ Headaches	Rarely.
☐ Insertion of foreign body	No.
☐ Nausea/vomiting	No.
☐ Neurologic problems, loss of sensation, muscle weakness, numbness or tingling anywhere in the body	No.
☐ Current medications	Hydrochlorothiazide. For the past 25 years, I have also taken aspirin daily to protect my heart.
☐ Past medical history	Hypertension. I take my blood pressure every day and it's well-controlled.
☐ Past surgical history	None.
☐ Family history of hearing loss	No.
☐ Occupation	Retired military veteran.
☐ Alcohol use	Never.
☐ Illicit drug use	Never.
☐ Tobacco	Never.
☐ Sexual activity	Only with my wife.
☐ Drug allergies	I develop a rash when I take penicillin.

Connecting with the Patient

☐ Examinee recognized the SP's emotions and responded with PEARLS.

Physical Examination

☐ Examinee washed his/her hands.

☐ Examinee asked permission to start the exam.

☐ Examinee used respectful draping.

☐ Examinee did not repeat painful maneuvers.

☑ Exam Component	Maneuver
☐ HEENT exam	Tested hearing by speaking with back turned; inspected sinuses, nose, mouth, and throat; funduscopic exam and otoscopy; assessed hearing with Rinne and Weber tests and whisper test
☐ CV/pulmonary exam	Auscultation
☐ Neurologic exam	Cranial nerves, sensation, motor, reflexes, cerebellar—finger to nose, heel to shin

Closure

☐ Examinee discussed initial diagnostic impressions.

☐ Examinee discussed initial management plans:

    ☐ Follow-up tests.

☐ Examinee asked if the SP had any other questions or concerns.

Sample Closure

Mr. Stout, I know that you are concerned about your problem. I can confirm that you do have some hearing loss. I would like to run several tests, including some blood tests. I would also like you to stop taking aspirin, because this may be contributing to your hearing loss. I will refer you to an audiometrist, who will assess you for a hearing aid. Do you have any questions for me?

Patient Note

History

_____
_____
_____
_____
_____
_____
_____
_____
_____

Physical Examination

_____
_____
_____
_____
_____
_____
_____
_____
_____
_____
_____
_____
_____

Differential Diagnosis

1. _____
2. _____
3. _____
4. _____
5. _____

Diagnostic Workup

1. _____
2. _____
3. _____
4. _____
5. _____

History

HPI: 75 yo M c/o bilateral hearing loss for all sounds; started 1 year ago and is progressively worsening. He had cerumen removal 1 month ago with no improvement. He reports occasional tinnitus and rare headaches. He notes that words sound jumbled in crowded places or when he is watching TV. He denies inserting any foreign body in the ear canal. No ear pain, no ear discharge, no vertigo, no loss of balance. No history of trauma to the ears; no difficulty comprehending or locating the source of sounds.

ROS: Negative.

Allergies: Penicillin, causes rash.

Medications: HCTZ, aspirin (for 25 years).

PMH: Hypertension. UTI 1 year ago, treated with antibiotics.

PSH: None.

SH: No smoking, no EtOH, no illicit drugs. Retired veteran. Sexually active with wife only.

FH: No history of hearing loss.

Physical Examination

Patient is in no acute distress.

VS: WNL.

HEENT: NC/AT, PERRLA, EOMI, no nystagmus, no papilledema, no cerumen. TMs with light reflex, no stigmata of infection, no redness to ear canal, no tenderness of auricle or periauricle, no lymphadenopathy, oropharynx normal. Weber test without lateralization; ⊕ Rinne test (revealed air conduction > bone conduction).

Chest: Clear breath sounds bilaterally.

Heart: RRR; S1/S2; no murmurs, rubs, or gallops.

Neuro: Cranial nerves: 2–12 grossly intact except for decreased hearing. Motor: Strength 5/5 throughout. DTRs: 2+ throughout. Sensation: Intact. Gait: Normal; no past pointing and ⊖ heel to shin.

Differential Diagnosis

1. Presbycusis
2. Cochlear nerve damage due to loud noise
3. Otosclerosis
4. Ménière disease
5. Ototoxicity
6. Acoustic neuroma

Diagnostic Workup

1. Audiometry
2. Tympanography
3. Brain stem auditory evoked potentials
4. CT—head
5. VDRL/RPR

CASE DISCUSSION

Differential Diagnosis

- **Presbycusis:** This is a process of the inner ear in which bone loss is greater than air loss, leading to a gradual loss of hearing. Presbycusis is a common diagnosis as people age and can be detected by performing the Rinne test. This patient should be referred to an audiologist who works in conjunction with an ENT specialist. He will likely need a hearing aid.

- **Cochlear nerve damage:** The cochlear nerve can become damaged as a result of loud noise. This patient is a military veteran and admits to a history of exposure to loud noises. Cochlear nerve damage would present in a manner similar to presbycusis. As with presbycusis, patients with suspected damage should be referred to an audiologist working in conjunction with an ENT specialist. Such patients will likely need hearing aids as well.

- **Otosclerosis:** This is a disease of the elderly that presents as gradual hearing loss. It is a conductive hearing loss, so air loss exceeds bone loss. In this case, the Weber test would lateralize to the affected side.

- **Ménière disease:** This condition usually presents with hearing loss, tinnitus, and episodic vertigo. It is caused by endolymphatic disruption in the inner ear. Causes include head trauma and syphilis.

- **Ototoxicity:** Hearing loss caused by antibiotics will become more pronounced and may even continue to worsen for a time after the drug is discontinued. Any sensorineural hearing loss associated with these drugs is permanent. Aspirin can also cause hearing loss, but such loss is reversible with discontinuation of the drug. While workup is pending in this patient, aspirin should be withheld.

- **Acoustic neuroma:** It is unlikely that the patient has an intracranial lesion such as a brain tumor in the absence of any other signs; however, this diagnosis should be considered if evidence of focal neurologic deficits is found.

Diagnostic Workup

- **Audiometry:** To assess hearing function and deafness to specific frequencies.

- **Tympanography:** A graphic display that represents the conduction of sound in the middle ear. It may help distinguish middle ear from inner ear dysfunction.

- **Brain stem auditory evoked potentials:** Used to diagnose auditory neuropathy.

- **CT—head:** Used to rule out any intracranial process, tumor, bleed, or CVA. An MRI of the brain would be better for an acoustic neuroma or a schwannoma.

- **VDRL/RPR:** To rule out syphilis associated with Ménière disease.

CASE 30
DOORWAY INFORMATION

Opening Scenario

The mother of Adam Davidson, an 8-year-old male child, comes to the office concerned that her son continues to wet the bed.

Examinee Tasks

1. Take a focused history.

2. Explain your clinical impression and workup plan to the mother.

3. Write the patient note after leaving the room.

Checklist/SP Sheet

Patient Description

The patient's mother offers the history; her son is in the waiting room.

Notes for the SP

None.

Challenging Questions to Ask

- "Did I do something wrong to cause this problem?"
- "Is my child going to get better?"

Sample Examinee Response

"There are a few medical problems that can lead to your child's condition, but it's just as likely to be an isolated symptom. Bed-wetting is much more common than most people believe, and there is no reason for you or your child to feel embarrassed or guilty. There are a number of treatment options available for this condition, and after we have run a few tests to rule out any physiologic abnormalities, I will discuss them with you."

Examinee Checklist

Building the Doctor-Patient Relationship

Entrance

☐ Examinee knocked on the door before entering.

☐ Examinee introduced self by name.

☐ Examinee identified his/her role or position.

☐ Examinee correctly used patient's name.

☐ Examinee made eye contact with the SP.

Reflective Listening

☐ Examinee asked an open-ended question and actively listened to the response.

☐ Examinee asked the SP to list his/her concerns and listened to the response without interrupting.

☐ Examinee summarized the SP's concerns, often using the SP's own words.

Information Gathering

☐ Examinee elicited data efficiently and accurately.

☑ Question	Patient Response
☐ Chief complaint	My child wets his bed.
☐ Frequency	Two or three times a week.
☐ Time of day	Only at night.
☐ Onset	I guess he has always had trouble at night. I don't think he has ever gone more than a few nights without an accident.
☐ Have you tried any interventions or drugs in the past?	We ordered one of those nighttime alarms, but everyone in the house could hear it, so we didn't use it for long.
☐ How has the behavior affected the child?	He is ashamed of himself. He avoids school trips because of it.
☐ How has the behavior affected you?	It bothers me. I'm afraid he has some underlying disease or abnormality.
☐ Have you ever punished or rewarded him?	I feel irritated sometimes, but I've never punished him. I try to encourage him by rewarding him on dry nights.
☐ Alleviating/exacerbating factors	None that I can think of.
☐ Does the problem increase in times of stress?	I'm not sure, but it probably does.
☐ Late-night eating or drinking	No.
☐ Volume of urine	I don't think it's a large amount but I'm not sure.
☐ Dysuria	No.
☐ Urinary urgency	No.
☐ Fever	No.
☐ Urine color	Yellow.
☐ Hematuria	No.
☐ Abdominal pain	No.
☐ Constipation	No.
☐ Snoring	No.
☐ Nighttime awakening	No.
☐ Environmental changes related to wetting	No, I can't think of anything. We haven't moved or had any family problems.
☐ Any major stresses?	No, he does well in school and has great friends. I think the only hard thing for him is not being able to attend sleepovers.
☐ Family history of enuresis	Actually, his father had the same trouble as a kid. From my understanding, his father didn't gain full control until he was about 10 years old.

✓ Question	Patient Response
☐ Neurologic history	As far as I know, he has never had any problems of this kind.
☐ Birth history	Normal.
☐ Child weight, height, and language development	He was always on time with his development. He walked early, talked on time, and is reading at a third-grade level.
☐ Current medications	None.
☐ Past medical history	None.
☐ Past surgical history	None.
☐ Drug allergies	No.

Connecting with the Patient

☐ Examinee recognized the SP's emotions and responded with PEARLS.

Physical Examination

None.

Closure

☐ Examinee discussed initial diagnostic impressions.

☐ Examinee discussed initial management plans:

    ☐ Further examination.

    ☐ Follow-up tests.

☐ Examinee asked if the SP had any other questions or concerns.

Sample Closure

Mrs. Davidson, your son's condition is probably an isolated symptom, but I would still like to examine your son and run some tests to make sure he does not have an underlying infection or a more serious medical problem. We can then discuss his treatment options. Do you have any questions for me?

Patient Note

History

Physical Examination

Differential Diagnosis

1.
2.
3.
4.
5.

Diagnostic Workup

1.
2.
3.
4.
5.

Patient Note

History

HPI: *The source of the information is the patient's mother. The mother of an 8 yo M c/o her child continuing to wet the bed several times a week. The child has never had a significant period of continence. He has no dysuria, hematuria, fever, or urgency. The mother denies that the child c/o abdominal pain or constipation. The child does not snore or wake up multiple times during the night. There are no exacerbating factors, and there have been no major lifestyle changes or stresses in the family. The problem is causing distress for the child, who has been avoiding school trips, as well as for the mother, who is worried about the possibility of an underlying medical condition.*

ROS: *Negative.*

Allergies: *NKDA.*

Medications: *None.*

PMH: *None.*

PSH: *None.*

Birth history: *Normal.*

Developmental history: *Normal.*

FH: *Positive family history of male nocturnal enuresis.*

Physical Examination

None.

Differential Diagnosis

1. *Monosymptomatic primary nocturnal enuresis*
2. *Secondary enuresis*
3. *Urinary tract infection*
4. *Constipation*
5. *Sleep apnea*
6. *Functional bladder disorder*

Diagnostic Workup

1. *Genital exam*
2. *UA*
3. *Urine culture*
4. *First-morning urine specific gravity*
5. *U/S—renal*
6. *BUN/Cr*

CASE DISCUSSION

Differential Diagnosis

- **Monosymptomatic primary nocturnal enuresis:** This is a diagnosis of exclusion. This patient's lifetime history indicates a primary problem as opposed to a secondary one. The history and physical exam do not provide any related signs or symptoms, suggesting a monosymptomatic pathology. A urine sample must be taken to rule out infection, and old records should be evaluated to ensure that the presentation is not part of a global delay.

- **Secondary enuresis:** The patient's mother does not report a major trauma or life or environmental change such as the divorce of parents, a major illness, or an abuse that might result in regression to incontinence. This diagnosis is further unlikely because the child has not been continent for any significant period.

- **Urinary tract infection (UTI):** Asymptomatic UTIs are common in children and should be screened for at annual visits. This patient does not have dysuria, frequency, or urgency, but incontinence alone should trigger an evaluation. A positive UA is diagnostic, and culturing can direct treatment.

- **Constipation:** Infrequent or hard stools may indicate chronic constipation, which can put pressure on the bladder and decrease capacity. This may delay continence and look like a primary disorder. Physical examination can reveal impacted stool on the left side.

- **Sleep apnea:** Wetting occurs in all stages of sleep but is associated with particular disorders, such as sleep apnea and narcolepsy. This patient does not present with snoring or upper airway obstruction, and thus there is no indication of apnea that might warrant further evaluation.

- **Functional bladder disorder:** Children with functional disorders void several times a day, hold urine until the last moment, and wet small volumes almost every night, sometimes multiple times a night. This patient has normal voiding patterns during the day and remains continent a majority of nights.

Diagnostic Workup

- **Genital exam:** To evaluate for disorders such as abnormalities of the meatus, epispadias, and phimosis.

- **UA:** Clear urine, a negative dipstick, and a negative microscopic examination combined have a negative predictive value between 95% and 98%.

- **Urine culture:** The only 100% specific test for infection.

- **First morning urine specific gravity:** An early-morning urine concentration of < 1.015 may indicate a lack of nighttime and early-morning ADH surges, which may predict a positive response to pharmacologic therapy with DDAVP.

- **U/S—renal:** Should be pursued if wetting continues with multiple treatments, abnormal voiding patterns, or recurrent UTIs confirmed by UA.

- **BUN/Cr:** Should be obtained before U/S—renal to evaluate renal function. To avoid unnecessary blood draws in children, blood for BUN/Cr testing should not be drawn until results from a urine sample are obtained.

CASE 31
DOORWAY INFORMATION

Opening Scenario

John Matthews, a 25-year-old male, comes to the ED following a motor vehicle accident.

Vital Signs

BP: 123/88 mm Hg

Temp: 100°F (38°C)

RR: 22/minute

HR: 85/minute, regular

Examinee Tasks

1. Take a focused history.

2. Perform a focused physical exam (do not perform rectal, genitourinary, or female breast exam).

3. Explain your clinical impression and workup plan to the patient.

4. Write the patient note after leaving the room.

Checklist/SP Sheet

Patient Description

Patient is a 25 yo M.

Notes for the SP

- Exhibit pain in the left chest that worsens during inspiration and movement (ie, when you breathe in, hold your side, and stop your breathing with a short gasp).
- Exhibit pain when your left chest is being palpated.
- Exhibit pain when your left upper abdomen is being palpated.
- Take fast, shallow breaths.
- Occasionally cough hard into a tissue.
- Moan occasionally and answer questions in short sentences.

Challenging Questions to Ask

"Do you think I am going to die?"

Sample Examinee Response

"Your condition raises concern and is obviously urgent. We will start by taking some images of your chest. Then, once we have a better idea of what is wrong, we can give you some medication to help you with your pain. If there is air or blood around your lungs, there is a procedure we can perform that can release the pressure. We will be monitoring you very closely from this point on, and if you have any significant problems, we will be available to help."

Examinee Checklist

Building the Doctor-Patient Relationship

Entrance

☐ Examinee knocked on the door before entering.

☐ Examinee introduced self by name.

☐ Examinee identified his/her role or position.

☐ Examinee correctly used patient's name.

☐ Examinee made eye contact with the SP.

Reflective Listening

☐ Examinee asked an open-ended question and actively listened to the response.

☐ Examinee asked the SP to list his/her concerns and listened to the response without interrupting.

☐ Examinee summarized the SP's concerns, often using the SP's own words.

Information Gathering

☐ Examinee elicited data efficiently and accurately.

☑ Question	Patient Response
☐ Chief complaint	I'm having trouble breathing and have this excruciating pain (holds left side).
☐ Onset	It started last night.
☐ Severity on a scale	It's some of the worst pain I've ever had; I guess I would say 8/10.
☐ Context	I was driving my car and was trying to answer my cell phone. When I looked up, I found that I had veered off the road. I immediately tried to slow down but hit a tree. I wasn't going very fast, and my car was basically okay. I was embarrassed, so I didn't call the police. I was wearing my seat belt and felt okay at first, so I didn't think I needed to come to the hospital.
☐ Alleviating factors	Nothing I do makes it better.
☐ Exacerbating factors	It gets even worse when I take a deep breath or try to move.
☐ Cough	I have been coughing for a couple of days, I guess.
☐ Sputum production	I have to use a tissue because I keep bringing up all this yellow junk.
☐ Fever/chills	I have been feeling a little warm and have noticed that my muscles ache, but I don't think I've had any shaking or chills.
☐ Other injuries	I have a few scratches on my arms from the car accident.
☐ Head trauma	No.
☐ Discharge from the ears, mouth, or nose (clear or bloody)	No.
☐ Loss of consciousness	No.

☑ *Question*	*Patient Response*
☐ Convulsions	No.
☐ Headache	No.
☐ Change in vision	No.
☐ Confusion, memory loss, or change in personality	No.
☐ Weakness or numbness in the extremities	No.
☐ Heart symptoms (palpitations)	No.
☐ Abdominal pain	Yes, I have sharp pain right here (point to the LUQ).
☐ Nausea/vomiting or stiff neck	No.
☐ Last meal/drink	I had breakfast this morning, about five hours ago. I didn't have any trouble keeping it down.
☐ Were you under the influence of alcohol or recreational drugs?	No.
☐ Pain on urination	No.
☐ Current medications	None.
☐ Past medical history	I had a sore throat, mild fever, and fatigue two weeks ago, and my doctor told me I had infectious mononucleosis, but it is gone now.
☐ Past surgical history	None.
☐ Family history	My mother and father are both healthy and living.
☐ Occupation	I'm a banker.
☐ Alcohol use	Occasionally, on the weekends.
☐ Illicit drug use	No.
☐ Tobacco	No.
☐ Drug allergies	No.

Connecting with the Patient

☐ Examinee recognized the SP's emotions and responded with PEARLS.

Physical Examination

☐ Examinee washed his/her hands.

☐ Examinee asked permission to start the exam.

☐ Examinee used respectful draping.

☐ Examinee did not repeat painful maneuvers.

☑ Exam Component	Maneuver
☐ Head and neck exam	Inspection
☐ CV exam	Auscultation
☐ Pulmonary exam	Inspection, auscultation, palpation, percussion
☐ Abdominal exam	Inspection, auscultation, palpation (examined specifically for organomegaly such as splenomegaly)
☐ Neurologic exam	Mental status, cranial nerves, gross motor
☐ Skin exam	Inspection for abrasion, lacerations, bruising

Closure

☐ Examinee discussed initial diagnostic impressions.

☐ Examinee discussed initial management plans:

    ☐ Follow-up tests.

☐ Examinee asked if the SP had any other questions or concerns.

Sample Closure

Mr. Matthews, you should always seek medical treatment after an accident like this. We must now observe you closely until we can determine what is causing your pain. We are going to run a few tests and take some x-rays of your chest. We will also give you something for your pain and will observe your breathing to make sure you are getting enough oxygen. Do you have any questions for me?

Patient Note

History

_____
_____
_____
_____
_____
_____
_____
_____

Physical Examination

_____
_____
_____
_____
_____
_____
_____
_____
_____
_____
_____

Differential Diagnosis

1. _____
2. _____
3. _____
4. _____
5. _____

Diagnostic Workup

1. _____
2. _____
3. _____
4. _____
5. _____

History

HPI: *25 yo M c/o left chest pain and LUQ pain following a MVA. The patient struck a tree with his car at a slow speed. The chest pain is 8/10. It is exacerbated with movement or when he takes a deep breath, and nothing relieves it. He reports dyspnea and a productive cough with a low-grade fever but denies LOC, headache, change in mental status, or change in vision. No cardiovascular or neurologic symptoms. No nausea, vomiting, neck stiffness, or unusual fluid from mouth or nose. No dysuria. Last meal was 5 hours ago. Denies being under the influence of alcohol or drugs.*

ROS: *As per HPI.*

Allergies: *NKDA.*

Medications: *None.*

PMH: *Infectious mononucleosis.*

PSH: *None.*

SH: *No smoking, occasional EtOH, no illicit drugs.*

FH: *Noncontributory.*

Physical Examination

Patient is in acute distress, dyspneic.

VS: *Temp 100°F, RR 22/minute.*

HEENT: *No JVD, no bruises, PERRLA, EOMI, no pharyngeal edema or exudates.*

Chest: *Two large bruises on left chest, left rib tenderness, decreased breath sounds over all of left lung field, right lung fields clear.*

Heart: *RRR; normal S1/S2; no murmurs, rubs, or gallops.*

Abdomen: *Soft, nondistended, ⊕ BS, LUQ tenderness, no rebound or guarding, no organomegaly.*

Skin: *No bruises or lacerations.*

Neuro: *Mental status: Alert and oriented × 3. Cranial nerves: 2–12 grossly intact. Motor: Strength 5/5 in all muscle groups. Sensation: Intact to pinprick and soft touch.*

Differential Diagnosis

1. *Pneumothorax*
2. *Hemothorax*
3. *Pneumonia*
4. *Rib fracture*
5. *Splenic rupture*
6. *Pleuritis*

Diagnostic Workup

1. *CXR*
2. *XR/CT—abdomen*
3. *Pulse oximetry*
4. *Urine toxicology*
5. *Blood alcohol level*
6. *Sputum and blood Gram stain and culture*

CASE DISCUSSION

Differential Diagnosis

The most important steps in any trauma are to assess the **ABCDEs**: **A**irway, **B**reathing, **C**irculation, **D**isability (neurologic), and **E**xposure. In this case, the exam is separated from the trauma by several hours and the patient is able to walk and talk, somewhat negating the urgency of a typical ED evaluation. At the same time, chest pain and dyspnea are serious symptoms that require swift evaluation and intervention.

- **Pneumothorax:** A pneumothorax forms when air collects between the pleural and visceral layers of the thorax. Physical findings include a unilateral loss of breath sounds with hyperresonance, shift of the trachea away from the injured side, and JVD. This patient's acute onset and distress suggest pneumothorax. CXR is the fastest diagnostic tool available.

- **Hemothorax:** This is defined by the presence of blood in the pleural space and is most commonly due to trauma. It presents with chest pain, shortness of breath, cough, and occasionally signs and symptoms of hypovolemic shock. The final diagnosis can be made by pleurocentesis or chest tube placement.

- **Pneumonia:** Most commonly caused by *Streptococcus pneumoniae*, bacterial pneumonia can present with acute respiratory distress, fever, cough, pleuritic pain, and shaking chills. This patient has a productive cough, low-grade fever, and unilateral chest pain suggestive of pneumonia. However, traumatic causes should be ruled out first. Physical signs include tachypnea, crackles, and dullness to percussion. The CXR will show a lobar infiltrate, and sputum cultures may help identify the bacterial pathogen.

- **Rib fracture:** Rib fractures are the most common chest injury and can result from almost any insult to the chest wall. A simple fracture could cause this patient's pain on inspiration and cough. Rib fractures can be diagnosed with a CXR.

- **Splenic rupture:** Splenic injuries are always of great concern following a trauma because they can cause significant blood loss very quickly. If this patient was exposed to infectious mononucleosis, his chances of splenic injury or bleeding are greater. As this patient's pain is primarily left-sided, the spleen should be evaluated with an ultrasound exam followed by further imaging with CT-abdomen. On physical exam, it is important to evaluate for any signs or symptoms of organomegaly.

- **Pleuritis:** Inflammation of the pleural membrane can cause severe pain that increases with inspiration or movement. The physical exam is generally negative with the exception of the chest pain. This patient may have a simple viral pleuritis, but more emergent causes need to be ruled out first.

Diagnostic Workup

- **CXR:** On CXR, lobar consolidation may indicate pneumonia; hemothorax may cause linear consolidation; and tension pneumothorax will show mediastinal shift. Rib fractures can also be diagnosed from the CXR if they are present.

- **XR/CT—abdomen:** Although a CT scan may offer a better evaluation for internal abdominal injury, a Focused Assessment with Sonography for Trauma (FAST) is an ultrasound exam which can quickly assess for any intra-abdominal bleeding given the history of infectious mononucleosis. An AXR remains a quick way to rule out free air in the abdomen.

- **Pulse oximetry:** Although not as sensitive as ABG analysis, pulse oximetry is a fast, noninvasive measure of respiratory distress. Remember that a patient with long-standing lung disease such as chronic obstructive pulmonary disease may have chronically suppressed oxygenation, which is necessary to maintain respiratory drive.

- **Urine toxicology and blood alcohol level:** These tests should be considered for any driver following a motor vehicle accident. Even though this patient's car accident occurred a while ago, it is still necessary to evaluate his current situation.

- **Sputum and blood Gram stain and culture:** Used to screen sputum samples for identification of bacterial pathogens such as *S. pneumoniae*. Other stains, such as acid-fast stains and monoclonal antibodies, can identify tuberculosis and *Pneumocystis jiroveci* (formerly *P. carinii*). A blood culture and Gram stain would also be useful given that the patient has a low-grade fever.

Opening Scenario

Julia Melton, a 25-year-old female, comes to the ED after being assaulted.

Vital Signs

BP: 120/85 mm Hg

Temp: 98.0°F (36.7°C)

RR: 17/minute

HR: 90/minute, regular

Examinee Tasks

1. Take a focused history.

2. Perform a focused physical exam (do not perform rectal, genitourinary, or female breast exam).

3. Explain your clinical impression and workup plan to the patient.

4. Write the patient note after leaving the room.

Checklist/SP Sheet

Patient Description

Patient is a 25 yo F.

Notes for the SP

- Look depressed and tearful.

- Start weeping when asked about physical and/or sexual assaults.

- Pretend to have right chest pain with deep inspiration, cough, and palpation.

Challenging Questions to Ask

"This is all my fault, doctor. Do you think my friends will ever accept me again?"

Sample Examinee Response

"I am so sorry for what happened to you; it is horrific and must be very difficult for you to handle. However, it is not your fault by any means. Whoever did this to you should be held accountable."

Examinee Checklist

Building the Doctor-Patient Relationship

Entrance

☐ Examinee knocked on the door before entering.

☐ Examinee introduced self by name.

☐ Examinee identified his/her role or position.

☐ Examinee correctly used patient's name.

☐ Examinee made eye contact with the SP.

Reflective Listening

☐ Examinee asked an open-ended question and actively listened to the response.

☐ Examinee asked the SP to list his/her concerns and listened to the response without interrupting.

☐ Examinee summarized the SP's concerns, often using the SP's own words.

Information Gathering

☐ Examinee elicited data efficiently and accurately.

☑ Question	Patient Response
☐ Chief complaint	I was attacked by two men.
☐ Onset	About three hours ago. I came to the ED right away.
☐ Incident location	It happened outside the bar that I usually go to.
☐ Did you recognize the assailants?	I have seen them in the bar but never talked to them.
☐ Did you report the incident?	No.
☐ Description of the assault	I was walking toward my car, and then all of a sudden I was pulled into a storage room. I started screaming, but the men started to slap me and beat me up with their fists.
☐ Assault objects	They used their fists and their bodies to hold me down. I couldn't move at all even though I tried to struggle against them.
☐ Sexual assault	Yes.
☐ Did they use condoms?	No.
☐ Did ejaculation occur?	I don't know.
☐ Type of intercourse (oral, vaginal, anal)	Vaginal.
☐ Foreign objects used	None.
☐ Last menstrual period	Three weeks ago.
☐ Contraceptives	I'm not on the pill or anything.
☐ Pain	Yes, I feel sore all over, especially on the right side of my chest.
☐ Location of the worst pain	The right chest.
☐ Radiation	No.
☐ Severity on a scale	About 8/10.
☐ Alleviating factors	It improves when I sit still.
☐ Exacerbating factors	It gets worse whenever I move or take a deep breath.
☐ Bleeding or bruises	No.

☑ Question	Patient Response
☐ Loss of consciousness	No.
☐ Headache	No.
☐ Change in vision	No.
☐ Dizziness	No.
☐ Weakness	No, I am just tired.
☐ Numbness	No.
☐ Shortness of breath	Yes, I feel that I can't get enough air.
☐ Palpitations	Yes.
☐ Blood in stool/urine	No, but I haven't gone to the bathroom since the incident.
☐ Vaginal bleeding	No.
☐ Nausea/vomiting	No.
☐ Abdominal pain	Yes, it hurts everywhere.
☐ Joint pain	My wrists hurt where they were holding me down.
☐ Current medications	None.
☐ Past medical history	None.
☐ Past surgical history	None.
☐ Family history	None.
☐ Occupation	Student.
☐ Alcohol use	Occasionally.
☐ Illicit drug use	Never.
☐ Tobacco	No.
☐ Drug allergies	No.

Connecting with the Patient

☐ Examinee recognized the SP's emotions and responded with PEARLS.

Physical Examination

☐ Examinee washed his/her hands.

☐ Examinee asked permission to start the exam.

☐ Examinee used respectful draping.

☐ Examinee did not repeat painful maneuvers.

☑ Exam Component	Maneuver
☐ Head and neck exam	Inspection, palpation
☐ Mouth exam	Inspection
☐ CV exam	Auscultation
☐ Pulmonary exam	Inspection, auscultation, palpation, percussion
☐ Abdominal exam	Inspection, auscultation, palpation
☐ Neurologic exam	Mental status, cranial nerves, gross motor
☐ Musculoskeletal exam	Inspection, palpation

Closure

☐ Examinee discussed initial diagnostic impressions.

☐ Examinee discussed initial management plans:

    ☐ Follow-up tests: Examinee mentioned the need for a pelvic exam.

☐ Examinee asked if the SP had any other questions or concerns.

Sample Closure

Ms. Melton, I am really sorry for what happened to you. I want to emphasize that it is not your fault, and you should not feel guilty about it. I recommend that you report the incident to the police. In the meantime, I will need to do a pelvic examination to make sure that you have no injuries in the genital area. I will also need to collect some specimens and swabs from your body and genital area so that they can be used as evidence if you choose to file charges, and also to look for STDs. We will run some blood tests for potential STDs, a pregnancy test, and some x-rays. If your pregnancy test is negative, we will offer you some options for emergency contraception. It would also be prudent to give you some antibiotics to protect you from infections. Finally, I can have our social worker come talk to you and provide you with phone numbers for support groups and other resources. Do you have any questions for me?

History

_____
_____
_____
_____
_____
_____
_____
_____

Physical Examination

_____
_____
_____
_____
_____
_____
_____
_____
_____
_____

Differential Diagnosis

1. _____

2. _____

3. _____

4. _____

5. _____

Diagnostic Workup

1. _____

2. _____

3. _____

4. _____

5. _____

Patient Note

History

HPI: 25 yo F comes to the ED after being sexually and physically assaulted. The event happened about 3 hours ago as she was leaving a bar. She was beaten and raped by two unknown men. They had vaginal intercourse with her without using condoms, and she is unsure if ejaculation occurred. She also c/o shortness of breath, palpitations, and right chest pain that is nonradiating. The chest pain is exacerbated by movement and deep breaths and is relieved by sitting still. No nausea or vomiting. No dizziness or headache. No weakness or numbness in her extremities; no vaginal, rectal, or urinary bleeding.

ROS: Negative except as above.

Allergies: NKDA.

Medications: None.

PMH: None.

PSH: None.

SH: No smoking, occasional EtOH, no illicit drugs.

FH: Noncontributory.

Physical Examination

Patient is anxious and in acute distress.

VS: WNL.

HEENT: No JVD, PERRLA, EOMI.

Chest: Clear breath sounds bilaterally; tenderness on palpation of right chest wall.

Heart: Normal S1/S2; no murmurs, rubs, or gallops.

Abdomen: Soft, nontender, nondistended, ⊕ BS, no rebound or organomegaly.

Neuro: Mental status: Alert and oriented × 3. Cranial nerves: 2–12 grossly intact. Motor: Strength 5/5 in all muscle groups.

Differential Diagnosis

1. Rib/bone fracture
2. Pneumothorax/hemothorax
3. STDs
4. Pregnancy

Diagnostic Workup

1. Pelvic exam
2. Urine hCG
3. Wet mount, KOH prep, cervical culture
4. XR—skeletal survey
5. HIV antibody, VDRL, HBV antigen
6. CXR
7. Evidence collection using rape kit

CASE DISCUSSION

Differential Diagnosis

- **Rib fracture:** Can result from any insult to the chest wall. A simple fracture can cause pain on inspiration and cough.

- **Pneumothorax/hemothorax:** Defined as the presence of air or blood in the pleural space between the visceral and parietal pleurae. Physical findings include unilateral loss of breath sounds with hyperresonance, shifting of the trachea away from the injured side, and JVD. Because she suffered physical trauma, this patient may have a traumatic pneumothorax. A CXR is a fast and easy tool with which to evaluate patients for a pneumothorax.

- **STDs:** Sexual assault victims may acquire a variety of pathogens during the incident, including trichomoniasis, chlamydia, gonorrhea, HIV, and hepatitis B.

- **Pregnancy:** All sexual assault victims should be evaluated for possible existing pregnancy and should be offered emergency contraception.

Diagnostic Workup

- **Pelvic exam:** To evaluate for any possible physical injury of the genital or anal area and to collect specimens for medical and forensic purposes.

- **Urine hCG:** To rule out pregnancy.

- **Wet mount, KOH prep, cervical culture:** The vaginal discharge is examined microscopically to evaluate for infection. The presence of epithelial cells covered with bacteria (clue cells) suggests bacterial vaginosis, and the presence of hyphae and spores points to candidal infection. Motile organisms are seen in trichomonal infection. A "fishy" odor after the addition of KOH to the discharge is indicative of bacterial vaginosis. If sperm are detected in the victim, testing of sperm DNA may aid in the identification of the assailants.

- **XR—skeletal survey:** To detect possible bone or rib fractures.

- **HIV antibody, VDRL, HBV antigen:** To rule out HIV, syphilis, and hepatitis B infection.

- **CXR:** To detect pneumothorax, pleural effusions, and rib fractures.

- **Evidence collection using rape kit:** Rape kits are available to facilitate and guide the evidence collection process. Tissue swabs should be collected as soon as possible from the victim to assist with the evidence collection process.

Opening Scenario

Tanya Parker, a 28-year-old female, comes to the clinic with a positive pregnancy test.

Vital Signs

BP: 120/70 mm Hg

Temp: 98.6°F (37°C)

RR: 14/minute

HR: 76/minute

Examinee Tasks

1. Take a focused history.

2. Perform a focused physical exam (do not perform rectal, genitourinary, or female breast exam).

3. Explain your clinical impression and workup plan to the patient.

4. Write the patient note after leaving the room.

Checklist/SP Sheet

Patient Description

Patient is a 28 yo F, married with no children.

Notes for the SP

If asked, tell the doctor that you feel tired all the time.

Challenging Questions to Ask

"We had not planned to have a baby so soon after marriage. What should I do, doctor?"

Sample Examinee Response

"I understand your anxiety about this unplanned pregnancy. I suggest that you discuss this with your husband. As your physician, I want to assure you that I am here to support and advise you in whatever decision you make. If you wish, I would be happy to discuss your options with both of you."

Examinee Checklist

Building the Doctor-Patient Relationship

Entrance

☐ Examinee knocked on the door before entering.

☐ Examinee introduced self by name.

☐ Examinee identified his/her role or position.

☐ Examinee correctly used patient's name.

☐ Examinee made eye contact with the SP.

Reflective Listening

☐ Examinee asked an open-ended question and actively listened to the response.

☐ Examinee asked the SP to list his/her concerns and listened to the response without interrupting.

☐ Examinee summarized the SP's concerns, often using the SP's own words.

Information Gathering

☐ Examinee elicited data efficiently and accurately.

☑ Question	Patient Response
☐ Chief complaint	Positive pregnancy test.
☐ Onset/duration	My periods have always been regular, but last month it was very light, and this month I haven't had one yet. So I checked a pregnancy test, and it was positive.
☐ Last menstrual period	Six weeks ago and it was only light spotting.
☐ Menarche	At the age of 14.
☐ Menstrual history	My periods last 3–4 days and occur at the same time every month. Last month I had some spotting for only a day or two. Usually I have moderate flow and use 4–5 pads per day.
☐ Pain with periods	No.
☐ Spotting between periods	No.
☐ Contraception	My husband withdraws before ejaculation.
☐ Pregnancy/miscarriages	None.
☐ Sexual activity/partners	I am sexually active only with my husband.
☐ History of STDs	None.
☐ Nausea/vomiting	I do feel nauseated lately, but I have not been vomiting.
☐ Postcoital bleeding	No.
☐ Abdominal pain	No.
☐ Appetite changes	I don't feel like eating anything because of the nausea, especially with some smells of food.
☐ Weight changes	I haven't checked my weight recently, but I have been feeling bloated all the time.
☐ Fatigue	Yes. I'm really easily tired out by doing my daily activities.
☐ Breast discharge/tenderness	My breasts are a little fuller than before.
☐ Last Pap smear	Eight months ago, and it was normal.
☐ Fever	No.
☐ Bowel habits	Once a day.
☐ Urinary habits	I feel I have to use the bathroom frequently now. I have no burning or itching.

☑ Question	Patient Response
☐ Shortness of breath	No.
☐ Skin changes	I have not noticed anything.
☐ Exercise	I normally run five miles a day, but lately I've had to cut back because I feel so tired all the time.
☐ Current medications	Multivitamins.
☐ Past medical history	None.
☐ Past surgical history	My appendix was removed when I was 20.
☐ Family history	My father is a diabetic. My mom has thyroid and obesity problems.
☐ Occupation	Graduate student.
☐ Alcohol use	Occasionally a beer or two a week.
☐ Illicit drug use	None.
☐ Tobacco	None.
☐ Drug allergies	None.
☐ Planned pregnancy	No.
☐ Desired pregnancy	Unsure.
☐ Domestic abuse	No.

Connecting with the Patient

☐ Examinee recognized the SP's emotions and responded with PEARLS.

Physical Examination

☐ Examinee washed his/her hands.

☐ Examinee asked permission to start the exam.

☐ Examinee used respectful draping.

☐ Examinee did not repeat painful maneuvers.

☑ Exam Component	Maneuver
☐ HEENT exam	Inspection/palpation of thyroid
☐ CV exam	Auscultation
☐ Pulmonary exam	Auscultation
☐ Abdominal exam	Inspection, auscultation, palpation
☐ Skin exam	Inspected for pigmentation or pallor

Closure

☐ Examinee discussed initial diagnostic impressions.

☐ Examinee discussed initial management plans.

  ☐ Follow-up tests: Examinee mentioned the need for a pelvic/breast exam.

☐ Examinee asked if the SP had any other questions or concerns.

Sample Closure

Mrs. Parker, on the basis of my observations and what you have told me, it appears that you are pregnant. I will have to repeat a urine pregnancy test to confirm the diagnosis. Your last period may not have been a real menstrual period, as spotting can frequently occur in the first trimester. Unfortunately, natural methods of contraception such as pulling out before ejaculation are not very effective. We will also need to perform a pelvic ultrasound to estimate the age of the fetus and the expected date of delivery. If you are pregnant, we will check some more blood tests, a Pap smear, and some vaginal cultures that we routinely perform in every pregnancy. For now, I recommend stopping alcohol consumption and avoiding intense exercises and excess caffeine. I will be giving you some prenatal multivitamins to take orally, and we will schedule your future prenatal visits. I will be able to advise you further as soon as we receive these tests. Do you have any questions or concerns?

☐ Examinee used respectful draping.

☐ Examinee did not repeat painful maneuvers.

☑ Exam Component	Maneuver
☐ HEENT exam	Inspection, palpation, auscultation of thyroid for lymphadenopathy
☐ CV exam	Auscultation
☐ Pulmonary exam	Auscultation
☐ Abdominal exam	Inspection, auscultation, palpation
☐ Extremities	Checked for tremor on outstretched fingertips; looked for edema
☐ Skin exam	Inspection
☐ Neurologic exam	Looked for brisk reflexes

Closure

☐ Examinee discussed initial diagnostic impressions.

☐ Examinee discussed initial management plans.

    ☐ Follow-up tests.

☐ Examinee asked if the SP had any other questions or concerns.

Sample Closure

Ms. Potter, on the basis of your history and my examination, I think there are a few factors that might be contributing to your sleeping problems. The first is the anxiety and stress you've been experiencing over performing well in college. Although this is perfectly understandable, you may not be able to perform at your best if you don't get a good night's sleep. On the other hand, your problems could stem from your caffeine use, which I urge you to reduce or stop completely. Another possibility has to do with your thyroid function. Sometimes hyperactivity of the thyroid gland can cause some of the symptoms you describe, and the only way to rule this out is through a blood test. I will also check a urine drug screen, and in light of your history of snoring, we may need to do a sleep study in the future to rule out sleep apnea. At this point, I encourage you to proceed with the lifestyle changes I have recommended, and I will see you for follow-up to see how you are doing. Do you have any questions or concerns?

Patient Note

History

_____
_____
_____
_____
_____
_____
_____
_____
_____
_____

Physical Examination

_____
_____
_____
_____
_____
_____
_____
_____
_____
_____
_____

Differential Diagnosis

1. _____
2. _____
3. _____
4. _____
5. _____

Diagnostic Workup

1. _____
2. _____
3. _____
4. _____
5. _____

History

HPI: *20 yo F college student c/o inability to sleep. She has difficulty falling asleep until 2 AM and also has difficulty staying asleep. She used to get 8 hours of sleep, but for the past month she has been getting a total of only 4 hours per night. She has difficulty getting up after hearing the alarm and feels tired while at school. She notes inability to concentrate during classes and while driving. The patient appears to be stressed about her coursework and about her performance at school. She has also been snoring for the past few months and has had palpitations, especially after drinking caffeine. She has a history of drinking 4–5 cups of coffee per day. She has lost weight (6 lbs in 1 month) and has sweaty palms. There is an increase in frequency of bowel movements. She lives with her boyfriend, and they use condoms and OCPs for contraception. There is no history of sexual abuse, recent infection, or recent tragic events in her life.*

ROS: *Negative except as above.*

Allergies: *NKDA.*

Medications: *Multivitamins, OCPs.*

PMH: *None.*

PSH: *Tonsillectomy at age 12.*

SH: *No smoking, 1–2 beers/week, no illicit drugs.*

FH: *Not significant.*

Physical Examination

Patient appears anxious and restless.

Chest: *Clear breath sounds bilaterally.*

Heart: *Tachycardic; normal S1/S2; no murmurs, rubs, or gallops.*

Abdomen: *Soft, nontender, nondistended, ⊕ BS, no guarding, no hepatosplenomegaly.*

Skin: *Normal, no rashes, palms moist.*

Neuro: *Brisk reflexes.*

Extremities: *Tremor on outstretched fingertips.*

Differential Diagnosis

1. *Anxiety*
2. *Caffeine-induced insomnia*
3. *Hyperthyroidism*
4. *Insomnia related to depression*
5. *Adjustment insomnia*
6. *Illicit drug abuse*
7. *Obstructive sleep apnea*

Diagnostic Workup

1. *TSH, free T_4*
2. *CBC with differential, chem 8*
3. *Urine toxicology*
4. *Polysomnography*
5. *ECG*

CASE DISCUSSION

Differential Diagnosis

- **Anxiety:** Fatigue and sleep disturbances are common in anxiety states. The clinical manifestations of anxiety can be both psychological (eg, tension, fears, difficulty concentrating) and somatic (eg, tachycardia, sweating, hyperventilation, palpitations, tremor). The patient is mildly tachycardic, further supporting this diagnosis.

- **Caffeine-induced insomnia:** The most common pharmacologic cause of insomnia, caffeine use produces increased latency to sleep onset, more frequent arousals during sleep, and a reduction in total sleep time several hours after ingestion. Even small amounts of caffeine can significantly disturb sleep in some patients.

- **Hyperthyroidism:** Clinical hyperthyroidism is associated with anxiety, tremor, palpitations, sweating, frequent bowel movements, fatigue, menstrual irregularities, and heat intolerance. The patient presented in this case has some of these symptoms, suggesting the need to rule out hyperthyroidism.

- **Insomnia due to depression:** Several mood disorders are associated with insomnia. Depression can be associated with sleep onset insomnia, sleep maintenance insomnia, or early-morning wakefulness. Hypersomnia occurs in some depressed patients, especially adolescents and those with either bipolar or seasonal (fall/winter) depression.

- **Adjustment insomnia:** Any significant life event, such as a change of occupation, loss of a loved one, illness, or anxiety over a deadline or an examination, can cause adjustment insomnia. Increased sleep latency, frequent awakenings from sleep, and early-morning awakening can all result. Recovery is rapid, usually occurring within a few weeks.

- **Illicit drug use:** Drugs such as cocaine and amphetamine increase sympathetic activity and can thus cause insomnia.

- **Obstructive sleep apnea (OSA):** More than 50% of patients evaluated for OSA complain of symptoms of insomnia, including difficulty in initiating and maintaining sleep and early-morning awakening.

Diagnostic Workup

- **TSH, free T$_4$:** The patient gives a history of weight loss, increased frequency of bowel movements, palpitations, and sweaty palms, all of which suggest hyperthyroidism. An elevated free T$_4$ with suppressed TSH is diagnostic.

- **CBC:** Can help detect anemia, hidden infection, or malignancy, all of which can cause the fatigue and weight loss seen in this patient.

- **Urine toxicology:** Although this patient denies illicit drug use, a toxicology screen will help rule out the use of CNS stimulants that can cause insomnia (eg, cocaine, amphetamine).

- **Polysomnography:** A diagnostic test for OSA syndrome that can also help assess the severity of the disease as well as any comorbidities with which it might be associated.

- **ECG:** Nonspecific changes can be seen with hyperthyroidism and anxiety disorders.

Opening Scenario

Jack Edwards, a 27-year-old male, comes to the ED complaining of seeing strange writing on the wall.

Vital Signs

BP: 140/80 mm Hg

Temp: 98.3°F (36.8°C)

RR: 15/minute

HR: 98/minute, regular

Examinee Tasks

1. Take a focused history.

2. Perform a focused physical exam (do not perform rectal, genitourinary, or female breast exam).

3. Explain your clinical impression and workup plan to the patient.

4. Write the patient note after leaving the room.

Checklist/SP Sheet

Patient Description

Patient is a 27 yo M.

Notes for the SP

- Sit up on the bed.
- Give the impression that you are staring at the wall.

Challenging Questions to Ask

"Do you think someone is trying to give me instructions through the writing I see on the wall?"

Sample Examinee Response

"I don't think anyone is trying to give you instructions. If you have been taking illicit drugs, it may be that the drugs are causing you to see this writing. In any case, we are going to do some tests to try to figure out what's going on."

Examinee Checklist

Building the Doctor-Patient Relationship

Entrance

☐ Examinee knocked on the door before entering.

☐ Examinee introduced self by name.

☐ Examinee identified his/her role or position.

☐ Examinee correctly used patient's name.

☐ Examinee made eye contact with the SP.

Reflective Listening

☐ Examinee asked an open-ended question and actively listened to the response.

☐ Examinee asked the SP to list his/her concerns and listened to the response without interrupting.

☐ Examinee summarized the SP's concerns, often using the SP's own words.

Information Gathering

☐ Examinee elicited data efficiently and accurately.

☑ Question	Patient Response
☐ Chief complaint	I have been seeing strange writing on the wall.
☐ Onset	It started yesterday.
☐ Content	It is not clear, and I can't read it most of the time.
☐ Duration	It lasts less than a minute.
☐ Constant/intermittent	It comes and goes.
☐ Frequency	It has happened 3–4 times since yesterday.
☐ Do you see the writing while your eyes are closed?	Sometimes.
☐ Alleviating factors	None.
☐ Exacerbating factors	None.
☐ Major life changes or stressors	Not really.
☐ Headache	None.
☐ Visual changes or vision loss	None.
☐ Hearing changes	I feel as though I hear strange voices when I see the writing.
☐ Hearing loss	No.
☐ Content of the voices	I can't understand them; the voices seem distant.
☐ Feeling of being controlled	No.
☐ Do the voices/writing order you to harm yourself or others?	No.
☐ Do you think about harming yourself or others?	No.
☐ Enjoyment of daily activities	Yes.
☐ Mental illness in family	No.
☐ Sleeping problems	No, but sometimes I find it difficult to wake up in the morning.
☐ Do you fall asleep suddenly during the day?	No, but sometimes I feel very sleepy during the day.

☑ Question	Patient Response
☐ Fever	No.
☐ Weight changes	None.
☐ Current medications	None.
☐ Past medical history	None.
☐ Head trauma	No.
☐ Past surgical history	None.
☐ Family history	My father had high blood pressure.
☐ Occupation	I work as a bartender.
☐ Alcohol use	No.
☐ Illicit drug use	Occasionally.
☐ Which illicit drugs do you use?	Angel dust; sometimes Ecstasy.
☐ Last use of illicit drugs	Two days ago at a party at my friend's house.
☐ Tobacco	Yes, I have smoked one pack a day for six years.
☐ Exercise	No.
☐ Sexual activity	Yes, with my girlfriend.
☐ Use of condoms	Yes, I use them.
☐ Drug allergies	No.

Connecting with the Patient

☐ Examinee recognized the SP's emotions and responded with PEARLS.

Physical Examination

☐ Examinee washed his/her hands.

☐ Examinee asked permission to start the exam.

☐ Examinee used respectful draping.

☐ Examinee did not repeat painful maneuvers.

☑ Exam Component	Maneuver
☐ Eye exam	Inspected pupils; checked for reactivity
☐ CV exam	Auscultation, vital signs
☐ Pulmonary exam	Auscultation
☐ Abdominal exam	Palpation
☐ Neurologic exam	Mini-mental status exam, cranial nerves, motor exam, DTRs, gait, sensory exam

Closure

☐ Examinee discussed initial diagnostic impressions.

☐ Examinee discussed initial management plans.

    ☐ Follow-up tests.

☐ Examinee asked if the SP had any other questions or concerns.

Sample Closure

Mr. Edwards, your symptoms could be caused by your illicit drug use, or they may be the result of a mental problem or even a medical condition. We will run some tests to try to clarify your condition. In addition, I recommend that you stop using illicit drugs and quit smoking. Do you have any questions for me?

Patient Note

History

Physical Examination

Differential Diagnosis

1.
2.
3.
4.
5.

Diagnostic Workup

1.
2.
3.
4.
5.

Patient Note

History

HPI: *27 yo M c/o episodes of seeing strange writing on the wall since yesterday. These episodes last less than a minute and have happened 3–4 times. The patient states that the writing is not clear and he cannot read the messages, but he thinks he might be getting instructions from them. He denies any other visual changes or visual loss. The patient also mentions hearing strange voices associated with the writing, adding that he cannot understand them either. He admits to having used illicit drugs 2 days before these events. He denies any headache, seizures, head trauma, or previous similar episodes. No appetite or weight changes, fever, or sleep problems.*

ROS: *Negative except as above.*

Allergies: *NKDA.*

Medications: *None.*

PMH: *None.*

PSH: *None.*

SH: *1 PPD for 6 years; uses PCP ("angel dust") and MDMA (Ecstasy) occasionally; no EtOH. Works as a bartender.*

FH: *Noncontributory.*

Physical Examination

Patient seems anxious and in mild distress.

VS: *WNL.*

HEENT: *Pupils reactive to light.*

Chest: *Clear breath sounds bilaterally.*

Heart: *RRR; normal S1/S2; no murmurs, rubs, or gallops.*

Abdomen: *Soft, nontender, nondistended, no hepatosplenomegaly.*

Neuro: *Mental status: Alert and oriented × 3, spells backward and recalls 3 objects. Cranial nerves: 2–12 intact. Motor: Strength 5/5 in all muscle groups. DTRs: Symmetric. Gait: Normal.*

Differential Diagnosis

1. Substance-induced psychosis
2. Brief psychotic disorder
3. Psychosis secondary to a medical condition
4. Narcolepsy
5. Seizure

Diagnostic Workup

1. Urine toxicology
2. Mental status exam
3. Electrolytes
4. Liver function tests
5. TSH, free T_4
6. EEG
7. Polysomnogram

CASE DISCUSSION

Differential Diagnosis

- **Substance-induced psychosis:** Psychosis may result from the ingestion of medications, alcohol, or illicit drugs, or it may stem from the withdrawal of alcohol or sedative drugs such as benzodiazepines. The presence of offending substances is usually detectable and points to the diagnosis.

- **Brief psychotic disorder:** Symptoms of psychosis may be induced by stressful events and may resolve with removal of the stressor. Auditory hallucinations are more common and typically accompany visual hallucinations. The content of the hallucinations is usually disturbing and antagonistic. The duration and frequency of hallucinations are highly variable.

- **Psychosis secondary to a medical condition:** A variety of medical conditions can lead to hallucination. These include neurologic problems such as CNS infections and neoplasms; endocrine conditions such as thyroid, parathyroid, or adrenal abnormalities; and hepatic and renal disorders.

- **Narcolepsy:** The visual hallucinations of narcolepsy are complex, generally occurring immediately before falling asleep (hypnagogic) or just after waking up (hypnopompic). Auditory or tactile sensations can be associated with visual hallucinations as well. The duration and frequency are variable. Associated symptoms of narcolepsy include excessive daytime sleepiness, sleep paralysis, and cataplexy.

- **Seizure:** Visual hallucinations of epileptic origin can be simple or complex. They are variable in frequency and usually last for a few seconds. An example would be idiopathic occipital epilepsy.

Diagnostic Workup

- **Urine toxicology:** To detect commonly used illicit drugs, such as amphetamines, barbiturates, benzodiazepines, cannabinoids, cocaine, opioids, and phencyclidine (PCP).

- **Mental status exam:** To evaluate for any possible neurologic disorder.

- **Electrolytes, liver function tests, TSH, free T$_4$:** To detect any medical condition that may cause neurologic or mental changes.

- **EEG:** To detect any seizure activity.

- **Polysomnogram:** A polysomnogram and the MSLT (multiple sleep latency test) are diagnostic tests for narcolepsy.

CASE 36
DOORWAY INFORMATION

Opening Scenario

The mother of Louise Johnson, a 10-year-old female child, comes to the office because she is concerned that her daughter was recently diagnosed with diabetes.

Examinee Tasks

1. Take a focused history.

2. Explain your clinical impression and workup plan to the mother.

3. Write the patient note after leaving the room.

Checklist/SP Sheet

Patient Description

The patient's mother offers the history; her daughter is in the waiting room.

Notes for the SP

None.

Challenging Questions to Ask

- "Doctor, I have no history of diabetes in my family. Why is this happening to my daughter?"

- "Will my child ever be able to eat sweets again?"

Sample Examinee Response

"Your daughter probably had a genetic tendency to develop diabetes. Then certain unknown environmental factors led her to get full-blown diabetes. Your daughter may have either type 1 or type 2 diabetes. In type 1 diabetes, the immune system attacks the pancreas and destroys the cells that are responsible for making insulin. Since insulin regulates and maintains blood sugar, a deficiency of insulin will lead to high levels of blood sugar. On the other hand, if your child is overweight and is not physically active, she may have type 2 diabetes, which is a combination of insulin deficiency and resistance to the action of insulin resulting from being overweight. In either case, it is not essential to have a positive family history. As far as sweets are concerned, this is a myth. Your daughter can still eat sweets, but in moderation. She will need to see a dietitian to develop healthy meal plans and to learn to recognize which foods contain carbohydrates."

Examinee Checklist

Building the Doctor-Patient Relationship

Entrance

☐ Examinee knocked on the door before entering.

☐ Examinee introduced self by name.

☐ Examinee identified his/her role or position.

☐ Examinee correctly used patient's name.

☐ Examinee made eye contact with the SP.

Reflective Listening

☐ Examinee asked an open-ended question and actively listened to the response.

☐ Examinee asked the SP to list his/her concerns and listened to the response without interrupting.

☐ Examinee summarized the SP's concerns, often using the SP's own words.

Information Gathering

☐ Examinee elicited data efficiently and accurately.

☑ Question	Patient Response
☐ Chief complaint	My child was recently diagnosed with diabetes.
☐ Type of diabetes	I am not sure.
☐ Onset	A month ago.
☐ Presenting symptoms at the time of diagnosis	Excessive thirst and urination.
☐ Effect on child	She is concerned about the effect this will have on her normal activities, such as playing tennis and attending school.
☐ Depression	I'm not sure, but she seems more concerned than depressed.
☐ Irritability	No.
☐ Effect on parents	We were shocked.
☐ Medication	Insulin injections.
☐ Site of injection	In the tummy.
☐ Insulin injector	I do it when she is at home, but when she is away from me, she does the injections herself.
☐ Compliance with insulin	Yes.
☐ Schedule of insulin	Two types: one with meals and one at bedtime.
☐ Measuring glucose at home	Yes, before each meal and at bedtime.
☐ Ranges of blood glucose readings	Her blood sugar levels are normally in the low 100s in the morning and in the high 100s before meals.
☐ Recent level of glucose	Today her morning glucose was 96 in the fasting state.
☐ Hypoglycemia	Not really; the lowest blood glucose reading was 80 in the morning.
☐ Urination	Normal.
☐ Abnormal thirst or extreme hunger	No, but she was excessively thirsty earlier.
☐ Weakness or fatigue	No.
☐ Vision problems (blurring of vision)	No.
☐ Weight changes	She has lost about nine pounds within the past three months, but now her weight is stable.
☐ Patient's weight and height	She weighs 180 pounds and has been on the heavy side for a long time. She is 5 feet, 1 inch tall.

☑ Question	Patient Response
☐ Tingling or numbness in limbs	No.
☐ Infections of skin or gums	No.
☐ Itchy skin	No.
☐ Any specific diet	We are trying to give her a balanced diet as suggested previously by a dietitian.
☐ Exercise and playful activities	Yes, she is active and plays tennis.
☐ When does she play?	Evenings.
☐ Loss of consciousness while playing	No.
☐ Last menstrual period	She has not yet started menstruating.
☐ Sleeping problems	No.
☐ Birth history	Normal.
☐ Child weight, height, and language development	She was always on time with her development. She walked early, talked on time, and is doing well in school.
☐ Past medical history	None.
☐ Past surgical history	None.
☐ Drug allergies	No.

Connecting with the Patient

☐ Examinee recognized SP's emotions and responded with PEARLS.

Physical Examination

None.

Closure

☐ Examinee discussed initial diagnostic impressions.

☐ Examinee discussed initial management plans.

    ☐ Further examination.

    ☐ Follow-up tests.

☐ Examinee asked if the SP had any other questions or concerns.

Sample Closure

Mrs. Johnson, I can understand how you have felt since your daughter was diagnosed with diabetes. Diabetes may alter the dynamics of the entire family and affects everyone, so your life is going to be a little different now. But believe me, we can manage this disease very well through a combination of insulin, a balanced diet, and regular exercise. First of all, you should understand the disease and know how to manage it. You will need to attend diabetes classes with your daughter. Second, everyone in your family, including your daughter, should learn to recognize signs of low glucose levels, such as confusion, disorientation, or fainting, and should know how to provide appropriate care. Your daughter should always carry glucose tablets or juices as an "emergency kit." Her teachers and friends should also be aware of her disease. I hope you understood what we discussed today. Do you have any additional questions or concerns?

Patient Note

History

Physical Examination

Differential Diagnosis

1. _____
2. _____
3. _____
4. _____
5. _____

Diagnostic Workup

1. _____
2. _____
3. _____
4. _____
5. _____

Patient Note

History

HPI: The source of the information is the patient's mother. The mother of a 10 yo F states that her child was diagnosed with DM 1 month ago, when she presented with excessive thirst and frequent urination. The parents were shocked after the diagnosis was made. The child seems concerned but not irritable or depressed. She is active, plays tennis, and is currently on a diet prescribed by a dietitian. She is on insulin injections and regularly monitors her blood glucose levels at home. Her compliance is good; she checks her blood glucose before each meal and at bedtime. Fasting glucose levels are usually 80 to the low 100s and in the high 100s before meals. She has not had any episodes of hypoglycemia. She has lost 9 lb in the past 3 months, but her weight is stable now at about 180 lb. She denies any weakness, fatigue, tingling over limbs, visual symptoms, or rash/itch at the injection sites. She has not yet started menstruating.

ROS: Negative.

Allergies: NKDA.

Medications: Insulin.

PMH: None.

PSH: None.

Birth history: Normal.

Developmental history: Normal.

FH: No family history of diabetes.

Physical Examination

None.

Differential Diagnosis

1. Type 1 diabetes mellitus
2. Type 2 diabetes mellitus
3. Secondary causes of diabetes (such as Cushing syndrome)

Diagnostic Workup

1. Basal metabolic profile
2. Glycosylated hemoglobin/HbA$_{1c}$
3. UA, urine microalbumin
4. Insulin and C-peptide levels
5. Islet cell antibodies
6. 24-hour urine free cortisol

CASE DISCUSSION

Differential Diagnosis

- **Diabetes mellitus (DM):** Although most cases of DM in the pediatric population are type 1, the increasing prevalence of obesity and physical inactivity in the urban population has led to a growing incidence of type 2 DM among children. In every suspected case of DM, it is mandatory to rule out other causes.

- **Secondary causes of diabetes (hyperglycemia):** DM can be secondary to other factors or medical conditions, such as drugs (eg, thiazide diuretics, glucocorticoids), Cushing syndrome, pancreatitis, cystic fibrosis, hemochromatosis, and acromegaly.

Diagnostic Workup

- **Basal metabolic profile:** To evaluate serum electrolytes and glucose levels.

- **Glycosylated hemoglobin/HbA$_{1c}$:** Not a test to diagnose DM, but conducted to estimate blood glucose control during the preceding 2–3 months. Elevated levels suggest existing DM as well as lack of control of blood glucose levels within the past 2–3 months.

- **UA, urine microalbumin:** To screen for diabetic nephropathy.

- **Insulin and C-peptide levels:** When combined, can be a useful tool in identifying type 1 DM.

- **Islet cell antibodies:** This finding will support the diagnosis of type 1 DM.

- **24-hour urine free cortisol:** To rule out coexisting Cushing syndrome.

Opening Scenario

Riva George, a 35-year-old female, comes to the hospital complaining of pain in her right calf.

Vital Signs

BP: 130/70 mm Hg

Temp: 98.2°F (36.8°C)

RR: 13/minute

HR: 74/minute

Examinee Tasks

1. Take a focused history.

2. Perform a focused physical exam (do not perform rectal, genitourinary, or female breast exam).

3. Explain your clinical impression and workup plan to the patient.

4. Write the patient note after leaving the room.

Checklist/SP Sheet

Patient Description

Patient is a 35 yo F, married with two children.

Notes for the SP

- Exhibit pain in your calf when the doctor dorsiflexes your right ankle.
- Place a bandage on your right leg to cover the cuts that you got after a fall.

Challenging Questions to Ask

"My father had a clot in his leg. What do you think I should do to make sure I don't get one too?"

Sample Examinee Response

"There are several measures you can take that may prevent you from having a clot. Above all, you should avoid immobilization for long periods of time—for example, while sitting at your computer desk or on long-distance plane trips. Try to move in place and perhaps take a short walk. If you are on oral contraceptive pills, I strongly recommend that you stop taking them, as they are known to precipitate clotting. Studies have also shown that obesity increases your risk of having a clot, so I suggest that you exercise regularly and manage your diet."

Examinee Checklist

Building the Doctor-Patient Relationship

Entrance

☐ Examinee knocked on the door before entering.

☐ Examinee introduced self by name.

☐ Examinee identified his/her role or position.

☐ Examinee correctly used patient's name.

☐ Examinee made eye contact with the SP.

Reflective Listening

☐ Examinee asked an open-ended question and actively listened to the response.

☐ Examinee asked the SP to list his/her concerns and listened to the response without interrupting.

☐ Examinee summarized the SP's concerns, often using the SP's own words.

Information Gathering

☐ Examinee elicited data efficiently and accurately.

☑ Question	Patient Response
☐ Chief complaint	Pain in my right calf muscle.
☐ Onset	The pain started a few days ago and has gotten worse.
☐ Frequency	It is present all the time.
☐ Progression	The pain was mild in the beginning, but now it hurts even when I take just one step.
☐ Severity on a scale	8/10.
☐ Radiation	No.
☐ Quality	Pressure, spasms.
☐ Alleviating factors	Pain medication (ibuprofen). It also helps if I prop up my leg with a pillow.
☐ Exacerbating factors	Walking and extending my knee.
☐ Swelling	At the end of the day, my legs feel heavy and pit on pressure.
☐ Injury	Yes, I fell down and scratched my right leg (points to bandage).
☐ Redness	Yes.
☐ Warmth	My right leg feels warmer than my left.
☐ Varicose veins	No.
☐ Shortness of breath	No.
☐ Chest pain	No.
☐ Recent immobilization	I travel frequently as part of my consulting business, and a week ago I took a 15-hour flight to meet an important client.
☐ Fever	No.
☐ Last menstrual period	Two weeks ago.
☐ Contraceptives	I have been taking oral contraceptives for two years.
☐ Frequency of menstrual periods	Regular. My periods last three days, and I use 3–4 pads. They are not accompanied by pain.

☑ Question	Patient Response
☐ Obstetric history	I have had two kids, both with a normal delivery.
☐ Last Pap smear	One year ago; it was normal.
☐ Weight changes	I gained 50 pounds after having my last child three years ago.
☐ Past medical history	None.
☐ Past surgical history	None.
☐ Family history	My dad had a clot in his leg.
☐ Occupation	Executive consultant.
☐ Alcohol use	No.
☐ Illicit drug use	No.
☐ Tobacco	No.
☐ Sexual activity	With my husband.
☐ Drug allergies/herbal medication	No.

Connecting with the Patient

☐ Examinee recognized the SP's emotions and responded with PEARLS.

Physical Examination

☐ Examinee washed his/her hands.

☐ Examinee asked permission to start the exam.

☐ Examinee used respectful draping.

☐ Examinee did not repeat painful maneuvers.

☑ Exam Component	Maneuver
☐ CV/pulmonary exam	Inspection, auscultation, palpation; compared pulses (femoral, popliteal, dorsalis pedis) on both sides
☐ Joint exam	Inspection, palpation, range of motion (knee, ankle, hip joint on both sides)
☐ Extremities	Inspection, palpation; checked for Homans sign
☐ Neurologic exam	Sensory and motor reflexes (knee, ankle)

Closure

☐ Examinee discussed initial diagnostic impressions.

☐ Examinee discussed initial management plans:

   ☐ Follow-up tests.

☐ Examinee asked if the SP had any other questions or concerns.

Sample Closure

Mrs. George, on the basis of your history and my physical examination, I believe it is possible that you had a blood clot. However, we will also look for other possible causes of your symptoms, such as an infection or a ruptured cyst. We will be running a few blood tests as well as some imaging studies that should help us make a final diagnosis. If your test results show a clot, we will start you on blood thinners, which should prevent further complications such as the possibility of a clot traveling to your lungs. Do you have any questions for me?

Patient Note

History

_____
_____
_____
_____
_____
_____
_____
_____

Physical Examination

_____
_____
_____
_____
_____
_____
_____
_____
_____
_____
_____

Differential Diagnosis

1. _____
2. _____
3. _____
4. _____
5. _____

Diagnostic Workup

1. _____
2. _____
3. _____
4. _____
5. _____

History

HPI: 35 yo F c/o calf pain of a few days' duration. The pain is constant, 8/10 in intensity, not radiating, aggravated on walking and extending the knee, and associated with swelling, redness, and warmth. It is alleviated on elevation of the foot and with ibuprofen. The patient took a 15-hour flight 1 week ago. She has a history of weight gain postpartum and cuts to the right leg secondary to a fall. She has 2 children, both normal deliveries. LMP was 2 weeks ago. The patient says she has gained 50 lb in the past 3 years. She has been on OCPs for 2 years. No history of chest pain or shortness of breath.

ROS: Negative except as above.

Allergies: NKDA.

Medications: OCPs, ibuprofen.

PMH: None.

PSH: None.

SH: No smoking, no EtOH, no illicit drugs.

FH: Father had DVT. No history of sudden deaths in the family.

Physical Examination

Patient is in severe pain.

VS: WNL.

Chest: Clear breath sounds bilaterally; no rales or rhonchi.

Heart: RRR; normal S1/S2; no murmurs, rubs, or gallops.

Abdomen: Soft, nontender, nondistended, ⊕ BS.

Extremities: Inspection: Right calf appears red and swollen compared to left; contours of the muscles appear normal; no ulcers or pigmentation. Palpation: Right leg is warmer compared to left; pitting pedal edema ⊕ on right side; multiple healing cuts covered with bandage on right leg; dorsalis pedis pulse felt and equal on both sides; mobility normal at ankle joint, knee, and hip joint; ⊕ Homans sign on right side.

Neuro: Mental status: Alert and oriented. DTRs: Symmetric 2+. Motor/sensation: Normal. Cranial nerves: 2–12 intact. Gait: Normal.

Differential Diagnosis

1. Deep venous thrombosis
2. Cellulitis/myositis
3. Rupture of Baker's cyst
4. Hematoma
5. Rupture of the medial head of the gastrocnemius
6. Spasm due to injury or sprain

Diagnostic Workup

1. Doppler U/S
2. D-dimer
3. Hypercoagulability testing
4. CBC with differential
5. CPK and myoglobin level
6. CT venography
7. MRI

CASE DISCUSSION

Differential Diagnosis

- **Deep venous thrombosis (DVT):** DVT is common in the lower limbs and may arise under conditions of stasis, hypercoagulability, and venous endothelial injury. Conditions that result in prolonged immobilization (eg, post-surgery, trauma, sedentary jobs, long hours of airplane or car travel) are predisposing factors. DVT may produce pain and edema of the affected limb or may be asymptomatic. A positive Homans sign (pain on dorsiflexion of the ankle) is indicative of DVT.

- **Cellulitis/myositis:** Trauma can lead to cellulitis of the skin and subcutaneous tissue or to myositis of the calf muscle. All the classic signs of inflammation associated with fever may point to the diagnosis. Myositis ossificans may occur as a complication of this disorder, causing hardening of the muscle and pain on contraction. Radiographs may show ossification in the muscle.

- **Rupture of Baker's cyst:** Baker's cysts (also known as popliteal cysts) are seen in the popliteal fossa. Arthritis or a cartilage tear of the knee joint may cause excess fluid to be accumulated, forming a cyst. Ruptures can present with tightness and swelling behind the knee, pain on knee extension, and stiffness of the calf muscle.

- **Hematoma:** Injuries can cause bleeding intramuscularly (in which no bruising occurs) or intermuscularly (in which bruising is usually present). Patients present with pain, swelling, and restricted movement. The condition may lead to posterior compartment syndrome.

- **Rupture of the gastrocnemius muscle:** Presents with sudden pain associated with rupture at the musculotendinous junction of the gastrocnemius muscle, halfway between the knee and the heel. There may be bruising and pain on standing on the tips of the toes. Patients also present with pain on dorsiflexion of the ankle against resistance.

- **Spasm/sprain:** Undue strain may cause physical tearing of muscles or tendons, inducing spasm and pain. Ligaments can be ruptured or torn due to overstretching or injuries.

Diagnostic Workup

- **Doppler U/S:** An initial diagnostic test that is noninvasive and can visualize clots in the veins of the leg.

- **D-dimer:** A cross-linked fibrin degradation product that may be increased in DVT. This is usually indicated in cases with a low to intermediate probability of thromboembolism. The negative predictive value of this test is sufficiently high to rule out DVT.

- **Hypercoagulability testing:** Several autoantibodies are implicated in thrombophilic states. Proteins C and S deficiency, partial antithrombin deficiency, hyperhomocysteinemia, antiphospholipid antibody syndrome, and paroxysmal nocturnal hemoglobinuria may all lead to increased coagulability.

- **CBC with differential:** To detect infections such as cellulitis.

- **CPK and myoglobin:** Both can be elevated in muscle injury (myositis).

- **CT/MRI:** CT venography is used to diagnose DVT in conjunction with contrast-enhanced spiral CT to rule out pulmonary embolism. MRI is noninvasive and can detect acute, symptomatic proximal DVTs as well as muscle or tendon rupture.

CASE 38
DOORWAY INFORMATION

Opening Scenario

Will Foreman, a 31-year-old male, comes to his primary care physician complaining of heel pain.

Vital Signs

BP: 125/80 mm Hg

Temp: 99.5°F (37.5°C)

RR: 14/minute

HR: 69/minute, regular

Examinee Tasks

1. Take a focused history.

2. Perform a focused physical exam (do not perform rectal, genitourinary, or female breast exam).

3. Explain your clinical impression and workup plan to the patient.

4. Write the patient note after leaving the room.

Checklist/SP Sheet

Patient Description

Patient is a 31 yo M.

Notes for the SP

- Pretend to have pain on the bottom of your right heel and into the arch of your right foot when the examinee extends your toes (moves them up).
- Exhibit pain when the examinee palpates the arch of your right foot and the bottom of your right heel.
- Give the appearance of pain with the first few steps you take after sitting.

Challenging Questions to Ask

"Doctor, can you just give me some powerful pain meds so that I can keep running? I am training for a marathon."

Sample Examinee Response

"First we need to do a complete evaluation to determine the cause of your pain, and from that point we can discuss the nature of your treatment."

Examinee Checklist

Building the Doctor-Patient Relationship

Entrance

☐ Examinee knocked on the door before entering.

☐ Examinee introduced self by name.

☐ Examinee identified his/her role or position.

☐ Examinee correctly used patient's name.

☐ Examinee made eye contact with the SP.

Reflective Listening

☐ Examinee asked an open-ended question and actively listened to the response.

☐ Examinee asked the SP to list his/her concerns and listened to the response without interrupting.

☐ Examinee summarized the SP's concerns, often using the SP's own words.

Information Gathering

☐ Examinee elicited data efficiently and accurately.

☑ Question	Patient Response
☐ Chief complaint	Right heel pain.
☐ Location	It hurts the most on the bottom of my heel.
☐ Onset	It came on gradually over the past two weeks.
☐ Precipitating events	Not really, but I have been training for a marathon.
☐ Constant/intermittent	Intermittent.
☐ Frequency	It usually hurts every day. It seems to be the worst in the morning.
☐ When does it hurt in the morning?	It hurts the most with the first few steps I take after I get out of bed.
☐ Progression	It has stayed about the same.
☐ Severity on a scale	When it hurts, it can get up to a 7/10.
☐ Radiation	It occasionally radiates into the arch of my foot.
☐ Radiation proximally (up the leg or down from the back)	No.
☐ Quality	Stretching/tearing pain.
☐ Burning, tingling, numbness	No.
☐ Alleviating factors	Massaging the arch of my foot and applying ice.
☐ Exacerbating factors	Walking barefoot or walking after sitting for a prolonged period of time.
☐ Other joint pain	No.
☐ Previous episodes of similar pain	No.
☐ Previous injury to your feet or ankles.	No.
☐ Constitutional symptoms (nausea/vomiting, weight/appetite changes, fever/chills, diarrhea/constipation, fatigue)	No.
☐ Current medications	Occasionally I take ibuprofen for the pain.

☑ Question	Patient Response
☐ Past medical history (be sure to address diabetes, rheumatologic disorders, and cancer)	No.
☐ Past surgical history	None.
☐ Family history (be sure to address diabetes, rheumatologic disorders, and cancer)	My father has arthritis.
☐ Occupation	I work as an accountant.
☐ Avocation	Runner.
☐ Alcohol use	I have approximately 1–2 beers a week.
☐ Illicit drug use	No.
☐ Tobacco	No.
☐ Sexual activity	I am sexually active with my wife of 10 years.
☐ Drug allergies	No.

Connecting with the Patient

☐ Examinee recognized the SP's emotions and responded with PEARLS.

Physical Examination

☐ Examinee washed his/her hands.

☐ Examinee asked permission to start the exam.

☐ Examinee used respectful draping.

☐ Examinee did not repeat painful maneuvers.

☑ Exam Component	Maneuver
☐ CV exam	Auscultation, distal pulses (posterior tibialis, dorsalis pedis), capillary refill of the toes
☐ Pulmonary exam	Auscultation
☐ Abdominal exam	Auscultation, palpation
☐ Extremities	■ Inspection of both feet and ankles—non–weight bearing, weight bearing, and with ambulation ■ Palpation of medial calcaneal tuberosity, Achilles tendon, plantar fascia, retrocalcaneal bursae ■ Passive range of motion and general strength of ipsilateral knee and hip ■ Ankle dorsiflexion and great toe extension and passive range of motion; strength testing of ankle dorsiflexion and plantar flexion
☐ Neurologic exam	Checked sensation to light touch for dermatomes of foot and ankle; assessed Achilles tendon reflex

Closure

☐ Examinee discussed initial diagnostic impressions.

☐ Examinee discussed initial management plans:

   ☐ Follow-up tests: X-ray of right ankle.

☐ Examinee asked if the SP had any other questions or concerns.

Sample Closure

Mr. Foreman, the most likely cause of your heel pain is plantar fasciitis, which is the most common cause of pain on the bottom of the heel. It typically resolves over a few months, with conservative treatment consisting of stretching, massage, NSAIDs, and avoidance of painful activities. We will get an x-ray today to help confirm that there is no obvious fracture or foreign body and to look for possible bone spurs. If you would like, I can send you to physical therapy to help you get started on these exercises. If your symptoms are not responsive to this treatment over the next two months, we may consider a bone scan to rule out a stress fracture. Do you have any questions for me?

Patient Note

History

Physical Examination

Differential Diagnosis

1.
2.
3.
4.
5.

Diagnostic Workup

1.
2.
3.
4.
5.

History

HPI: *31 yo M c/o pain on the plantar surface of his right heel. The pain started insidiously about 2 weeks ago and has not progressed. The patient denies trauma or a specific inciting event but does admit to training for a marathon. He states that the pain is worse with the first few steps after getting out of bed in the morning and after prolonged sitting. He reports that the pain has a tearing/stretching quality and that it can get as high as 7/10. He has used ice, massage, and occasional ibuprofen for pain, with minor relief. The patient denies any tingling, burning, or numbness. He denies proximally radiating symptoms but does report occasional pain radiating into his arch.*

ROS: *Denies nausea/vomiting, weight/appetite changes, fever/chills, diarrhea/constipation, or fatigue.*

Allergies: *NKDA.*

Medications: *Occasional ibuprofen.*

PMH: *None. Denies cancer, rheumatologic disorders, diabetes.*

PSH: *None.*

SH: *No smoking, 1–2 beers/week, no illicit drugs. Works as an accountant; sexually active only with wife of 10 years. Marathon runner.*

FH: *Father with arthritis, probable osteoarthritis. Denies FH of cancer, rheumatologic disorders, or diabetes.*

Physical Examination

Patient is pleasant and in no acute distress.

VS: *WNL.*

Chest: *Clear to auscultation bilaterally.*

Heart: *RRR; normal S1/S2; no murmurs, rubs, or gallops.*

Abdomen: *Soft, nontender, nondistended, ⊕ BS.*

Extremities: *Posterior tibialis and dorsalis pedis pulses 2+ bilaterally; mild bilateral rear/midfoot pronation; range of motion WNL for hip/knee/ankle and foot. Tender to palpation over medial calcaneal tuberosity and plantar fascia; plantar heel and arch pain with passive extension of toes.*

Neuro: *Motor: Strength 5/5 in hip/knee/ankle/foot. Sensation: Intact to light touch in saphenous, sural, and deep/superficial peroneal nerve distribution (dermatomes L4–S1). DTRs: 1+ in Achilles tendon. Gait: Nonantalgic gait pattern.*

Differential Diagnosis

1. Plantar fasciitis
2. Calcaneal stress fracture
3. Achilles tendinitis
4. Retrocalcaneal bursitis
5. Tarsal tunnel syndrome
6. Foreign body
7. Ankle sprain

Diagnostic Workup

1. XR—right ankle
2. Bone scan
3. MRI

CASE DISCUSSION

Differential Diagnosis

Heel pain in adults can be caused by several distinct entities. For this reason, it is essential that the examiner ascertain the precise location of the symptoms, as this is the first step in determining the most likely diagnosis.

- **Plantar fasciitis:** The most common cause of plantar heel pain in adults, plantar fasciitis typically results from repetitive use or excessive loading (eg, training for a marathon). Pes planus, pes cavus, decreased subtalar joint mobility, and a tight Achilles tendon can all predispose to plantar fasciitis. The pain is typically gradual in onset and worse with the first few steps in the morning and after prolonged sitting. Examination reveals marked tenderness over the medial calcaneal tuberosity and increased pain with passive dorsiflexion of the toes. Conservative management includes analgesics, stretching, exercise, orthotics, and night splinting.

- **Calcaneal stress fracture:** The calcaneus is second only to the metatarsals in terms of stress fractures of the foot. Stress fractures are common in athletes who are involved in running or jumping sports, as well as in patients who have risk factors for osteopenia. Patients typically have diffuse heel pain that is made worse by medial and lateral compression. A calcaneal stress fracture may be considered in this patient if his symptoms prove refractory to conservative management. Follow-up diagnostic testing (eg, x-ray, bone scan) may then be warranted.

- **Achilles tendinitis:** Patients with Achilles tendinitis typically complain of posterior heel pain either on the Achilles tendon insertion site or on the tendon itself during running, jumping, and harsh activities. Tenderness to palpation and swelling along the Achilles tendon are common. Pain may also increase with passive dorsiflexion of the ankle. Again, this is commonly due to overuse or to poor biomechanics. Conservative management includes rest, analgesics, and stretching/strengthening exercises.

- **Retrocalcaneal bursitis:** Patients with this condition usually complain of posterior heel pain secondary to chronic irritation of the underlying bursae. The bursae are located between the posterior calcaneus and the Achilles tendon, and between the Achilles tendon and the skin. The condition is commonly caused by ill-fitting footwear that has a poorly fitting, rigid heel cup. It can also be associated with Haglund deformity (a bony spur on the posterosuperior aspect of the calcaneus), which may exacerbate the condition. Conservative management includes analgesics, proper shoe wear, and heel padding.

- **Tarsal tunnel syndrome:** The tarsal tunnel is on the medial aspect of the heel and is formed by the flexor retinaculum traversing over the talus and calcaneus. Compression of the tibial nerve in the tunnel can lead to pain, burning, tingling, or numbness that can radiate to the plantar heel and even to the distal sole and toes. Symptoms may be exacerbated by percussion of the tarsal tunnel or with dorsiflexion and eversion of the foot. Conservative management includes analgesics and correction of foot mechanics with orthotics.

- **Foreign body:** If a foreign body is suspected, the foot should be inspected for signs of an entrance wound. The patient may or may not describe a mechanism of injury. Signs of local infection such as warmth, erythema, pain, induration, or a fluctuant mass should also be sought. Conservative management includes foreign body removal, topical antimicrobials, and appropriate dressing.

- **Ankle sprain:** Ankle ligament injuries are the most common musculoskeletal injury, with the lateral collateral ligament complex most commonly involved. Patients typically describe an injury pattern consistent with "rolling" the ankle, often in the plantar flexed and inverted position. Examination reveals tenderness to palpation over the involved ligaments and increased laxity on stress testing. Significant edema and ecchymosis are often present in the acute/subacute stages. Conservative treatment involves rest, ice, compression, elevation, NSAIDs, and bracing.

Diagnostic Workup

- **XR—right ankle:** X-rays in this region may demonstrate calcaneal spur formation (calcification) at the proximal plantar fascia (as in this patient) or at the Achilles tendon insertion. Care must be taken to correlate these findings with symptoms and with the physical examination, as such calcification can also be seen in asymptomatic patients. Increased prominence of the posterosuperior calcaneus (Haglund deformity) may also be demonstrated.

- **Bone scan:** If conservative treatment fails in this patient, follow-up with a bone scan is recommended in 2 months to rule out calcaneal stress fracture, as would be demonstrated by an increased area of uptake.

- **MRI:** Reserved for suspected soft tissue involvement, which could include the degree of Achilles tendon degeneration, rupture of the Achilles tendon, or articular cartilage defects.

CASE 39
DOORWAY INFORMATION

Opening Scenario

The mother of David Whitestone, a 5-day-old male child, calls the office complaining that her child has yellow skin and eyes.

Examinee Tasks

1. Take a focused history.

2. Explain your clinical impression and workup plan to the mother.

3. Write the patient note after leaving the room.

Checklist/SP Sheet

Patient Description

The patient's mother offers the history.

Notes for the SP

Show concern about your child's health, but add that you do not want to come to the office unless you have to because you do not have transportation.

Challenging Questions to Ask

"Can this jaundice hurt my baby?"

Sample Examinee Response

"Newborns often develop a mild case of natural jaundice after birth. This type of jaundice will resolve and rarely poses a threat to the baby. However, if your newborn has a more severe type of jaundice, his pigment levels may rise too high and cause damage to his brain. To determine the severity of your child's illness, I must examine him in the office and then obtain some blood tests. After seeing him, I should be able to give you a more accurate assessment of his condition."

Examinee Checklist

Building the Doctor-Patient Relationship

Entrance

☐ Examinee introduced self by name.

☐ Examinee identified his/her role or position.

☐ Examinee correctly used patient's name and identified caller and relationship of caller to patient.

Reflective Listening

☐ Examinee asked an open-ended question and actively listened to the response.

☐ Examinee asked the SP to list his/her concerns and listened to the response without interrupting.

☐ Examinee summarized the SP's concerns, often using the SP's own words.

Information Gathering

☐ Examinee elicited data efficiently and accurately.

☑ Question	Patient Response
☐ Chief complaint	My baby has yellow skin and eyes.
☐ Onset	I noticed it yesterday.
☐ Progression	It is not getting worse, but I'm still concerned.
☐ Parts of body involved	It is mainly visible on his face and hands.
☐ Age of child	Five days old.
☐ Vomiting	None.
☐ Abdominal distention	No.
☐ Frequency of bowel movements	He has 2–3 bowel movements a day.
☐ Color of stool	Brown.
☐ Blood in stool	No.
☐ Urinary frequency	Every 3–4 hours.
☐ Number of wet diapers	About 7–8 diapers per day.
☐ Breast-feeding and frequency	Started soon after birth. Every 4–5 hours.
☐ Sucking well	Yes.
☐ Activities and cry	Yes, he is playful and active. He cries occasionally.
☐ Awake and responsive	Yes.
☐ Recent URI	No.
☐ Fever	No.
☐ Breathing fast	No.
☐ Dry mouth	No.
☐ Cough, pulling ear	No.
☐ Shaking (seizures)	No.
☐ Your own blood group and the blood groups of your husband and baby	I'm B Rh positive and my husband is A Rh positive. My baby is also B Rh positive.
☐ Ill contacts	Not to my knowledge.
☐ Other pregnancies and miscarriages	I have a three-year-old daughter and have had no miscarriages.
☐ Birth history	It was an uncomplicated vaginal delivery.
☐ Complications during pregnancy	Yes, I had a positive culture for some bacteria and received antibiotics before delivery.
☐ Delivery at term or premature	At term.
☐ Smoking, alcohol, or recreational drugs during pregnancy	No.

☑ Question	Patient Response
☐ First bowel movement of baby	Soon after delivery.
☐ Discharge from hospital	Uneventful.
☐ Current medications	None.
☐ Past medical history	None.
☐ Past surgical history	None.
☐ Family history	My daughter also had jaundice after the first week of birth. She was admitted to the hospital.
☐ Drug allergies	Not known.

Connecting with the Patient

☐ Examinee recognized the SP's emotions and responded with PEARLS.

Physical Examination

None.

Closure

☐ Examinee discussed initial diagnostic impressions.

☐ Examinee discussed initial management plans:

    ☐ Follow-up tests.

☐ Examinee asked if the SP had any other questions or concerns.

Sample Closure

Mrs. Whitestone, given the information you have provided, I'm considering the possibility of physiologic or natural jaundice. This condition usually peaks on day 4 or 5 and then gradually disappears within 1–2 weeks. However, breast-feeding, some other pathologic conditions, and certain birth defects can also cause jaundice in infants, and these need to be ruled out. I suggest that you bring your child to the medical center for further evaluation. I hope you understood what we discussed today. Do you have any concerns or questions?

Patient Note

History

Physical Examination

Differential Diagnosis

1.
2.
3.
4.
5.

Diagnostic Workup

1.
2.
3.
4.
5.

Patient Note

History

HPI: *The source of information is the patient's mother. The mother of a 5-day-old M c/o her child having yellow discoloration of the eyes and skin for 2 days. It has not worsened. The child is awake, responsive, playful, and active. He is breast-fed. His stomach is soft and he has 2–3 daily bowel movements. The color of the stools is brown. She denies any h/o recent fever, vomiting, seizure, URI, or breathlessness. There is no noticeable dryness of the mouth. He is wetting 7–8 diapers per day every 3–4 hours. He was delivered vaginally at full term. The mother did receive antibiotics for a positive culture before delivery. The blood group of both mother and neonate is B positive, while that of the father is A positive.*

ROS: *Negative.*

Allergies: *NKDA.*

Medications: *None.*

PMH: *None.*

PSH: *None.*

FH: *His elder sister was hospitalized after the first week of birth for jaundice.*

Physical Examination

None.

Differential Diagnosis

1. *Physiologic jaundice*
2. *ABO or Rh incompatibility*
3. *Neonatal sepsis*
4. *Cephalohematoma*
5. *Breast-feeding jaundice*
6. *Polycythemia*
7. *Familial neonatal hyperbilirubinemia*

Diagnostic Workup

1. *Total and indirect bilirubin*
2. *Blood typing*
3. *Direct Coombs test*
4. *C-reactive protein*
5. *CBC*
6. *Titers for CMV, toxoplasmosis, and rubella (if required)*

CASE DISCUSSION

Differential Diagnosis

Early-onset neonatal jaundice (within one week):

- **Physiologic jaundice:** A condition that peaks between the third and seventh days of life. Underlying causes include accelerated destruction of erythrocytes, decreased excretory capacity, and decreased activity of the bilirubin-conjugating enzymes in hepatic cells. It is predominantly seen in preterm infants.

- **ABO or Rh incompatibility:** The hemolysis that results from blood group incompatibility may also cause clinically significant jaundice in neonates.

- **Neonatal sepsis:** Signs of infection such as lethargy, vomiting, poor feeding, fever, and/or abnormally colored urine are often present in neonatal sepsis. A history of maternal infections, particularly TORCH and group B streptococcus, yields an additional clue to this diagnosis.

- **Cephalohematoma:** As this scalp hemorrhage reabsorbs, it can also serve as a source of increased bilirubin production.

- **Breast-feeding jaundice:** This is usually seen toward the end of the first week of life in an infant who is otherwise thriving.

- **Polycythemia:** A condition that may also lead to abnormal levels of bilirubin.

- **Familial neonatal hyperbilirubinemia:** Look for a positive history of a sibling who had neonatal jaundice requiring phototherapy.

Late-onset neonatal jaundice (after one week):

- **Breast milk jaundice.**

- **Biliary atresia.**

- **Metabolic disorders:** Hypothyroidism, galactosemia, or hereditary hemolytic disorders such as spherocytosis or G6PD deficiency.

Diagnostic Workup

- **Total and indirect bilirubin:** The first step in determining the severity and type of jaundice. Phototherapy is usually indicated when bilirubin levels exceed 15 mg/dL.

- **Blood typing and direct Coombs testing:** To evaluate for jaundice stemming from blood group incompatibility. All infants who are born to mothers with type O blood should routinely receive direct Coombs testing to check for maternal-fetal incompatibility. Such children should also be closely followed for evidence of jaundice from hemolysis.

- **C-reactive protein:** For early assessment and to monitor for signs of infection.

- **CBC:** To evaluate the status of blood parameters such as hematocrit and hemoglobin due to suspected underlying hemolysis. Differential counts may provide additional clues about infections causing sepsis.

- **Titers for CMV, toxoplasmosis, and rubella:** In suspected maternal TORCH infections.

DOORWAY INFORMATION

Opening Scenario

The mother of Angelina Harvey, a 2-year-old female child, calls the office complaining that her child has noisy and strange breathing.

Examinee Tasks

1. Take a focused history.

2. Explain your clinical impression and workup plan to the mother.

3. Write the patient note after leaving the room.

Checklist/SP Sheet

Patient Description

The patient's mother offers the history.

Notes for the SP

Show concern about your child's health, but add that you don't want to come to the office unless you have to because you do not have transportation.

Challenging Questions to Ask

"Can you explain to me exactly what is going on with my child and what can be done for it?"

Sample Examinee Response

"It is hard for me to give you an accurate answer over the phone. I would like you to bring your baby here so that I can examine her and perhaps run some tests. After that, I will be able to give you a more accurate assessment of her condition."

Examinee Checklist

Building the Doctor-Patient Relationship

Entrance

☐ Examinee introduced self by name.

☐ Examinee identified his/her role or position.

☐ Examinee correctly used patient's name and identified caller and relationship of caller to patient.

Reflective Listening

☐ Examinee asked an open-ended question and actively listened to the response.

☐ Examinee asked the SP to list his/her concerns and listened to the response without interrupting.

☐ Examinee summarized the SP's concerns, often using the SP's own words.

Information Gathering

☐ Examinee elicited data efficiently and accurately.

☑ Question	Patient Response
☐ Chief complaint	My baby has noisy and strange breathing.
☐ Onset	It started suddenly about an hour ago.
☐ Progression	It is getting worse.
☐ Description of the activity that preceded the event	She was playing with toys.
☐ Description of the sound	It is a noisy sound, as if she swallowed a washing machine.
☐ Consistency	The sound is always the same.
☐ Best heard on inhalation or exhaling air	On inhalation.
☐ Can you identify anything that may have caused it?	None.
☐ Alleviating/exacerbating factors (feeding, crying, supine position, sleep)	None.
☐ Associated problems (cough, fever)	Yes, there is some coughing, but it was present earlier. She has no fever.
☐ Is the cough barking in nature?	No.
☐ Is it productive?	No.
☐ Any blood in cough?	No.
☐ Is she crying?	Yes.
☐ Is her crying muffled or weak?	Weak.
☐ Breathing fast	No.
☐ Nausea/vomiting	No.
☐ Drooling	No.
☐ Blueness of skin or fingers	No.
☐ Difficulty in swallowing food	No.
☐ Similar episodes in the past	No.
☐ Hoarseness of voice	No.
☐ Snoring at night	No.
☐ History of allergies in the family	No.
☐ Psychological or social stress in the recent past	No.
☐ Day care center	Yes.
☐ Ill contacts in day care center	Not to my knowledge.
☐ Vaccinations	Up to date.
☐ Last checkup	Two weeks ago, and everything was normal.

☑ Question	Patient Response
☐ Growth, development, and milestones	All were fine. She met all milestones in a timely manner.
☐ Birth history	It was an uncomplicated spontaneous vaginal delivery.
☐ Eating habits	Normal.
☐ Current medications	None.
☐ Past medical history	Nothing of note.
☐ Past surgical history	None.
☐ Family history	None.

Connecting with the Patient

☐ Examinee recognized the SP's emotions and responded with PEARLS.

Physical Examination

None.

Closure

☐ Examinee discussed initial diagnostic impressions.

☐ Examinee discussed initial management plans:

   ☐ Follow-up tests.

☐ Examinee asked if the SP had any other questions or concerns.

Sample Closure

Mrs. Harvey, on the basis of the information I have gathered from you, I'm considering the possibility that your daughter might have aspirated a foreign body. However, the possibility that an infection might be causing her problem needs to be ruled out. Right now, I feel that your daughter needs emergency medical attention. Since you do not have access to transportation, I strongly suggest that you call 911 immediately and bring her to the medical center. In the meantime, I suggest that you avoid putting a finger in her mouth or performing any blind finger sweep, as doing so may cause the foreign body to become more deeply lodged if it is actually present. If you observe significant respiratory compromise or choking, perform the Heimlich maneuver by thrusting your daughter's tummy with sudden pressure. I hope you understood what we have discussed. Do you have any questions or concerns? Alright, I will see you once you get to the hospital.

Patient Note

History

_____
_____
_____
_____
_____
_____
_____
_____

Physical Examination

_____
_____
_____
_____
_____
_____
_____
_____
_____
_____

Differential Diagnosis

1. _____

2. _____

3. _____

4. _____

5. _____

Diagnostic Workup

1. _____

2. _____

3. _____

4. _____

5. _____

Patient Note

History

HPI: *The source of information is the patient's mother. The mother of a 2 yo F c/o her child suddenly developing noisy breathing that is getting progressively worse. The child was playing with her toys when she developed the noisy breathing. The sound is consistent, best heard on inhalation, and similar to that of a washing machine. There is no relation to posture. It is associated with a nonproductive cough without any associated fever, hemoptysis, tachypnea, hoarseness of voice, drooling, or bluish discoloration of the skin. Her vaccinations are up to date.*

ROS: *Negative.*

Allergies: *NKDA.*

Medications: *None.*

PMH: *Uncomplicated spontaneous vaginal delivery.*

PSH: *None.*

FH: *Noncontributory.*

Physical Examination

None.

Differential Diagnosis

1. *Foreign body aspiration*
2. *Croup*
3. *Laryngitis*
4. *Epiglottitis*
5. *Retropharyngeal abscess*
6. *Angioedema*
7. *Peritonsillar abscess*
8. *Laryngeal papilloma*

Diagnostic Workup

1. *ABG*
2. *CXR—PA and lateral*
3. *XR—neck, AP and lateral*
4. *CBC with differential*
5. *Direct laryngoscopy*
6. *Bronchoscopy*

CASE DISCUSSION

Differential Diagnosis

- There are three types of stridor:
    - **Inspiratory stridor:** Indicates obstruction at the level of larynx or superior to it.
    - **Expiratory stridor:** Points to obstruction inferior to the larynx.
    - **Biphasic stridor:** Suggests obstruction in the trachea.
- Stridor that presents with hoarseness suggests involvement of the vocal cords.
- **Aspiration of a foreign body:** The sudden and dramatic onset of symptoms, especially when a foreign body (usually a toy or peanuts) is in the vicinity before the patient develops symptoms, helps support this diagnosis.
- **Croup:** Common in children six months to three years of age; develops insidiously as an URI. A characteristic barking cough is often present.
- **Laryngitis:** Occurs in children older than five years of age. The absence of stridor and the presence of a hoarse voice are characteristic.
- **Epiglottitis:** Occurs more frequently in children 2–6 years of age and begins with a short prodrome. Significant drooling, with symptomatic relief while bending forward, is the hallmark feature. A history of incomplete vaccinations is often present.
- **Retropharyngeal abscess:** Patients are usually younger than six years of age. They lack stridor, their voice is muffled, and drooling is often present.
- **Angioedema:** Can occur at any age. Onset is sudden, and the clinical features of stridor and facial edema are found. Respiration is laborious.
- **Peritonsillar abscess:** Occurs in children older than 10 years of age. Onset is gradual, with a history of a sore throat and tonsillitis. There is no stridor.
- **Laryngeal papilloma:** A chronic condition characterized by a hoarse voice; most commonly diagnosed in children three months to three years of age.

Diagnostic Workup

- **ABG:** It is essential to determine blood gas concentrations in order to indirectly assess ventilation and gaseous exchange in the lung.
- **CXR—PA and lateral:** It is noteworthy that the majority of foreign bodies are not visible on CXR PA plain films. Therefore, a normal radiograph cannot rule out an aspirated foreign body. However, when a foreign body obstructs the lower airway and causes air trapping, the expiratory film may sometimes reveal air trapping as a result of the ball-and-valve effect.
- **XR—neck, lateral:** May show narrowing of the trachea (steeple sign), extrinsic pressure, or a classic swollen glottis (thumbprint sign), which may assist with the specific diagnosis of croup or epiglottitis, respectively.
- **CBC with differential:** To rule out or rule in an underlying infective pathology.
- **Direct laryngoscopy:** Useful when differentials of laryngomalacia or laryngeal lesions such as papilloma are suspected.
- **Bronchoscopy:** Used as a diagnostic and therapeutic modality in cases of foreign body aspiration.

CASE 41
DOORWAY INFORMATION

Opening Scenario

Frank Emanuel, a 32-year-old male, comes to the office for a preemployment medical checkup as requested by his prospective employer.

Vital Signs

BP: 130/85 mm Hg

Temp: 98.3°F (36.8°C)

RR: 15/minute

HR: 70/minute, regular

Examinee Tasks

1. Take a focused history.

2. Perform a focused physical exam (do not perform rectal, genitourinary, or female breast exam).

3. Explain your clinical impression and workup plan to the patient.

4. Write the patient note after leaving the room.

Checklist/SP Sheet

Patient Description

Patient is a 32 yo M.

Notes for the SP

- Sit up on the bed.
- Hold the physical exam request form in your hand.

Challenging Questions to Ask

"Do you think they are going to give me the job?"

Sample Examinee Response

"Employers routinely request medical examinations to ensure that potential employees are fit for the job, as well as to determine if they have any medical conditions that may prove hazardous to others in the work environment. I will ask you few questions and perform a physical examination, and on the basis of what I find, I may or may not order further tests. Hopefully everything will be fine."

Examinee Checklist

Building the Doctor-Patient Relationship

Entrance

☐ Examinee knocked on the door before entering.

☐ Examinee introduced self by name.

☐ Examinee identified his/her role or position.

411

☐ Examinee correctly used patient's name.

☐ Examinee made eye contact with the SP.

Reflective Listening

☐ Examinee asked an open-ended question and actively listened to the response.

☐ Examinee asked the SP to list his/her concerns and listened to the response without interrupting.

☐ Examinee summarized the SP's concerns, often using the SP's own words.

Information Gathering

☐ Examinee elicited data efficiently and accurately.

☑ Question	Patient Response
☐ Medical complaints or problems	No.
☐ Chest pain (current and past)	No.
☐ Shortness of breath (current and past)	No.
☐ Palpitations or slow heart rate	No.
☐ Swelling in legs	No.
☐ Loss of consciousness/seizures	No.
☐ Headache	No.
☐ Weakness/numbness	No.
☐ Cough	Yes.
☐ Onset of cough	I've had this cough for years.
☐ Changes in the cough during the day	None.
☐ Progression of the cough	It is the same.
☐ Wheezing	No.
☐ Do you cough at night?	No.
☐ Sputum production	Yes.
☐ Amount of sputum	I am not sure. Around half a teaspoonful; stable.
☐ Color	White mucus.
☐ Odor	None.
☐ Blood in sputum	No.
☐ Fever/chills	None.
☐ Night sweats	No.
☐ Exposure to TB	No.
☐ Recent travel	I emigrated from Africa one month ago.
☐ Last PPD	I have never had this test.

☑ Question	Patient Response
☐ Joint pain or swelling	No.
☐ Nausea/vomiting	No.
☐ Abdominal pain	No.
☐ Diarrhea/constipation	No.
☐ Weight changes	No.
☐ Appetite changes	No.
☐ Change in stool color	No.
☐ Current medications	None.
☐ Past medical history	None.
☐ Past surgical history	None.
☐ Medical problems or diseases in your family	None.
☐ Vaccinations	My immunizations are up to date. I have my papers at home; I can fax them to you.
☐ Occupation	I used to work in a coal mine back home. I am applying for a new job.
☐ Alcohol use	No.
☐ Illicit drug use	No.
☐ Tobacco	Yes, one pack a day for 10 years.
☐ Sexual activity	Yes, with my wife.
☐ Drug allergies	None.

Connecting with the Patient

☐ Examinee recognized the SP's emotions and responded with PEARLS.

Physical Examination

☐ Examinee washed his/her hands.

☐ Examinee asked permission to start the exam.

☐ Examinee used respectful draping.

☐ Examinee did not repeat painful maneuvers.

☑ Exam Component	Maneuver
☐ Head and neck exam	Inspected mouth, throat; palpated lymph nodes
☐ CV exam	Auscultation
☐ Pulmonary exam	Auscultation, palpation, percussion
☐ Abdominal exam	Auscultation, palpation
☐ Extremities	Inspection
☐ Neurologic exam	Cranial nerves, motor exam, DTRs, gait

Closure

☐ Examinee discussed initial diagnostic impressions.

☐ Examinee discussed initial management plans:

    ☐ Follow-up tests.

☐ Examinee asked if the SP had any other questions or concerns.

Sample Closure

Mr. Emanuel, your physical examination is normal, but your cough may raise concern for some possible medical problems. We need to order some tests to make sure you are free of any serious medical conditions, and if we find anything, we will treat it right away. Since you just came here from Africa and you have never been tested for TB, we need to rule out pulmonary tuberculosis, not only because it is harmful to you but also because you may transmit it to your future coworkers. The other issue I want to talk to you about is your smoking. It puts you at increased risk of heart and lung disease, and I strongly urge you to quit. Do you have any questions?

Patient Note

History

_____
_____
_____
_____
_____
_____
_____
_____
_____

Physical Examination

_____
_____
_____
_____
_____
_____
_____
_____
_____
_____
_____

Differential Diagnosis

1. _____
2. _____
3. _____
4. _____
5. _____

Diagnostic Workup

1. _____
2. _____
3. _____
4. _____
5. _____

History

HPI: *32 yo M with no PMH presents for a preemployment medical examination. He has no medical complaints or problems. Nevertheless, he mentioned having a chronic cough for many years with no recent change in frequency or severity. The cough is productive of half a teaspoonful of white mucus with no blood. The patient denies any dyspnea, fever or chills, chest pain, or wheezing and has had no appetite or weight changes. The patient is an African immigrant who came to the United States 1 month ago and reports no TB exposure. He has never had a PPD test. However, he states that his immunizations are up to date, and he will be faxing us the report to review.*

ROS: *Negative except as above.*

Allergies: *NKDA.*

Medications: *None.*

PMH: *Per HPI.*

PSH: *None.*

SH: *1 PPD for 10 years, no EtOH, no illicit drugs. Sexually active with wife only.*

FH: *Noncontributory.*

Physical Examination

VS: *WNL.*

HEENT: *Mouth and pharynx WNL.*

Neck: *No JVD, no lymphadenopathy.*

Chest: *Clear breath sounds bilaterally; no rhonchi, rales, or wheezing; tactile fremitus normal.*

Heart: *RRR; normal S1/S2; no murmurs, rubs, or gallops.*

Abdomen: *Soft, nontender, nondistended, ⊕ BS, no hepatosplenomegaly.*

Extremities: *No clubbing, cyanosis, or edema.*

Neuro: *Cranial nerves: 2–12 intact. Motor: Strength 5/5 in all muscle groups. DTRs: Symmetric. Gait: Normal.*

Differential Diagnosis

1. *Pulmonary tuberculosis*
2. *COPD/chronic bronchitis*
3. *Pulmonary silicosis*
4. *Asthma*
5. *GERD*

Diagnostic Workup

1. *CXR—PA and lateral*
2. *PPD test*
3. *Sputum Gram stain, AFB smear, routine and mycobacterial sputum cultures*
4. *CBC*

CASE DISCUSSION

Differential Diagnosis

- **Pulmonary tuberculosis:** TB should be ruled out in this patient before he starts a new job, since he is an immigrant and has never been tested for TB.

- **COPD/chronic bronchitis:** This patient's chronic cough and sputum production might be due to COPD/chronic bronchitis secondary to his smoking history.

- **Pulmonary silicosis:** Considering his occupational history as a coal miner, this patient is at increased risk of pulmonary silicosis, which might predispose him to pulmonary tuberculosis.

- **Other possible causes:** There are other possible causes of the patient's chronic cough that may be benign, such as GERD and asthma.

Diagnostic Workup

- **CXR—PA and lateral:** A good initial test in evaluating chronic cough. It may demonstrate cavitary lesions in TB or may show nodular calcification in silicosis. It is usually normal in benign causes of cough, such as asthma or GERD.

- **PPD (tuberculin skin test):** Used as a screening tool to identify individuals who have been infected with *Mycobacterium tuberculosis*, but does not distinguish between active and latent infection.

- **Sputum Gram stain, AFB smear, routine and mycobacterial sputum cultures:** To identify a causative agent of possible infection.

- **CBC:** To identify leukocytosis in infection (nonspecific).

Opening Scenario

Oliver Jefferson, a 62-year-old male, comes to the office complaining of hoarseness.

Vital Signs

BP: 115/75 mm Hg

Temp: 98.0°F (36.7°C)

RR: 16/minute

HR: 74/minute, regular

Examinee Tasks

1. Take a focused history.

2. Perform a focused physical exam (do not perform rectal, genitourinary, or female breast exam).

3. Explain your clinical impression and workup plan to the patient.

4. Write the patient note after leaving the room.

Checklist/SP Sheet

Patient Description

Patient is a 62 yo M, married with 4 children.

Notes for the SP

Speak slowly, and in a hoarse voice.

Challenging Questions to Ask

"Am I going to get my voice back?"

Sample Examinee Response

"I see that you are very concerned about your voice, and I am concerned, too. I am not sure right now what has caused your hoarseness. We will need to do some tests to find out what the problem is and decide on your treatment."

Examinee Checklist

Building the Doctor-Patient Relationship

Entrance

☐ Examinee knocked on the door before entering.

☐ Examinee introduced self by name.

☐ Examinee identified his/her role or position.

☐ Examinee correctly used patient's name.

☐ Examinee made eye contact with the SP.

Reflective Listening

☐ Examinee asked an open-ended question and actively listened to the response.

☐ Examinee asked the SP to list his/her concerns and listened to the response without interrupting.

☐ Examinee summarized the SP's concerns, often using the SP's own words.

Information Gathering

☐ Examinee elicited data efficiently and accurately.

☑ Question	Patient Response
☐ Chief complaint	Hoarseness.
☐ Onset	Three months ago.
☐ Suddenly or gradually	It started gradually.
☐ Constant or intermittent	It is all the time.
☐ Progression	It is getting worse.
☐ Similar episodes in the past	No.
☐ Pain during speaking	No.
☐ Voice overuse recently	I was a teacher for 20 years, but now I am retired.
☐ Exposure to cold weather or dust	No.
☐ Recent upper infection (eg, sore throat, runny nose)	I had the flu four weeks ago.
☐ Alleviating factors	Nothing.
☐ Exacerbating factors	Nothing.
☐ Heartburn	Yes, I have heartburn all the time, but I don't take any medication for it.
☐ History of CVA or TIA	No.
☐ Weight changes	I lost 10 pounds during the past three months.
☐ Appetite changes	I have a poor appetite.
☐ Swollen glands or lymph nodes	Yes, I feel like there's a lump in my throat.
☐ Fever, night sweats	I feel hot a little bit, but I didn't measure my temperature and I don't have chills or night sweats.
☐ Fatigue	Yes, I don't have the same energy as before.
☐ GI symptom (eg, N/V, constipation)	No.
☐ Cardiac symptoms (eg, palpitation)	No.
☐ Pulmonary symptoms (eg, SOB, hemoptysis, cough)	No.
☐ Past medical history	High cholesterol, but I don't take any medication for it.
☐ Past surgical history	None.

☑ Question	Patient Response
☐ Diet	The usual. No change in my diet. Just eating less.
☐ Current medications	None.
☐ Family history	My mother had thyroid disease and my father had lung cancer.
☐ Occupation	Retired teacher.
☐ Alcohol use	Three glasses of wine every day.
☐ CAGE questionnaire	0/4.
☐ Tobacco	Yes, I have been smoking one pack a day for the past 30 years.
☐ Illicit drug use	None.
☐ Drug allergies	None.

Connecting with the Patient

☐ Examinee recognized the SP's emotions and responded with PEARLS.

Physical Examination

☐ Examinee washed his/her hands.

☐ Examinee asked permission to start the exam.

☐ Examinee used respectful draping.

☐ Examinee did not repeat painful maneuvers.

☑ Exam Component	Maneuver
☐ HEENT	Inspected conjunctivae, mouth and throat, lymph nodes; examined thyroid gland
☐ CV exam	Auscultation
☐ Pulmonary exam	Auscultation
☐ Abdominal exam	Auscultation, palpation, percussion
☐ Extremities	Inspection, DTRs

Closure

☐ Examinee discussed initial diagnostic impressions.

☐ Examinee discussed initial management plans:

    ☐ Follow-up tests.

☐ Examinee asked if the SP had any other questions or concerns.

Sample Closure

Mr. Jefferson, there are a few things that could be causing your hoarseness, such as an infection or a growth caused by either a benign polyp or a cancer. To find out, I need to do a laryngoscopy, which is a procedure to view the inside of your throat, and a CT scan of your neck. These tests will likely reveal the underlying problem. Since cigarette smoking is dangerous to your health, I advise you to quit smoking; we have many ways to help you if you are interested. I also recommend that you stop drinking, as alcohol and smoking are associated with laryngeal cancer. Do you have any questions for me?

Patient Note

History

_____
_____
_____
_____
_____
_____
_____
_____
_____

Physical Examination

_____
_____
_____
_____
_____
_____
_____
_____
_____
_____
_____

Differential Diagnosis

1. _____
2. _____
3. _____
4. _____
5. _____

Diagnostic Workup

1. _____
2. _____
3. _____
4. _____
5. _____

Patient Note

History

HPI: *62 yo M c/o hoarseness × 3 months.*

- *Painless, gradually getting worse.*
- *Mild fever, fatigue, and "lump in my throat."*
- *Poor appetite; lost 10 lb in 3 months.*
- *History of flu 4 weeks ago.*

ROS: *Negative, except as above.*

Allergies: *None.*

Medications: *None.*

PMH: *High cholesterol*

PSH: *None.*

SH: *Drinks 3 glasses wine/day/30 years; smoked 30 pack/year; CAGE (0/4). History of voice overuse (worked as a teacher for 20 years).*

FH: *Mother (hypothyroid), father (lung cancer).*

Physical Examination

Patient is in no acute distress.

NAD, VS: *WNL.*

HEENT: *Nose, mouth, and pharynx WNL.*

Neck: *WNL.*

Chest: *Nontender, bilateral clear BS.*

Heart: *PMI not displaced, regular rhythm, no M or rubs.*

ABD: *⊕ BS, nondistended, no organomegaly.*

Extremities: *DTRs are equal.*

Differential Diagnosis

1. *Laryngeal cancer*
2. *Vocal cord polyps/nodules*
3. *Laryngitis*
4. *Hypothyroidism*
5. *Mitral valve stenosis*

Diagnostic Workup

1. *CBC*
2. *Laryngoscopy*
3. *TSH*
4. *CT—chest and neck*
5. *Cardiac echocardiography*

CASE DISCUSSION

Differential Diagnosis

- **Laryngeal cancer:** This is the most likely diagnosis given the constitutional symptoms and long period of smoking and drinking.

- **Laryngitis:** This is a common condition of the larynx and can be acute or chronic. The acute form is most likely viral and is self-limited. The common causes of the chronic form are cigarette smoke, polluted air, and GERD. This patient has long history of untreated GERD so it could be a sign of chronic laryngitis.

- **Vocal cord polyps/nodules:** Benign vocal fold lesions are sometimes related to overuse of the voice and can be identified easily by laryngoscopy. However, this diagnosis does not explain the constitutional symptoms in this patient.

- **Hypothyroidism:** Hoarseness is one of the symptoms of hypothyroidism. Hypothyroidism can explain some of the patient's complaints, such as loss of appetite and fatigue, but does not explain all his symptoms.

- **Mitral valve stenosis (MVS):** Hoarseness in MVS is due to enlargement of the left atrium and compression of the recurrent laryngeal nerve. MVS is more common in women and usually presents with a history of rheumatoid fever. Other symptoms of MVS include palpitation and easy fatigue. The physical exam findings include diastolic murmur and tachycardia.

Diagnostic Workup

- **CBC:** Anemia can be associated with hypothyroidism, and elevated white blood cell count is common in infections.

- **TSH:** To diagnose thyroid disease.

- **Cardiac echocardiography:** Essential in diagnosing cardiac valvular diseases.

- **CT—chest and neck:** Can identify the location and extent of most laryngeal lesions.

- **Laryngoscopy:** The gold standard for evaluating the larynx. It allows direct visualization of the vocal cords. It also allows biopsy of suspicious lesions for pathologic evaluation.

Opening Scenario

Carol Holland, a 67-year-old female, comes to the office complaining of neck pain.

Vital Signs

BP: 115/75 mm Hg

Temp: 98.0°F (36.7°C)

RR: 16/minute

HR: 74/minute, regular

Examinee Tasks

1. Take a focused history.

2. Perform a focused physical exam (do not perform rectal, genitourinary, or female breast exam).

3. Explain your clinical impression and workup plan to the patient.

4. Write the patient note after leaving the room.

Checklist/SP Sheet

Patient Description

Patient is a 67 yo F who lives with her husband.

Notes for the SP

- Sit still with your back slightly hunched and head straight ahead; avoid turning your neck and instead just move your eyes to make eye contact with the examinee.

- Show pain when moving your neck and when the examinee palpates your neck.

- Pretend to have numbness in the back of your left forearm.

Challenging Questions to Ask

"I'm supposed to visit my sister in Florida in three days. Will I still be able to go?"

Sample Examinee Response

"Before I am comfortable with you traveling, I want to make sure you don't have a serious injury, like a broken bone or a nerve compression in your spine. I would like to see the results of some tests first to make sure you'll be safe."

Examinee Checklist

Building the Doctor-Patient Relationship

Entrance

☐ Examinee knocked on the door before entering.

☐ Examinee introduced self by name.

☐ Examinee identified his/her role or position.

☐ Examinee correctly used patient's name.

☐ Examinee made eye contact with the SP.

Reflective Listening

☐ Examinee asked an open-ended question and actively listened to the response.

☐ Examinee asked the SP to list his/her concerns and listened to the response without interrupting.

☐ Examinee summarized the SP's concerns, often using the SP's own words.

Information Gathering

☐ Examinee elicited data efficiently and accurately.

☑ Question	Patient Response
☐ Chief complaint	Pain in my neck.
☐ Onset	Two days ago.
☐ Associated/precipitating events	Someone called my name and I turned my head to the left to look—since then it hurts to move.
☐ Progression	It has stayed the same.
☐ Severity on a scale	2/10 at rest, 8/10 with motion.
☐ Location	The whole neck, but worst on the left.
☐ Radiation	It radiates down my left arm.
☐ Quality	Sharp.
☐ Alleviating factors	Holding my head still.
☐ Exacerbating factors	Turning my head in either direction.
☐ Weakness/numbness	No weakness, but my left arm tingles.
☐ Recent trauma	No.
☐ Recent heavy lifting	No.
☐ History of neck pain/trauma	I have thrown my neck out before, but not like this.
☐ Trouble breathing	No.
☐ Fever, night sweats, weight loss	I've lost about 10 pounds in the past six months, and my appetite has decreased.
☐ Headaches, dizziness, photophobia, nausea, vomiting	No.
☐ Past medical history	None.
☐ Past surgical history	None.
☐ Health maintenance	I am up to date on mammograms and had a normal colonoscopy last year. I was found to have osteopenia at my last osteoporosis screening.

☑ Question	Patient Response
☐ Current medications	I take calcium and vitamin D supplements.
☐ Family history	My mother had osteoporosis and my father had a heart attack at 68.
☐ Occupation	Retired magazine editor.
☐ Travel history, sick contact	No.
☐ Alcohol use	Just a glass of wine with dinner on weekends.
☐ Illicit drug use	Never.
☐ Tobacco	Never.
☐ Drug allergies	None.

Connecting with the Patient

☐ Examinee recognized the SP's emotions and responded with PEARLS.

Physical Examination

☐ Examinee washed his/her hands.

☐ Examinee asked permission to start the exam.

☐ Examinee used respectful draping.

☐ Examinee did not repeat painful maneuvers.

☑ Exam Component	Maneuver
☐ Neck exam	Inspection, palpation, stiffness, range of motion, Lhermitte sign, Spurling test
☐ Extremities	Inspection, palpation of peripheral pulses, range of motion
☐ Neurologic exam	Motor, DTRs, sensory exam, Kernig and Brudzinski signs

Closure

☐ Examinee discussed initial diagnostic impressions.

☐ Examinee discussed initial management plans:

    ☐ Follow-up tests.

☐ Examinee asked if the SP had any other questions or concerns.

Sample Closure

Mrs. Holland, given your symptoms, I am concerned that you may have a pinched nerve in your neck. Since you have a history of low bone density, I want to make sure your symptoms weren't caused by a fracture. And, although it's unlikely, certain cancers may spread to the neck and spine and cause similar symptoms. I want to run some tests to rule out this possibility. I would like to start by getting an x-ray of your neck. Do you have any other questions for me?

Patient Note

History

Physical Examination

Differential Diagnosis

1.
2.
3.
4.
5.

Diagnostic Workup

1.
2.
3.
4.
5.

Patient Note

History

HPI: *67 yo F with 2 days of neck pain and left upper extremity numbness.*

- *Started after quick rotation to the left.*
- *Sharp pain 2/10 at rest, 8/10 with motion.*
- *Associated left arm numbness. Denies weakness.*
- *10-lb weight loss in past 6 months attributed to poor appetite.*
- *No recent trauma or heavy lifting.*
- *No dyspnea, fevers, night sweats.*
- *Screenings up to date.*

ROS: *Negative except as above.*

Allergies: *NKDA.*

Medications: *Calcium and vitamin D supplements.*

PMH: *Osteopenia on last DEXA.*

PSH: *None.*

SH: *Social alcohol use, no tobacco or drugs. Retired magazine editor.*

FH: *Mother with osteoporosis, father with MI at 68.*

Physical Examination

Patient sitting rigid and still, avoiding moving neck.

Neck: *No scars or deformities, limited ROM 2/2 pain. ⊕ Tenderness to palpation on cervical spinous processes. ⊖ Lhermitte and Spurling tests.*

Extremities: *No scars or deformities, brachial and radial pulses full. Full range of motion.*

Neuro: *Motor: Strength 5/5 throughout upper extremities. DTRs: 2+ symmetric, ⊖ Babinski bilaterally. Sensation: Loss of pinprick sensation noted on dorsum of left hand and posterior left arm and forearm—all other sensation normal.*

Differential Diagnosis

1. *Disk herniation*
2. *Cervical fracture*
3. *Neck muscle strain*
4. *Osteoarthritis*
5. *Cervical spondylosis*
6. *Metastatic cancer*
7. *Multiple myeloma*

Diagnostic Workup

1. *XR—C-spine*
2. *MRI—C-spine*
3. *Nerve conduction studies*
4. *CBC, calcium, BUN/Cr*
5. *Serum and urine protein electrophoresis*

CASE DISCUSSION

Differential Diagnosis

- **Disk herniation:** Much like in other areas of the spine, pain at the site of compression with the addition of signs of nerve compression suggests radiculopathy caused by a disk herniation. The most common areas for compression in the cervical spine are the lower vertebrae where the diameter of the vertebrae narrows.

- **Cervical fracture:** Cervical fractures are dangerous, acute findings that can compromise innervation to the diaphragm if they interrupt the phrenic nerve. The exam would presumably show tenderness to palpation, but it is critical to include this in the differential given the patient's osteopenic history.

- **Neck muscle strain:** Many people experience neck strains caused by quick turning of the head. This patient's radiculopathy suggests this is more than a simple strain.

- **Osteoarthritis:** Degenerative disease of the spine could cause the findings seen by the same routes as herniation and fracture—compression of the nerves.

- **Cervical spondylosis:** A spondylosis would be caused by the same channels as degenerative disk disease.

- **Metastatic cancer:** Cancers like breast and lung can metastasize to the bone. A possible spine lesion and weight loss in an older woman should raise concern for metastatic disease.

- **Multiple myeloma:** Although a rarer malignancy, multiple myeloma is a cause of spinal lesions in both men and women. Associated findings may include symptoms of anemia, renal failure, and hypercalcemia, in addition to the typical constitutional symptoms commonly found in malignancy.

Diagnostic Workup

- **XR—C-spine:** The first test to order in pain concerning for fracture or radiculopathy. Check for space narrowing or fractures.

- **MRI—C-spine:** The most sensitive method to diagnose disk, spine, and spinal cord pathology. Note that because of high sensitivity, MRI may detect clinically insignificant abnormalities.

- **Nerve conduction studies:** Nerve stimulation will determine if the patient's loss of sensation is due to a conduction issue in the peripheral nerve. Although they are specific, nerve conduction studies are not necessarily sensitive for cervical pathology.

- **CBC, calcium, BUN/Cr:** To detect anemia, hypercalcemia, and renal failure, all of which may be clues to underlying multiple myeloma.

- **Serum and urine protein electrophoresis:** To detect a monoclonal paraprotein in myeloma.

Opening Scenario

The mother of Michaela Weber, an 11-month-old female child, comes to the emergency department after her daughter has a seizure.

Examinee Tasks

1. Take a focused history.

2. Explain your clinical impression and workup plan to the mother.

3. Write the patient note after leaving the room.

Checklist/SP Sheet

Patient Description

The patient's mother offers the history; she is a good historian.

Notes for the SP

Express anxiety about your daughter's condition.

Challenging Questions to Ask

"Is my child going to have permanent brain damage from this?"

Sample Examinee Response

"The most likely explanation for your daughter's seizure is her fever, in which case there should be no permanent damage. There are some causes of seizures that are more serious, though. We will run all the necessary tests to make sure one of those is not the cause."

Examinee Checklist

Building the Doctor-Patient Relationship

Entrance

☐ Examinee knocked on the door before entering.

☐ Examinee introduced self by name.

☐ Examinee identified his/her role or position.

☐ Examinee correctly used patient's name.

☐ Examinee made eye contact with the SP.

Reflective Listening

☐ Examinee asked an open-ended question and actively listened to the response.

☐ Examinee asked the SP to list his/her concerns and listened to the response without interrupting.

☐ Examinee summarized the SP's concerns, often using the SP's own words.

Information Gathering

☐ Examinee elicited data efficiently and accurately.

☑ **Question**	**Patient Response**
☐ Chief complaint	My child had a seizure.
☐ Onset	This morning at 11 A.M.
☐ Description of event	We were laying her down for her nap and her whole body just started shaking.
☐ Duration	It lasted about a minute total.
☐ Postictal symptoms	She seemed sleepy afterward.
☐ Tongue/head trauma	No.
☐ Has this happened before?	No.
☐ Whole-body shaking	Yes.
☐ Family history of seizures	None.
☐ Recent illness	Yes, she has had a temperature and runny nose the past two days.
☐ Fevers/chills	Her temperature was 102.9°F last night; she hasn't had any chills.
☐ Rash	No.
☐ Medication for fever	I gave her some Children's Tylenol last night—it helped a little.
☐ Ear tugging	No.
☐ Nausea/vomiting	No.
☐ Change in bowel habits or in stool color or consistency	No.
☐ Change in urinary habits or in urine smell or color; change in number of wet diapers	Fewer wet diapers than usual.
☐ Appetite changes	She has had Pedialyte and some breast milk but not much else.
☐ Appearance/demeanor (lethargic, irritated, playful, etc)?	She has been more fussy the past couple days, but consolable.
☐ Ill contacts	No.
☐ Day care center	No.
☐ Home environment	She lives with me, my husband, and her three-year-old brother.
☐ Vaccinations	Up to date.
☐ Last checkup	Two months ago for nine-month checkup.
☐ Birth history	38-week vaginal delivery with no complications.
☐ Weight, height, and language development	Normal.
☐ Eating habits	She is breast-fed and eats some table food but hasn't been eating the table food the past couple days. She takes iron supplements that our pediatrician gave us.
☐ Sleeping habits	She has not slept well the past three nights.

☑ Question	Patient Response
☐ Current medications	Just the Tylenol.
☐ Past medical history	None.
☐ Past surgical history	None.
☐ Drug allergies	No.

Connecting with the Patient

☐ Examinee recognized the SP's emotions and responded with PEARLS.

Physical Examination

None.

Closure

☐ Examinee discussed initial diagnostic impressions.

☐ Examinee discussed initial management plans:

   ☐ Follow-up tests.

☐ Examinee asked if the SP had any other questions or concerns.

Sample Closure

Mrs. Weber, it sounds like your child has indeed had a seizure. The most likely cause is her high fevers; seizures caused by fevers happen in many young children. However, because there are many types of seizures, I would like to examine your child and also do some tests to make sure that the seizures are not being caused by something more serious, like meningitis. Do you have any questions for me?

Patient Note

History

Physical Examination

Differential Diagnosis

1. _____
2. _____
3. _____
4. _____
5. _____

Diagnostic Workup

1. _____
2. _____
3. _____
4. _____
5. _____

Patient Note

History

HPI: *The source of information is the patient's mother. Patient is an 11-month-old F with a tonic-clonic seizure.*

- *Witnessed this AM by parents, lasted approx. 1 min.*
- *No tongue or body trauma.*
- *Postictal drowsiness noted.*
- *No history of prior seizures.*
- *Patient has rhinorrhea for past 2 days, fevers to 102.9°F w/decreased PO intake, difficulty sleeping, and fewer wet diapers.*
- *No rash, nausea/vomiting, lethargy, or inconsolability.*
- *No sick contacts.*

ROS: *Negative except as above.*

Allergies: *NKDA.*

Medications: *Tylenol.*

PMH: *None.*

Birth history: *Term uncomplicated vaginal delivery.*

Dietary history: *Breast-feeding, table foods, and supplemental vitamins.*

Immunization history: *Up to date.*

Developmental history: *Last checkup was 2 months ago and showed normal weight, height, and development.*

Physical Examination

None.

Differential Diagnosis

1. *Simple febrile seizure*
2. *Meningitis*
3. *Hyponatremia*
4. *UTI*
5. *Occult bacteremia*

Diagnostic Workup

1. *Lumbar puncture*
2. *CBC, electrolytes*
3. *Blood culture, UA, and urine culture*
4. *CT—head*
5. *EEG*

CASE DISCUSSION

Differential Diagnosis

- **Simple febrile seizure:** The most common cause of an isolated seizure in a child with a common febrile illness is a febrile seizure. These tend to be familial and may recur with subsequent febrile illnesses but will disappear before adulthood. They do not require treatment and will not cause permanent neurologic damage.

- **Meningitis:** In children younger than 1 year of age, meningitis findings can often be limited to fever and clinical symptoms. The infant might be irritable but is usually easily consolable. Viral meningitis is common in infants and could be likely in this patient considering the baby's poor appetite, high fever, and decreased urine output. A seizure suggests neurologic involvement, and the most important cause to rule out is meningitis.

- **Hyponatremia:** Hyponatremia from various causes can result in pediatric seizures—the classic case occurs when a poor family waters down their infant's formula. There are also congenital causes of hyponatremia, such as congenital adrenal hyperplasia. The occurrence in the setting of fever makes this less likely than the infectious causes.

- **UTI:** Decreased urine output is not necessarily caused by a UTI in this patient. However, given the patient's high fever and gender, a UTI with subsequent pyelonephritis or bacteremia is a possibility.

- **Occult bacteremia:** This child has a fever > 102°F (38.9°C) and no clear source of infection. Bacteremia and sepsis may present in this manner in children younger than 1 year of age; the incidence is highest in neonates and decreases with age.

Diagnostic Workup

- **Lumbar puncture (LP):** A fever with seizures may be benign or it may suggest meningitis. An LP allows CSF analysis of cell count and differentials, glucose, protein, Gram stain, culture, viral cultures and PCR, and opening pressure.

- **CBC, electrolytes, glucose:** To test for hyponatremia caused by any source. The potassium and glucose levels help in assessing adrenal function. A WBC count > 15,000/μL might be suggestive of occult bacteremia.

- **Blood culture, UA, and urine culture:** These tests constitute the "septic" or occult bacteremia workup in children with unexplained high fever. UTI may be occult and must be investigated.

- **CT—head:** Used mainly to rule out brain abscess, encephalitis, or hemorrhage.

- **Electroencephalogram (EEG):** Used to identify epileptiform activity, although a single febrile seizure might not warrant an EEG.

Top-Rated Review Resources

HOW TO USE THE DATABASE

This section is a database of recommended clinical science review books, sample examination books, and commercial review courses marketed to medical students studying for the USMLE Step 2 CS. For each book, we list the **Title** of the book, the **First Author** (or editor), the **Current Publisher**, the **Copyright Year**, the **Edition**, the **Number of Pages**, the **ISBN Code**, the **Approximate List Price**, and the **Format** of the book. Most entries also include **Summary Comments** that describe their style and utility for studying. Finally, each book receives a **Rating.**

The rating scale is composed of six letter grades that reflect the detailed student evaluations. Each book receives one of the following ratings:

A+	Excellent for boards review.
A A–	Very good for boards review; choose among the group.
B+ B B–	Good, but use only after exhausting better sources.

The **Rating** is meant to reflect the overall usefulness of the book in preparing for the USMLE Step 2 CS examination. This is based on a number of factors, including the following:

- The cost of the book
- The readability of the text
- The appropriateness and accuracy of the book
- The quality and number of sample questions
- The quality of written answers to sample questions
- The quality and appropriateness of the illustrations (eg, graphs, diagrams, photographs)
- The length of the text (longer is not necessarily better)
- The quality and number of other books available in the same discipline
- The importance of the discipline on the USMLE Step 2 CS examination

Please note that **the rating does not reflect the quality of the book for purposes other than reviewing for the USMLE Step 2 CS examination.** Many books with low ratings are well written and informative but are not ideal for boards preparation. We have also avoided listing or commenting on the wide variety of general textbooks available in the clinical sciences.

Evaluations are based on the cumulative results of formal and informal surveys of hundreds of medical students from medical schools across the country. The summary comments and overall ratings represent a consensus opinion, but there may have been a large range of opinions or limited student feedback on any particular book.

Please note that the data listed are subject to change because:

- Publishers' prices change frequently.
- Individual bookstores often charge an additional markup.
- New editions come out frequently, and the quality of updating varies.
- The same book may be reissued through another publisher.

We actively encourage medical students and faculty to submit their opinions and ratings of these clinical science review books so that we may update our database (see "How to Contribute," p. xvii). In addition, we ask that publishers and authors submit review copies of clinical science review books, including new editions and books not included in our database, for evaluation. We also solicit reviews of new books or suggestions for alternate modes of study that may be useful in preparing for the examination, such as flash cards, computer-based tutorials, commercial review courses, and Internet Web sites.

Disclaimer/Conflict of Interest Statement

No material in this book, including the ratings, reflects the opinion or influence of the publisher. All errors and omissions will gladly be corrected if brought to the attention of the authors through the publisher.

A

USMLE Step 2 CS: Complex Cases: 35 Cases You Are Likely to See on the Exam

BROTTMAN

$40.00   Review

Kaplan, 2009, 312 pages, 2nd edition, ISBN 9781607140634

A thorough review book that is not presented in workbook format.

Pros: Features a lengthy section on exam basics, including high-yield tips on the physical exam, as well as 35 cases providing doorway information, suggested checklists for the history and physical exam, and a note with a differential diagnosis and follow-up exam. A discussion of history taking, the physical exam, and the patient note is included with each case. Also includes 96 flash cards featuring the chief complaint/patient scenario on one side and the differential/workup on the other. Additional online clinical cases are available with purchase of the book. International Medical Graduates (IMGs) may find this book especially helpful since it offers great tips and common phraseology for test takers not familiar with clinical exams.

Cons: If you need a workbook-style text, this is not the one for you.

Summary: A good text for examinees who are willing to put in the time but don't need the redundancy of a workbook-style text. May be especially useful for IMGs who need help with English phrases and wording.

A–

USMLE Step 2 Clinical Skills Triage

SCHWECHTEN

$39.95   Review

Oxford University Press, 2010, 288 pages, 1st edition, ISBN 9780195398236

An organized case-by-case presentation of patient encounters.

Pros: Has 40 cases that simulate actual examination scenarios covering the most common complaints and diagnoses. Information is organized linearly into "Symptoms," "Diagnosis," and "Treatment" sections and then summarized by "Take Home Points." Includes integrated tables and figures plus 100 full-color pictures that help to clarify and organize information.

Cons: Some may find that cases are not sufficiently detailed. The format of the practice cases does not facilitate practice with a partner.

Summary: A succinct but thorough review of the most common clinical conditions.

B+

Core Concepts for USMLE Step 2 CS: A focused and goal-oriented approach

SHARMA

$44.95   Review

Createspace, 2010, 380 pages, 1st edition, ISBN 97814053608043

A thorough text that reviews core clinical concepts in the context of the CS exam.

Pros: Incorporates solid clinical skills for evaluating a patient into preparation for the Step 2 CS exam. It thoroughly explains expectations of the standardized patients and examiners so test-takers are better prepared, which is especially helpful for IMGs. Also includes specific sections of the exam such as ethical dilemmas, counseling, and phone interviews.

Cons: If you are not used to the integrated format of the text, you may not find this text appropriate. The format of the practice cases makes it challenging to practice with a partner, especially one with no medical background.

Summary: A clear and thorough concept-oriented review book useful for all Step 2 CS test-takers.

B+

NMS Review for the USMLE Clinical Skills Exam
ARIAS

$44.95   Review

Lippincott Williams & Wilkins, 2007, 296 pages, 2nd edition, ISBN 9780781766937

A sleek review book presented in a non-workbook format.

Pros: Provides extensive coverage of physical exam techniques and signs and symptoms and includes a wealth of basic science information. Chapters devoted to the physical exam and note writing cover OB/GYN, neurology, psychology, pediatrics, and trauma medicine. Also features 91 review cases covering internal medicine and family practice, surgery and orthopedics, OB/GYN, the nervous system, pediatric and phone medicine, and trauma medicine.

Cons: Some of the material may not be sufficiently high yield for the Step 2 CS. Cases are compressed into a one-page format with a written patient note, a differential diagnosis, a diagnostic workup plan, and a short paragraph on clinical correlation. Some may find that there are not enough specific details about what is needed for the exam.

Summary: A great book for both Step 2 CS and Step 2 CK preparation that provides a large number of very concise cases. However, the text does not provide a step-by-step approach to the patient exam or patient note.

B+

The Ultimate Guide and Review for the USMLE Step 2 Clinical Skills Exam
SWARTZ

$39.95   Review

Saunders, 2006, 424 pages, 1st edition, ISBN 9781416037279

A large workbook-style review text.

Pros: Easy to read and printed in a large font. Includes a detailed chapter outlining the basics of the exam. Approximately 20 pages are devoted to communication skills, and an additional 10 pages are devoted to a guide to US culture.

Cons: Because the workbook format takes up a significant amount of space, only 30 review cases are provided.

Summary: A text that may be best suited to examinees who seek practice documenting checklists and patient notes. The lengthy sections on communication skills and US culture make it more suitable for IMGs. Those who seek a quick review might be better served by a more concise text.

B | ***CS Checklists: Portable Review for the USMLE Step 2 CS*** | ***$34.95*** Review

ROONEY

McGraw-Hill, 2007, 250 pages, 2nd edition, ISBN 9780071488235

A pocket-sized text presented in workbook format.

Pros: Provides detailed descriptions of the components of a complete health history, physical exam, and patient note write-up, presented in bullet-point format. Also features 55 cases organized by chief complaint along with a brief paragraph on history. A patient history checklist, a physical exam checklist, and physical exam findings are also provided. One-page "answers" listed at the end of the book include a differential diagnosis, an appropriate workup, and a brief paragraph on clinical correlation. Also features a case index with diagnoses and corresponding page numbers.

Cons: Offers limited general information on the physical exam and on how to perform and interpret exam findings. The formatting may be somewhat confusing.

Summary: A concise text that contains all the information needed for Step 2 CS review. Cases are streamlined to allow for practice without taking up copious amounts of space. However, may not be as accurate and detailed as more thorough sources. Overall, a high-yield book that may require additional texts if more in-depth information is needed on the physical exam.

B | ***Mastering the USMLE Step 2 CS*** | ***$45.95*** Review

RETEGUIZ

McGraw-Hill Medical, 2004, 420 pages, 3rd edition, ISBN 9780071443340

A large workbook-style text.

Pros: Easy to read, with a large font and a smattering of cartoon-like illustrations. Offers a detailed general discussion of the Step 2 CS exam. Also features 50 workbook-style cases covering a wide range of topics, with each case including doorway information, a standardized patient checklist, a patient note, a differential diagnosis, and a diagnostic workup. Learning objectives with "pearls" on history taking, the physical exam, and the patient note are also provided. High-yield chapters cover the top 10 reasons for failure and a quick review with commonly tested scenarios.

Cons: A large book with a lot of repetition, especially for examinees who don't need a workbook format. Some reviewers find that it does not cover all the key questions for patient interviews. Also, limited information is provided on physical exam techniques. This review is also more than seven years old and therefore may not fully reflect the most current clinical practice.

Summary: A highly comprehensive text that may be too detailed for quick review. May need more current supplemental material.

B

Blueprints USMLE Step 2 CS   ***$27.95***   Review
WAHL

Lippincott Williams & Wilkins, 2004, 160 pages, 1st edition, ISBN 9781405104388

A pocket-sized text presented in workbook format.

Pros: A highly concise review book that still allows space for practice. Makes good use of standard mnemonics to guide the history.

Cons: Printed in a small font. Provides sufficient but cursory information on the basics of the Step 2 CS exam. Includes only 20 cases, with no accompanying master list or categories. No clinical correlation is provided for the cases, and the discussion of physical exam techniques is limited. This review is also more than seven years old and therefore may not fully reflect the most current clinical practice.

Summary: A high-yield text that is ideal for examinees who are comfortable with the Step 2 CS format and seek only a quick review. May not be suitable for IMGs or for those who are less familiar with the exam. May need more current supplemental material.

USEFUL WEB SITES

The following is a collection of online resources and Web sites that may also help you prepare for the Step 2 CS exam:

Fee Subscription Resources:

http://www.usmleworld.com
http://www.kaptest.com/Medical-Licensing/Step2cs.html
http://usmlecsprep.com

Free Resources:

http://www.conntutorials.com

► **NOTES**

APPENDIX

ACRONYMS AND ABBREVIATIONS

Abbreviation	Meaning
AAMC	Association of American Medical Colleges
ABG	arterial blood gas
ACE	angiotensin-converting enzyme
ACh	acetylcholine
ACTH	adrenocorticotropic hormone
ADH	antidiuretic hormone
ADHD	attention-deficit hyperactivity disorder
ADLs	activities of daily living
AFB	acid-fast bacillus
AFP	α-fetoprotein
AIDS	acquired immunodeficiency syndrome
ALT	alanine aminotransferase
ANA	antinuclear antibody
AP	anteroposterior
AST	aspartate aminotransferase
AXR	abdominal x-ray
BP	blood pressure
BPH	benign prostatic hypertrophy
BPPV	benign paroxysmal positional vertigo
BS	bowel sounds
BUN	blood urea nitrogen
CABG	coronary artery bypass graft
C-ANCA	cytoplasmic antineutrophil cytoplasmic antibody
CBC	complete blood count
CC	chief complaint
CD	cluster of differentiation
CEA	carcinoembryonic antigen
CHF	congestive heart failure
CIS	communication/interpersonal skills [CSE score]
CMV	cytomegalovirus
CN	cranial nerve
CNS	central nervous system
c/o	complains of
COPD	chronic obstructive pulmonary disease
CPK	creatine phosphokinase
CPK-MB	creatine phosphokinase, MB fraction
Cr	creatinine

Abbreviation	Meaning
CREST	calcinosis, Raynaud's phenomenon, esophageal dysmotility, sclerodactyly, telangiectasia [syndrome]
CRP	C-reactive protein
CS	Clinical Skills
CSA	Clinical Skills Assessment
CSEC	Clinical Skills Evaluation Collaboration [center]
CSF	cerebrospinal fluid
CT	computed tomography
CV	cardiovascular
CVA	costovertebral angle, cerebrovascular accident
CXR	chest x-ray
D&C	dilatation and curettage
DDAVP	1-deamino (8-d-arginine) vasopressin
DEXA	dual-energy x-ray absorptiometry
DFA	direct fluorescent antibody [test]
DG	data gathering [CSE score]
DHEAS	dehydroepiandrosterone sulfate
DI	diabetes insipidus
DIC	disseminated intravascular coagulation
DM	diabetes mellitus
DNA	deoxyribonucleic acid
dsDNA	double-stranded deoxyribonucleic acid
DTR	deep tendon reflex
DVT	deep venous thrombosis
EBNA	Epstein-Barr nuclear antigen
EBV	Epstein-Barr virus
ECFMG	Educational Commission for Foreign Medical Graduates
ECG	electrocardiogram
ED	erectile dysfunction, emergency department
EEG	electroencephalogram
EMG	electromyogram
ENT	ear, nose, and throat
EOMI	extraocular movements intact

Abbreviation	Meaning
ERCP	endoscopic retrograde cholangiopancreatography
ESR	erythrocyte sedimentation rate
ET	essential tremor
EtOH	ethyl alcohol
FH	family history
FSH	follicle-stimulating hormone
FT_4	free thyroxine
GBS	group B *Streptococcus*
GC	gonorrhea and *Chlamydia*
GERD	gastroesophageal reflux disease
GI	gastrointestinal
HbA_{1c}	hemoglobin A_{1c}
HBsAg	hepatitis B surface antigen
HBV	hepatitis B virus
hCG	human chorionic gonadotropin
HCTZ	hydrochlorothiazide
HEENT	head, eyes, ears, nose, and throat
5-HIAA	5-hydroxyindoleacetic acid
HIDA	hepatobiliary iminodiacetic acid [scan]
HIV	human immunodeficiency virus
HPI	history of present illness
HR	heart rate
HRT	hormone replacement therapy
HSV	herpes simplex virus
IADLs	instrumental activities of daily living
ICE	integrated clinical encounter [CSE score]
Ig	immunoglobulin
IMED	International Medical Education Directory
IMG	international medical graduate
IPS	interpersonal skills [CSE score]
IV	intravenous
IVDU	intravenous drug use
IVP	intravenous pyelography
IWA	Interactive Web Application
JVD	jugular venous distention
KOH	potassium hydroxide
LDH	lactose dehydrogenase
LH	luteinizing hormone
LLQ	left lower quadrant
LMP	last menstrual period
LOC	loss of consciousness
LP	lumbar puncture
LUQ	left upper quadrant
LVH	left ventricular hypertrophy
MCP	metacarpophalangeal [joint]
MDI	metered-dose inhaler
MDMA	methylenedioxymethamphetamine ("ecstasy")
MI	myocardial infarction
MRA	magnetic resonance angiography
MRCP	magnetic resonance cholangiopancreatography
MRI	magnetic resonance imaging

Abbreviation	Meaning
MS	multiple sclerosis
MTP	metatarsophalangeal [joint]
MVA	motor vehicle accident
NBME	National Board of Medical Examiners
NC/AT	normocephalic/atraumatic
NKDA	no known drug allergies
NOS	not otherwise specified
NSAID	nonsteroidal anti-inflammatory drug
N/V	nausea or vomiting
OASIS	Online Applicant Status and Information System
OCP	oral contraceptive pill
OSA	obstructive sleep apnea
OTC	over the counter
PA	posteroanterior
PCI	patient-centered interview
PCOS	polycystic ovary syndrome
PCR	polymerase chain reaction
PD	Parkinson's disease
PERRLA	pupils equal, round, and reactive to light and accommodation
PFT	pulmonary function test
PID	pelvic inflammatory disease
PMH	past medical history
PMI	point of maximal impulse
PN	patient note
PPD	pack per day; purified protein derivative [tuberculin skin test]
prn	pro re nata [as needed]
PSA	prostate-specific antigen
PSH	past surgical history
PT	prothrombin time
PTSD	post-traumatic stress disorder
PTT	partial thromboplastin time
RBC	red blood cell
RF	rheumatoid factor
RLQ	right lower quadrant
ROS	review of systems
RPR	rapid plasma reagin
RR	respiratory rate
RRR	regular rate and rhythm
RUQ	right upper quadrant
SEP	spoken English proficiency [CSE score]
SH	social history
SIADH	syndrome of inappropriate antidiuretic hormone
SLE	systemic lupus erythematosus
SP	standardized patient
SPECT	single-photon emission computed tomography
SPEP	serum protein electrophoresis
STD	sexually transmitted disease
T_3	triiodothyronine
T_4	thyroxine
TB	tuberculosis

Abbreviation	Meaning
TCA	tricyclic antidepressant
TEE	transesophageal echocardiography
TIA	transient ischemic attack
TIBC	total iron-binding capacity
TM	tympanic membrane
TMJ	temporomandibular joint
TOEFL	Test of English as a Foreign Language
TSE	test of spoken English
TSH	thyroid-stimulating hormone
TTE	transthoracic echocardiography
UA	urinalysis
UPEP	urine protein electrophoresis
URI	upper respiratory infection

Abbreviation	Meaning
U/S	ultrasound
USMLE	United States Medical Licensing Examination
UTD	up to date [vaccinations]
UTI	urinary tract infection
VCA	virus capsid antigen
VDRL	Venereal Disease Research Laboratory
V/Q	ventilation-perfusion [scan]
VS	vital signs
WBC	white blood cell
WNL	within normal limits
XR	x-ray
yo	year old

ACRONYMS AND ABBREVIATIONS

A

Abdominal pain, 103–107, 132–146
  appendicitis, acute, 106, 145
  cholangitis, ascending, 104
  cholecystitis, acute, 104, 138
  diverticulitis, 106
  hepatitis, acute, 105
  intestinal obstruction, 105
  irritable bowel syndrome, 107
  key history, 103
  key physical exam, 103
  mesenteric ischemia/infarction, 106
  nephrolithiasis, 103
  ovarian torsion, 106
  pancreatic cancer, 104
  pancreatitis, acute, 104
  pelvic inflammatory disease, 107
  peptic ulcer
    disease, 105
    perforation, 105
  practice case, 132–146
    case discussion, 138, 145–146
    checklist/SP sheet, 132, 139
    closure, 134, 142
    examinee checklist, 132–134, 140–141
    examinee tasks, 132, 139
    opening scenario, 132, 139
    patient note, 136–137, 143–144
    physical examination, 134, 142
    sample closure, 135, 142
    vital signs, 132, 139
  splenic rupture, 105
ABO or Rh incompatibility, 404

Abortion, spontaneous, 116, 145
Abuse, 118–119
  domestic violence, 118
  key history, 118
  key physical exam, 118
  rape, 119
Acetaminophen liver toxicity, 208
Achalasia, 102
Achilles tendinitis, 397
Acoustic neuroma, 229, 334
Acute retroviral syndrome, 95
Adjustment disorder, 127
  with depressed mood, 236
Adnexal torsion, 145
Alzheimer disease, 84, 215
Amenorrhea, 114–115, 302–308
  anorexia nervosa, 115
  anxiety-induced, 115
  Asherman syndrome, 308
  hyperprolactinemia, 308
  key history, 114
  key physical exam, 114
  menopause, 115
  polycystic ovary syndrome (PCOS), 114, 308
  practice case, 302–308
    case discussion, 308
    checklist/SP sheet, 302
    closure, 305
    examinee checklist, 302–304
    examinee tasks, 302
    opening scenario, 302
    patient note, 306–307
    physical examination, 304
    sample closure, 305
    vital signs, 302
  pregnancy, 114, 308
  premature ovarian failure, 308

  secondary to prolactinoma, 115
  Sheehan syndrome, 115
  thyroid disease, 308
Anemia, 243
Angina, 98, 122
Angiodysplasia, 167
Angioedema, 410
Ankle sprain, 397
Anorexia nervosa, 115
Aortic dissection, 99, 174
Aortic stenosis, 294
Appendicitis, acute, 106, 145
Arm pain, 147–153
  elder abuse, 153
  humeral fracture, 153
  practice case
    case discussion, 153
    checklist/SP sheet, 147
    closure, 149
    examinee checklist, 147–149
    examinee tasks, 147
    opening scenario, 147
    patient note, 151–152
    physical examination, 149
    sample closure, 150
    vital signs, 147
  osteoporosis, 153
  rotator cuff tear, 153
  shoulder dislocation, 153
Arthritis
  degenerative, 321
  osteoarthritis, 121, 278, 430
  psoriatic, 120
  rheumatoid, 120, 278
  septic, 121
    gonococcal, 278
    nongonococcal, 278
Asherman syndrome, 308

Asthma, 95
Attention-deficit hyperactivity
    disorder (ADHD), 127

B

Back pain. *See* Low back pain
Bacteremia, 327
    occult, 180, 436
Bacterial vaginosis, 117
Baker's cyst, rupture of, 390
Bed-wetting, 335–340
    constipation, 340
    functional bladder disorder, 340
    monosymptomatic primary
        nocturnal, 340
    practice case
        case discussion, 340
        checklist/SP sheet, 335
        closure, 337
        examinee checklist, 335–337
        examinee tasks, 335
        opening scenario, 335
        patient note, 338–339
        physical examination, 337
        sample closure, 337
        vital signs, 335
    secondary, 340
    sleep apnea, 340
    urinary tract infection (UTI),
        340
Behavioral problems in childhood,
    127
    adjustment disorder, 127
    age-appropriate behavior, 127
    attention-deficit hyperactivity
        disorder (ADHD), 127
    key history, 127
    key physical exam, 127
    substance abuse, 127
Benign positional vertigo, 88, 229
Benign prostatic hyperplasia
    (BPH), 112, 264
Bereavement, normal, 85
Biliary obstruction, extrahepatic,
    208
Bipolar I disorder, 86
Bladder disorder, functional, 340

Bladder cancer, 111, 264
Blood in stool, 110–111, 161–167
    colorectal cancer, 110, 167
    diverticulosis, 111, 167
    key history, 110
    key physical exam, 110
    practice case, 161–167
        case discussion, 167
        checklist/SP sheet, 161
        closure, 163
        examinee checklist, 161–163
        examinee tasks, 161
        opening scenario, 161
        patient note, 165–166
        physical examination, 163
        sample closure, 164
        vital signs, 161
    ulcerative colitis, 111, 167
Breathing, noisy, 405–410
    abscess
        peritonsillar, 410
        retropharyngeal, 410
    angioedema, 410
    croup, 410
    epiglottitis, 410
    foreign body, aspiration of, 410
    laryngeal papilloma, 410
    laryngitis, 410
    practice case
        case discussion, 410
        checklist/SP sheet, 405
        closure, 407
        examinee checklist, 405–407
        examinee tasks, 405
        opening scenario, 405
        patient note, 408–409
        physical examination, 407
        sample closure, 407
    stridor
        biphasic, 410
        expiratory, 410
        inspiratory, 410
Brief psychotic disorder, 376
Bronchitis
    acute, 193
    chronic (COPD), 96
Bursitis, retrocalcaneal, 397

C

Calcaneal stress fracture, 397
Calf pain, 384–390
    Baker's cyst, rupture of, 390
    cellulitis/myositis, 390
    deep venous thrombosis (DVT),
        390
    gastrocnemius muscle, rupture
        of, 390
    hematoma, 390
    practice case
        case discussion, 390
        checklist/SP sheet, 384
        closure, 387
        examinee checklist, 384–386
        examinee tasks, 384
        opening scenario, 384
        patient note, 388–389
        physical examination, 386
        sample closure, 387
        vital signs, 384
    spasm/sprain, 390
Cardiac arrhythmia (causing syn-
    cope), 89, 294
Carpal tunnel syndrome, 119
Cellulitis, 390
Cephalohematoma, 404
Cervical cancer, 116
Cervical fracture, 430
Cervical spondylitis, 430
Cervicitis, 315
Chest pain, 97–99, 168–174
    angina, 98
    aortic dissection, 99, 174
    cocaine-induced, 174
    costochondritis, 99, 174
    gastroesophageal reflux disease
        (GERD), 98, 174
    key history, 97
    key physical exam, 97
    myocardial infarction (MI), 98,
        174
    pericarditis, 98, 174
    pneumothorax, 174
    practice case, 168–174
        case discussion, 174
        checklist/SP sheet, 168

closure, 171
examinee checklist, 168–170
examinee tasks, 168
opening scenario, 168
patient note, 172–173
physical examination, 170
sample closure, 171
vital signs, 168
pulmonary embolism, 99, 174
pulmonary infarction, due to
sickle cell disease, 98
Cholangitis, ascending, 104
Cholecystitis, acute, 104, 138
Chronic obstructive pulmonary disease (COPD), 200, 417
chronic bronchitis, 96, 417
Cirrhosis, primary biliary, 208
Clostridium difficile (pseudomembranous) colitis, 108, 167
Cluster headache, 81, 257
Cochlear nerve damage, 334
Colitis
pseudomembranous (Clostridium difficile), 108
ulcerative, 111, 167
Colon cancer, 92
Colorectal cancer, 108, 110, 167
Confusion/memory loss, 83–85, 209–215
Alzheimer disease, 84, 215
Creutzfeldt-Jakob disease, 84
depression with pseudodementia, 215
hypoglycemia, 85
hypothyroidism, 215
key history, 83
key physical exam, 83
normal pressure hydrocephalus, 84
practice case, 209–215
case discussion, 215
checklist/SP sheet, 209
closure, 212
examinee checklist, 209–211
examinee tasks, 209
opening scenario, 209
patient note, 213–214

physical examination, 211–212
sample closure, 212
vital signs, 209
subdural hematoma, 85, 215
vascular ("multi-infarct") dementia, 83, 215
vitamin B$_{12}$ deficiency, 215
Congestive heart failure (CHF), 97
Conjunctivitis, bacterial, 126
Constipation/diarrhea, 107–109, 340. See also Diarrhea
colorectal cancer, 108
Crohn disease, 109
infectious diarrhea (gastroenteritis), 108
irritable bowel syndrome, 108
key history, 107
key physical exam, 107
lactose intolerance, 109
low-fiber diet, 108
pseudomembranous (Clostridium difficile) colitis, 108
traveler's diarrhea, 109
Costochondritis, 99, 174
Cough/shortness of breath, 95–97, 187–201
asthma, 95
bronchitis, acute, 193
congestive heart failure (CHF), 97
COPD (chronic bronchitis), 96, 200
key history, 95
key physical exam, 95
lung abscess, 200
lung cancer, 96, 200
pleurodynia, 193
pneumonia, 96, 193
atypical, 96, 200
typical, 200
practice case, 187–201
case discussion, 193, 200–201
checklist/SP sheet, 187, 194
closure, 190, 197
examinee checklist, 188–189, 195–196

examinee tasks, 187, 194
opening scenario, 187, 194
patient note, 191–192, 198–199
physical examination, 189–190, 196–197
sample closure, 190, 197
vital signs, 187, 194
tuberculosis, 97, 200
URI-associated, 193
Wegener granulomatosis, 200
Creutzfeldt-Jakob disease, 84
Crohn disease, 109
Croup, 410
Cushing syndrome, 301

D
Deep venous thrombosis (DVT), 122, 390
Degenerative arthritis, 321
Dementia, vascular ("multi-infarct"), 83, 215
Depressed mood, 85–86, 92, 94
bereavement, normal, 85
bipolar I disorder, 86
key history, 85
key physical exam, 85
major depressive disorder, 86
insomnia related to, 94
Depression, 92, 236, 243, 250, 257, 271
and insomnia, 369
with pseudodementia, 215
Diabetes insipidus (DI), 243
Diabetes mellitus (DM), 92, 216–222, 243, 377–383
hyperglycemia, 383
practice case, 216–222, 377–383
case discussion, 222, 383
checklist/SP sheet, 216, 377
closure, 219, 379
examinee checklist, 216–218, 377–379
examinee tasks, 216, 377
opening scenario, 216, 377
patient note, 220–221, 381–382

Diabetes mellitus (DM) (*Continued*)
  practice case (*Continued*)
    physical examination, 219,
      379
    sample closure, 219, 380
    vital signs, 216, 377
Diabetic peripheral neuropathy, 91
Diarrhea, 322–327. *See also* Consti-
      pation/diarrhea
  bacteremia, 327
  bacterial, 327
  infectious (gastroenteritis), 108
  intussusception, 327
  malabsorption, 327
  practice case, 322–327
    case discussion, 327
    checklist/SP sheet, 322
    closure, 324
    examinee checklist, 322
    examinee tasks, 322–324
    opening scenario, 322
    patient note, 325–326
    physical examination, 324
    sample closure, 324
    vital signs, 322
  rotavirus, 327
  traveler's, 109
  urinary tract infection (UTI),
      327
Disk herniation, 123, 321, 430
Diverticulitis, 106
Diverticulosis, 111, 167
Dizziness, 87–88, 223–229
  acoustic neuroma, 229
  benign positional vertigo, 88,
      229
  hypotension, orthostatic
    drug-induced, 88
    due to dehydration, 88, 229
  key history, 87
  key physical exam, 87
  labyrinthitis, 88, 229
  Ménière disease, 87, 229
  perilymphatic fistula, 229
  practice case, 223–229
    case discussion, 229
    checklist/SP sheet, 223

closure, 225
examinee checklist, 223–225
examinee tasks, 223
opening scenario, 223
patient note, 227–228
physical examination, 225
sample closure, 226
vital signs, 223
vestibular neuronitis, 88
Domestic violence, 118, 119, 243,
    315
Dyspareunia, 118, 309–315
  atrophic vaginitis, 118
  cervicitis, 315
  domestic violence, 315
  endometriosis, 118, 315
  key history, 118
  key physical exam, 118
  pelvic tumor, 315
  practice case, 309–315
    case discussion,
    checklist/SP sheet, 309
    closure, 312
    examinee checklist, 309–311
    examinee tasks, 309
    opening scenario, 309
    patient note, 313–314
    physical examination, 311
    sample closure, 312
    vital signs, 309
  vaginismus, 315
  vulvodynia, 315
  vulvovaginitis, 315
Dyspepsia, functional or nonulcer,
    138
Dysphagia, 101–102
  achalasia, 102
  esophageal cancer, 102
  esophagitis, 102
  key history, 101
  key physical exam, 102
  Plummer-Vinson syndrome, 102

E

Ectopic pregnancy, 117, 362
  ruptured, 145
Elder abuse, 153

Endometrial cancer, 116
Endometriosis, 118, 145, 315
Enuresis. *See* Bed-wetting
Epicondylitis, lateral (tennis el-
      bow), 121
Epiglottitis, 410
Erectile dysfunction (ED), 113–
      114, 222
  alcohol-related, 271
  caused by vascular disease, 271
  drug-related, 114, 271
  key history, 113
  key physical exam, 113
Esophageal cancer, 102
Esophagitis, 102

F

Fatigue and sleepiness, 91–92,
      230–250
  adjustment disorder with de-
      pressed mood, 236
  anemia, 243
  colon cancer, 92
  depression, 92, 236, 243, 250
  diabetes insipidus (DI), 243
  diabetes mellitus (DM), 92, 243
  domestic violence, 243
  HIV infection, 236
  hypothyroidism, 92, 236, 243,
      250
  key history, 91
  key physical exam, 91
  myasthenia gravis, 243
  obstructive sleep apnea, 92, 236
  pancreatic cancer, 250
  pancreatitis, chronic, 250
  peptic ulcer disease, 250
  posttraumatic stress disorder, 92,
      236
  practice case, 230–250
    case discussion, 236, 243
    checklist/SP sheet, 230, 237,
      244
    closure, 233, 240, 247
    examinee checklist, 230–232,
      237–239, 244–246
    examinee tasks, 230, 237, 244

opening scenario, 230, 237,
244

patient note, 234–235, 241–
242, 248–249

physical examination, 232,
239–240, 246–247

sample closure, 233, 240, 247

vital signs, 230, 237, 244

sleep deprivation, 92

Fever, child with, 123–124, 175–
186

bacteremia, occult, 180

fifth disease, 186

gastroenteritis, 124, 180

key history, 123

key physical exam, 123

measles, 124

meningitis, 180, 186

neonatal sepsis, 124

otitis media, acute, 124, 180, 186

pneumonia, 180

practice case, 175–186

case discussion, 180, 186

checklist/SP sheet, 175, 181

closure, 177, 183

examinee checklist, 175–177,
181–183

examinee tasks, 175, 181

opening scenario, 175, 181

patient note, 178–179, 184–
185

physical examination, 177, 183

sample closure, 177, 183

scarlet fever, 186

URI, viral, 180

UTI, 180

varicella, 186

Fifth disease, 186

Foreign body, aspiration of, 410

G

Gastric cancer, 138

Gastritis, 110, 138

Gastrocnemius muscle, rupture of,
390

Gastroenteritis (infectious diarrhea), 108, 124, 145, 180

Gastroesophageal reflux disease
(GERD), 98, 174

Gastrointestinal bleeding. *See*
Blood in stool; Upper GI
bleeding

Gastrointestinal symptoms in child,
124–125

colic, 125

Hirschsprung disease, 125

intussusception, 125

key history, 124

key physical exam, 124

pyloric stenosis, 125

somatoform disorder, 125

Giant cell (temporal) arteritis, 81

Glomerulonephritis, 264

Gonorrhea, disseminated, 121

Gout, 278

Guillain-Barré syndrome, 90

H

Hallucinations, visual, 370–376

brief psychotic disorder, 376

narcolepsy, 376

practice case

case discussion, 376

checklist/SP sheet, 370

closure, 373

examinee checklist, 370–372

examinee tasks, 370

opening scenario, 370

patient note, 374–375

physical examination, 372

sample closure, 373

vital signs, 370

psychosis

secondary to medical condition, 376

substance-induced, 376

seizure, 376

Headache, 81–83, 251–257

key history, 81

key physical exam, 81

cluster, 81, 257

depression, 257

intracranial mass lesion, 257

meningitis (bacterial/HSV), 82

migraine, 81, 257

practice case, 251–257

case discussion, 257

checklist/SP sheet, 251

closure, 254

examinee checklist, 251–253

examinee tasks, 251

opening scenario, 251

patient note, 255–256

physical examination, 253

sample closure, 254

vital signs, 251

pseudotumor cerebri, 82, 257

sinusitis, 82, 257

subarachnoid hemorrhage, 82

temporal (giant cell) arteritis, 81

tension, 82, 257

trigeminal neuralgia, 83

Hearing loss, 328–334

acoustic neuroma, 334

cochlear nerve damage, 334

Ménière disease, 334

otosclerosis, 334

ototoxicity, 334

presbycusis, 334

practice case

case discussion, 334

checklist/SP sheet, 328–329

closure, 331

examinee checklist, 329–330

examinee tasks, 328

opening scenario, 328

patient note, 332–333

physical examination, 330–
331

sample closure, 331

vital signs, 328

Heel pain, 391–398

Achilles tendinitis, 397

ankle sprain, 397

calcaneal stress fracture, 397

foreign body, 397

plantar fasciitis, 397

practice case

case discussion, 397–398

checklist/SP sheet, 391

closure, 394

Heel pain (*Continued*)
  practice case (*Continued*)
    examinee checklist, 391–393
    examinee tasks, 391
    opening scenario, 391
    patient note, 395–396
    physical examination, 393–394
    sample closure, 394
    vital signs, 391
  retrocalcaneal bursitis, 397
  tarsal tunnel syndrome, 397
Hematoma, 390
Hematuria, 111–112
  bladder cancer, 111
  key history, 111
  key physical exam, 111
  polycystic kidney disease, 111
  renal cell carcinoma, 112
Hemorrhoids, 167
Hemothorax, 347, 355
Hepatitis
  acute, 105
  alcoholic, 208
  viral, 208
Hip
  dislocation, traumatic, 120
  fracture, 120
Hirschsprung disease, 125
HIV/acute retroviral syndrome, 95, 236
Hoarseness, 418–424
  hypothyroidism, 424
  laryngeal cancer, 424
  laryngitis, 424
  mitral valve stenosis (MVS), 424
  practice case
    case discussion, 424
    checklist/SP sheet, 418
    closure, 420
    examinee checklist, 418–420
    examinee tasks, 418
    opening scenario, 418
    patient note, 422–423
    physical examination, 420
    sample closure, 421
    vital signs, 418
  vocal cord polyps/nodules, 424

Humeral fracture, 153
Hydrocephalus, normal pressure, 84
Hyperbilirubinemia, familial neo-
  natal, 404
Hyperglycemia, 383
Hyperprolactinemia, 308
Hypertension, 265–271
  depression, 271
  erectile dysfunction (ED)
    alcohol-related, 271
    caused by vascular disease, 271
    drug-induced, 271
  hypogonadism, 271
  practice case
    case discussion, 271
    checklist/SP sheet, 265
    closure, 268
    examinee checklist, 265
    examinee tasks, 265
    opening scenario, 265
    patient note, 269–270
    physical examination, 267–268
    sample closure, 268
    vital signs, 265
  Peyronie disease, 271
Hyperthyroidism, 101, 286, 369
Hypogonadism, 271
Hypoglycemia, 85, 100
  insulin-induced, 222
Hyponatremia, 436
Hypotension, orthostatic
  drug-induced, 88
    causing syncope, 89, 294
  due to dehydration, 88, 229
Hypothyroidism, 92, 215, 236, 243,
  250, 301, 424

I

Incontinence
  stress, 113
  urge, 113
Insomnia, 93–94, 363–369
  adjustment, 369
  anxiety, 369
  caffeine-induced, 369
  due to depression, 369

hyperthyroidism, 369
illicit drug use, 369
key history, 93
key physical exam, 93
obstructive sleep apnea, 94, 369
practice case, 363–369
  case discussion,
  checklist/SP sheet, 363
  closure, 366
  examinee checklist, 363–365
  examinee tasks, 363
  opening scenario, 363
  patient note, 367–368
  physical examination, 365–366
  sample closure, 366
  vital signs, 363
  related to major depressive disor-
    der, 94
  stress-induced, 93
Intestinal obstruction, 105
Intracranial mass lesion, 257
Intussusception, 125, 327
Irritable bowel syndrome, 107, 108

J

Jaundice, 202–208, 399–404
  ABO or Rh incompatibility, 404
  acetaminophen liver toxicity,
    208
  biliary obstruction, extrahepatic,
    208
  breast-feeding, 404
  cephalohematoma, 404
  cirrhosis, primary biliary, 208
  hepatitis
    alcoholic, 208
    viral, 208
  hyperbilirubinemia, familial neo-
    natal, 404
  neonatal sepsis, 404
  physiologic, 404
  polycythemia, 404
  practice case, 202–208, 399–404
    case discussion, 208, 404
    checklist/SP sheet, 202, 399
    closure, 205, 401

examinee checklist, 202–204, 399–401

examinee tasks, 202, 399

opening scenario, 202, 399

patient note, 206–207, 402–403

physical examination, 205, 401

sample closure, 205, 401

vital signs, 202

Joint/limb pain, 119–122

angina/MI, 122

carpal tunnel syndrome, 119

deep venous thrombosis (DVT), 122

domestic violence, 119

arthritis

psoriatic, 120

rheumatoid, 120

septic, 121

gonorrhea, disseminated, 121

hip

dislocation, traumatic, 120

fracture, 120

osteoarthritis, 121

peripheral vascular disease, 122

plantar fasciitis, 121

rhabdomyolysis, due to simvastatin or clofibrate, 122

shoulder dislocation, 122

stress fracture, 121

systemic lupus erythematosus (SLE), 120

tennis elbow (lateral epicondylitis), 121

K

Kidney disease, polycystic, 111

Knee pain, 272–279

arthritis

rheumatoid, 278

septic, 278

gout, 278

osteoarthritis, 278

practice case

case discussion, 278–279

checklist/SP sheet, 272

closure, 275

examinee checklist, 272–274

examinee tasks, 272

opening scenario, 272

patient note, 276–277

physical examination, 275

sample closure, 275

vital signs, 272

pseudogout, 278

systemic lupus erythematosus (SLE), 278

L

Labyrinthitis, 88, 229

Lactose intolerance, 109

Laryngeal cancer, 424

Laryngeal papilloma, 410

Laryngitis, 410, 424

Limb pain. See Joint/limb pain

Loss of consciousness (LOC), 89, 288–294

aortic stenosis, 294

cardiac arrhythmia (causing syncope), 89, 294

convulsive, 294

hypotension, orthostatic (causing syncope), 89, 294

key history, 89

key physical exam, 89

practice case, 288–294

case discussion,

checklist/SP sheet, 288

closure, 291

examinee checklist, 288–290

examinee tasks, 288

opening scenario, 288

patient note, 292–293

physical examination, 290

sample closure, 291

vital signs, 288

seizure, complex tonic-clonic, 89, 294

vasovagal, 294

Low back pain, 122–123, 316–321

arthritis, degenerative, 321

disk herniation, 123, 321

key history, 122

key physical exam, 123

lumbar muscle strain, 123, 321

lumbar spinal stenosis, 321

malingering, 123, 321

multiple myeloma, 321

practice case, 316–321

case discussion, 321

checklist/SP sheet, 316

closure, 318

examinee checklist, 316–318

examinee tasks, 316

opening scenario, 316

patient note, 319–320

physical examination, 318

sample closure, 318

vital signs, 316

prostate cancer, metastatic, 321

Low-fiber diet, 108

Lumbar muscle strain, 123, 321

Lumbar spinal stenosis, 321

Lung abscess, 200

Lung cancer, 96, 200

M

Major depressive disorder, 86

insomnia related to, 94

Malabsorption, 327

Malingering, 123, 321

Measles, 124

Memory loss. See Confusion/memory loss

Ménière disease, 87, 229, 334

Meningitis, 180, 436

bacterial/HSV, 82

meningococcal, 186

Menopause, amenorrhea due to, 115

Mesenteric ischemia/infarction, 106

Midbrain lesion, 286

Migraine headache, 81, 257

Mitral valve stenosis (MVS), 424

Molar pregnancy, 362

Mononucleosis, infectious, 94, 160

Motor vehicle accident, 341–348

hemothorax, 347

pleuritis, 347

Motor vehicle accident (*Continued*)
pneumonia, 347
pneumothorax, 347
practice case
case discussion, 347
checklist/SP sheet, 341
closure, 344
examinee checklist, 342–343
examinee tasks, 341
opening scenario, 341
patient note, 345–346
physical examination, 343–344
sample closure, 344
vital signs, 341
rib fracture, 347
splenic rupture, 347
Multiple myeloma, 222, 321, 430
Multiple sclerosis, 90
Myasthenia gravis, 91, 243
Myocardial infarction (MI), 98, 122, 174
Myositis, 390

N

Narcolepsy, 376
Nausea/vomiting, 102–103
key history, 102
key physical exam, 103
pregnancy, 103
Neck pain, 425–430
cervical fracture, 430
cervical spondylitis, 430
disk herniation, 430
metastatic cancer, 430
multiple myeloma, 430
neck muscle strain, 430
osteoarthritis, 430
practice case
case discussion, 430
checklist/SP sheet, 425
closure, 427
examinee checklist, 425–427
examinee tasks, 425
opening scenario, 425
patient note, 428–429
physical examination, 427

sample closure, 427
vital signs, 425
Neonatal sepsis, 124, 404
Nephrolithiasis, 103
Neuronitis, vestibular, 88
Night sweats, 93
key history, 93
key physical exam, 93
tuberculosis, 93
Normal pressure hydrocephalus, 84
Numbness/weakness, 90–91
diabetic peripheral neuropathy, 91
Guillain-Barré syndrome, 90
key history, 90
key physical exam, 90
multiple sclerosis, 90
myasthenia gravis, 91
stroke, 90
Todd paralysis, 91
transient ischemic attack (TIA), 90

O

Obesity
familial, 301
lithium-related, 301
Obstructive sleep apnea, 92, 94, 236, 369
Osteoarthritis, 121, 278, 430
Osteoporosis, 153
Otitis media, acute, 124, 180, 186
Otosclerosis, 334
Ototoxicity, 334
Ovarian cyst, ruptured, 145
Ovarian failure, premature, 308
Ovarian torsion, 106

P

Palpitations, 99–100
hypoglycemia, 100
key history, 99
key physical exam, 99
panic attack, 100
social phobia, 100
Pancreatic cancer, 104, 250
Pancreatitis

acute, 104
chronic, 250
Panic attack, 100
Parkinson disease, 286
Patient encounter, 38–78
challenging questions and situations, 64–71
confidentiality/ethical issues, 65
disease-related issues, 69–71
patient belief/behavioral issues, 65–69
closure, 61–63
counseling, 71–74
alcoholic patient, 72
depressed patient, 73
sexually promiscuous patient, 73
smoker, 72
STD (trichomoniasis), patient with, 74
uncontrolled diabetes, patient with, 72–73
doorway information, 39–42
history, taking, 42–52
common questions to ask patient, 44–52
guidelines, 42
tips, 42–44
patient note, 74–78
preparing to write, 77
scoring, 77
writing, 74–77
physical exam, 52–61, 78
documenting, 78
guidelines, 52
review, 54
SP simulation of findings, 59–61
special challenges during, 59
special patients, how to interact with, 63–64
summary overview of, 75–76
Pelvic inflammatory disease (PID), 107, 145
Pelvic tumor, 315
Peptic ulcer
bleeding, 110

disease, 105, 138, 250
perforation, 105
Pericarditis, 98, 174
Perilymphatic fistula, 229
Peripheral neuropathy, 222
alcoholic, 222
diabetic, 91, 222
Peripheral vascular disease, 122
Peritonsillar abscess, 410
Peyronie disease, 271
Pharyngitis, 95
group A streptococcal, 160
Plantar fasciitis, 121, 397
Pleuritis, 347
Pleurodynia, 193
Plummer-Vinson syndrome, 102
Pneumonia, 96, 180, 193, 200, 347
atypical, 96, 200
bacterial, 347
typical, 200
Pneumothorax, 174, 347, 355
Polycystic kidney disease, 111
Polycystic ovary syndrome
(PCOS), 114, 308
Polycythemia, 404
Posttraumatic stress disorder, 92,
236
Preemployment physical, 411–417
COPD/chronic bronchitis, 417
practice case
case discussion, 417
checklist/SP sheet, 411
closure, 414
examinee checklist, 411–413
examinee tasks, 411
opening scenario, 411
patient note, 415–416
physical examination, 413–
414
sample closure, 414
vital signs, 411
pulmonary silicosis, 417
pulmonary tuberculosis, 417
Pregnancy
amenorrhea due to, 114, 308
ectopic, 117, 362
ruptured, 145

following sexual assault, 355
molar, 362
nausea/vomiting due to, 103
normal, 362
practice case, 356–362
case discussion, 362
checklist/SP sheet, 356
closure, 359
examinee checklist, 356–358
examinee tasks, 356
opening scenario, 356
patient note, 360–361
physical examination, 358
sample closure, 359
vital signs, 356
weight gain due to, 301
Presbycusis, 334
Prolactinoma, amenorrhea secondary to, 115
Prostate
benign prostatic hyperplasia
(BPH), 112, 264
cancer, 112, 264
metastatic, 321
Pseudogout, 278
Pseudomembranous (*Clostridium
difficile*) colitis, 108, 167
Pseudotumor cerebri, 82, 257
Psoriatic arthritis, 120
Psychosis, 86–87, 376
key history, 86
key physical exam, 86
schizoaffective disorder, 87
schizophrenia, 86
secondary to medical condition,
376
substance-induced, 87, 376
Pulmonary embolism, 99, 174
Pulmonary infarction, due to sickle
cell disease, 98
Pyelonephritis, acute, 113
Pyloric stenosis, 125

R

Rape, 119
Red eye, in child, 126
conjunctivitis, bacterial, 126

key history, 126
key physical exam, 126
Renal cell carcinoma, 112, 264
Retropharyngeal abscess, 410
Review resources, top-rated,
437–443
database, how to use, 438–439
Rhabdomyolysis, due to simvastatin
or clofibrate, 122
Rheumatoid arthritis, 120, 278
Rib fracture, 347, 355
Rotator cuff tear, 153
Rotavirus, 327

S

Scarlet fever, 186
Schizoaffective disorder, 87
Schizophrenia, 86
Seizure, 376, 431–436
bacteremia, occult, 436
complex tonic-clonic, 89, 294
hyponatremia, 436
meningitis, 436
practice case, 431–436
case discussion, 436
checklist/SP sheet, 431
closure, 433
examinee checklist, 431–433
examinee tasks, 431
opening scenario, 431
patient note, 434–435
physical examination, 433
sample closure, 433
simple febrile, 436
urinary tract infection (UTI),
436
Sepsis, neonatal, 124
Septic arthritis, 121
gonococcal, 278
nongonococcal, 278
Sexual assault, 349–355
pneumothorax/hemothorax,
355
practice case
case discussion, 355
checklist/SP sheet, 349
closure, 352

Sexual assault (*Continued*)
  practice case (*Continued*)
    examinee checklist, 349–351
    examinee tasks, 349
    opening scenario, 349
    patient note, 353–354
    physical examination, 351–352
    sample closure, 352
    vital signs, 349
  pregnancy, 355
  rib fracture, 355
  sexually transmitted diseases (STDs), 355
Sexually transmitted diseases (STDs), 355
Sheehan syndrome, 115
Short stature, child with, 126
  familial, 126
  key history, 126
  key physical exam, 126
Shortness of breath. *See* Cough/ shortness of breath
Shoulder dislocation, 122, 153
Silicosis, pulmonary, 417
Sinusitis, 82, 257
Sleep apnea, 340
  obstructive, 92, 94, 236, 369
Sleep deprivation, 92
Smoking cessation, 101, 301
Social phobia, 100
Somatoform disorder, in child with GI symptoms, 125
Sore throat, 94–95, 154–160
  HIV/acute retroviral syndrome, 95
  key history, 94
  key physical exam, 94
  mononucleosis, infectious, 94, 160
  pharyngitis, 95, 160
  practice case, 154–160
    case discussion, 160
    checklist/SP sheet, 154
    closure, 157
    examinee checklist, 154–156
    examinee tasks, 154

    opening scenario, 154
    patient note, 158–159
    physical examination, 156
    sample closure, 157
    vital signs, 154
Spinal stenosis, lumbar, 321
Splenic rupture, 105, 347
Spontaneous abortion, 116, 145
Stress fracture, 121
Stress incontinence, 113
Stridor
  biphasic, 410
  expiratory, 410
  inspiratory, 410
Stroke, 90
Subarachnoid hemorrhage, 82
Subdural hematoma, 85, 215
Substance abuse, 127
Substance-induced psychosis, 87
Syncope
  convulsive, 294
  due to cardiac arrhythmia, 89
  due to orthostatic hypotension, 89
  vasovagal, 294
Systemic lupus erythematosus (SLE), 120, 278

T

Tarsal tunnel syndrome, 397
Temporal (giant cell) arteritis, 81
Tennis elbow (lateral epicondylitis), 121
Tension headache, 82, 257
Thyroid disease, amenorrhea due to, 308
Todd paralysis, 91
Transient ischemic attack (TIA), 90
Traveler's diarrhea, 109
Tremor, 280–287
  drug-induced, 286
  essential (ET), 286
  hyperthyroidism, 286
  midbrain lesion, 286
  Parkinson disease, 286

physiologic, 286
  practice case
    case discussion, 286
    checklist/SP sheet, 280
    closure, 282
    examinee checklist, 280–282
    examinee tasks, 280
    opening scenario, 280
    patient note, 284–285
    physical examination, 282
    sample closure, 283
    vital signs, 280
  psychogenic, 286
  Wilson's disease, 286
Trigeminal neuralgia, 83
Tuberculosis, 93, 97, 200, 417

U

Ulcer, perforated, 138
Ulcerative colitis, 111, 167
Upper GI bleeding, 109–110
  gastritis, 110
  key history, 109
  key physical exam, 109
  peptic ulcer, 110
Upper respiratory infection (URI)
  cough associated with, 193
  viral, 180
Urethritis, 113
Urge incontinence, 113
Urinary symptoms, 112–113
  benign prostatic hyperplasia (BPH), 112, 264
  bladder cancer, 264
  glomerulonephritis, 264
  incontinence
    stress, 113
    urge, 113
  key history, 112
  key physical exam, 112
  practice case, 258–264
    case discussion, 264
    checklist/SP sheet, 258
    closure, 260
    examinee checklist, 258–260
    examinee tasks, 258

opening scenario, 258
patient note, 262–263
physical examination, 260
sample closure, 261
vital signs, 258
prostate cancer, 112, 264
pyelonephritis, acute, 113
renal cell carcinoma, 112, 264
urethritis, 113
urolithiasis, 264
UTI, 264
Urinary tract infection (UTI), 180, 264, 327, 340, 436
Urolithiasis, 264
USMLE Step 2 CS
guide to, 1–35
basics, 2–10
IMGs, 12–18
test-day tips, 10–11
travel guide, 19–35
Atlanta, 22–24
Chicago, 24–27
Houston, 27–30
Los Angeles, 30–32
Philadelphia, 32–35
United States, traveling to, 20–22
Web sites, 35
Uterine bleeding, dysfunctional, 116

V

Vaginal bleeding, 116–117
cervical cancer, 116
ectopic pregnancy, 117
endometrial cancer, 116
key history, 116
key physical exam, 116
spontaneous abortion, 116
uterine, dysfunctional, 116
Vaginal discharge, 117
bacterial vaginosis, 117
key history, 117
key physical exam, 117
vaginitis
candidal, 117
trichomonal, 117
Vaginismus, 315
Vaginitis
atrophic, 118
candidal, 117
trichomonal, 117
Varicella, 186
Vascular ("multi-infarct") dementia, 83, 215
Vertigo, benign positional, 88
Vestibular neuronitis, 88
Vitamin B_{12} deficiency, 215
Vocal cord polyps/nodules, 424
Vomiting. *See* Nausea/vomiting

Vulvodynia, 315
Vulvovaginitis, 315

W

Wegener granulomatosis, 200
Weight gain, 101
Cushing syndrome, 301
familial obesity, 301
hypothyroidism, 301
key history, 101
key physical exam, 101
lithium-related obesity, 301
practice case, 295–301
case discussion, 301
checklist/SP sheet, 295
closure, 298
examinee checklist, 295–297
examinee tasks, 295
opening scenario, 295
patient note, 299–300
physical examination, 297
sample closure, 298
vital signs, 295
pregnancy, 301
smoking cessation, 101, 301
Weight loss, 100–101
hyperthyroidism, 101
key history, 100
key physical exam, 101
Wilson's disease, 286

ABOUT THE AUTHORS

Tao Le, MD, MHS

Tao developed a passion for medical education while still a medical student. He currently edits over 15 titles in the *First Aid* series. In addition, he is the founder of the *USMLERx* online video and test bank series as well as a cofounder of the *Underground Clinical Vignettes* series. As a medical student, he was editor-in-chief of the University of California, San Francisco (UCSF) *Synapse*, a university newspaper with a weekly circulation of 9000. Tao earned his medical degree from UCSF in 1996 and completed his residency training in internal medicine at Yale University and fellowship training at Johns Hopkins University. At Yale, he was a regular guest lecturer on the USMLE review courses and an adviser to the Yale University School of Medicine curriculum committee. Dr. Le subsequently went on to cofound Medsn, a medical education technology venture, and served as its chief medical officer. He is currently conducting research in asthma education at the University of Louisville.

Vikas Bhushan, MD

Vikas is an author, editor, entrepreneur, and roaming teleradiologist who divides his days between Los Angeles, Maui, and balmy remote locales with abundant bandwidth. In 1992 he conceived and authored the original *First Aid for the USMLE Step 1*, and in 1998 he originated and coauthored the *Underground Clinical Vignettes* series. His entrepreneurial adventures include a successful software company; a medical publishing enterprise (S2S); an elearning company (Medsn); and, most recently, an ED teleradiology venture (24/7 Radiology). His eclectic interests include medical informatics, independent film, humanism, Urdu poetry, world music, South Asian diasporic culture, and avoiding a day job. He has also coproduced a music documentary on qawwali; coproduced and edited *Shabash 2.0: The Hip Guide to All Things South Asian in North America*; and is now completing a CD/book project on Sufi poetry translated into four languages. Vikas completed a bachelor's degree in biochemistry from the University of California, Berkeley; an MD with thesis from the University of California, San Francisco; and a radiology residency from the University of California, Los Angeles.

Mae Sheikh–Ali, MD

Mae is currently an assistant professor of medicine and an assistant program director for the Endocrinology Fellowship Program at the University of Florida College of Medicine, Jacksonville. She earned her medical degree from Damascus University School of Medicine in Syria. She completed her residency training in internal medicine at Drexel University College of Medicine in Philadelphia and endocrinology fellowship training at Mayo Clinic College of Medicine, Jacksonville, Florida. She is an editor and contributing author of several editions of the *First Aid for the USMLE* and the *Underground Clinical Vignettes series*. Mae is passionate about medical education. She is taking an active role in teaching and empowering medical students, residents, fellows, and patients. Mae is currently pursuing an academic career in endocrinology, with a focus on vitamin D, obesity, and diabetes research projects.

Fadi Abu Shahin, MD

Fadi is a distinguished graduate of Damascus University medical school in Syria. He subsequently moved to the United States and worked in the Department of Obstetrics and Gynecology at Yale University as a postdoctoral fellow where he did research focused on ovarian cancer and the effects of estrogen on the immune system. He received his residency training in obstetrics and gynecology at Northwestern University in Chicago where he served as a chief resident. Fadi then completed a fellowship in gynecologic oncology at the Cleveland Clinic in Cleveland, Ohio and is currently a gynecologic oncologist in private practice in Fort Myers, Florida. Fadi has been a contributor, an editor, and an author of several editions of the *First Aid for the USMLE* and the *Underground Clinical Vignettes* series.